369 0246565

KU-279-045

PREVENTION OF HEARING LOSS

OTOLARYNGOLOGY RESEARCH ADVANCES

Additional books in this series can be found on Nova's website
under the Series tab.

Additional e-books in this series can be found on Nova's website
under the e-book tab.

HUMAN ANATOMY AND PHYSIOLOGY

Additional books in this series can be found on Nova's website
under the Series tab.

Additional e-books in this series can be found on Nova's website
under the e-book tab.

OTOLARYNGOLOGY RESEARCH ADVANCES

PREVENTION OF HEARING LOSS

VALERIE NEWTON
PETER ALBERTI
AND
ANDREW SMITH
EDITORS

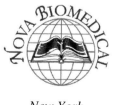

New York

Copyright © 2012 by Nova Science Publishers, Inc.

NOTICE TO THE READER

The Publisher has taken reasonable care in the preparation of this book, but makes no expressed or implied warranty of any kind and assumes no responsibility for any errors or omissions. No liability is assumed for incidental or consequential damages in connection with or arising out of information contained in this book. The Publisher shall not be liable for any special, consequential, or exemplary damages resulting, in whole or in part, from the readers' use of, or reliance upon, this material. Any parts of this book based on government reports are so indicated and copyright is claimed for those parts to the extent applicable to compilations of such works.

Independent verification should be sought for any data, advice or recommendations contained in this book. In addition, no responsibility is assumed by the publisher for any injury and/or damage to persons or property arising from any methods, products, instructions, ideas or otherwise contained in this publication.

This publication is designed to provide accurate and authoritative information with regard to the subject matter covered herein. It is sold with the clear understanding that the Publisher is not engaged in rendering legal or any other professional services. If legal or any other expert assistance is required, the services of a competent person should be sought. FROM A DECLARATION OF PARTICIPANTS JOINTLY ADOPTED BY A COMMITTEE OF THE AMERICAN BAR ASSOCIATION AND A COMMITTEE OF PUBLISHERS.

Additional color graphics may be available in the e-book version of this book.

Library of Congress Cataloging-in-Publication Data

ISBN: 978-1-61942-745-7

MONKLANDS HOSPITAL
LIBRARY
MONKSCOURT AVENUE
AIRDRIE ML60JS
☎ 01236712005

Published by Nova Science Publishers, Inc. † New York

Contents

Foreword

Hearing loss is a chronic and often lifelong disability that can cause profound damage to the development of speech, language, and cognitive skills in children, especially when commencing before the critical period of language development in infancy. That damage, in turn, affects the child's progress in school and, later, his or her ability to obtain, keep, and perform an occupation. At all ages and for both sexes, hearing loss causes difficulties with interpersonal communication and leads to significant individual social problems, especially isolation and stigmatization. All these difficulties are much magnified in developing countries, where there are generally limited services, few trained staff members, and little awareness about how to deal with these difficulties.

The size of the problem of hearing loss is increasing globally. WHO estimated that, in 2005, according to current WHO definitions, there were at least 278 million people world-wide (4.2% of the world population) with moderate or worse bilateral "disabling" hearing loss. A further 364 million had mild hearing impairment. These figures have increased substantially over the last 25 years due to better case-finding, ageing populations and rising incidence from noise-induced hearing loss, excessive use of ototoxic drugs, and untreated chronic otitis media. Eighty percent of people with disabling hearing loss live in low- and middle-income countries. Studies of the global burden of disease have shown that, in 2005, adult-onset hearing loss ranked third in terms of years live with disability (YLD) causing 4.8% of the total global estimate of YLD

In addition to its effects on individuals, data from several countries indicate that hearing loss has huge economic consequences. Thus, prevention of hearing loss, as well as being socially and morally justifiable, makes substantial economic sense as well.

In spite of this state of affairs, hearing loss is neglected and forgotten. Most people are not aware of the consequences of the loss of hearing, the size of the problem, or the opportunities for prevention. There are few national programmes to prevent and manage the disability, and it remains very difficult to mobilize resources in this field.

This dire situation is beginning to change. There is increasing knowledge of the burden of hearing loss, though much information remains to be gathered. Research is revealing fundamental biological processes causing hearing damage. New interventions are being developed for prevention and management of hearing loss that can be implemented on population-level scales using public-health methods.

Because of the awakening attention to these issues, there is an urgent need for an in-depth review of the processes and opportunities for prevention of hearing loss. This unique book fulfils that need because it is comprehensive, authoritative and ranges widely from covering basic science to practical applications in the field, and from the philosophical understanding of disability to how hearing loss and its prevention affects people's lives. It is also very timely, because there is no other book that covers this area. The book will help to raise awareness on prevention of hearing loss amongst policy makers, professionals, students and other workers in the field of hearing loss, and show that there are ways in which the incidence of hearing loss can be reduced, that some hearing loss can be effectively treated and that methods are available to reduce the impact upon individuals and upon society.

The book should be of great value to public health specialists in Government and other organizations, health planners and policy makers, students in University and related training establishments.

I heartily commend this book for your perusal, enjoyment, and use.

Dr. Ala Alwan
Assistant Director-General
The World Health Organization

Preface

Hearing loss is a major cause of disability which can affect the communication skills, educational prospects, and the social and occupational lives of those affected: it impacts on society as a whole, and has huge economic costs. Consequently, preventing hearing loss is a goal worth achieving. In this context the term "prevention" is used to include the detection, treatment and management of hearing loss.

This book aims to provide a comprehensive text for all those involved in planning or delivering services with the purpose of preventing hearing loss. The first four chapters are important for understanding the basis of hearing impairment. Starting with a consideration of the various ways hearing loss is described and classified, the book then provides newly acquired information on the global prevalence of hearing loss or impairment. This is significantly greater than previously suspected and indicates the size of the problem facing those seeking to re-/habilitate those affected, especially the many who live in developing economies where there are competing calls upon limited resources.

In recent years there have been significant advances in our understanding of the mechanisms underlying sensorineural hearing impairment, the main type of permanent hearing loss. The processes involved in cochlear hair cell damage and the methods currently being used to treat this are described in the third chapter. How hearing loss affects individuals is crucial to an appreciation of its prevention and the fourth chapter in this book describes the impact on children and adults, with different degrees of hearing loss and discusses listening and its importance.

Knowledge of the various strategies to prevent hearing loss are important for those charged with this task and the fifth chapter considers these from a global and public health perspective. Subsequent chapters give more detailed accounts of some of the various strategies that can be employed.

Immunisation has proved an effective means of preventing hearing loss as a result of infectious diseases acquired in pregnancy and in childhood. While it was not the primary goal of the programme, it has nevertheless been an effective means of reducing the incidence of both conductive and sensorineural hearing loss. The sixth chapter describes the role of immunisation as a preventative strategy.

Research indicating the potential role of nutrients in preventing hearing loss is considered in Chapter 7 as this could potentially be a cheap and available method of prevention. Genetic counselling, on the other hand is an established method of prevention, which depends upon the decision of parents, or those affected, to limit their families. The chapter on genetic counselling shows how advances made in genetic research can provide better information to facilitate this decision.

It is essential to detect congenital hearing loss early as habilitation in the first few months of life can significantly improve the language development of affected babies. Universal newborn hearing screening is advocated in Chapter 9 which also describes the surveillance procedures which can be employed to detect an impairment in those who missed screening or acquired a hearing loss subsequently.

Some hearing losses can be treated and the surgical and medical means available to accomplish this are described in this book. A subsequent chapter describes how hearing aids and cochlear implants can reduce the impact of a hearing loss for many children and adults.

Legislation is playing a large role in the prevention of some types of hearing loss. It is not always realised that noise in social and community environments can also be damaging to health in general. The various ways in which this can be eliminated or reduced is separately considered in the next chapter.

The acoustic environment in which hearing impaired children and adults live and work can affect their ability to make optimal use of the devices provided; in milder losses it may even eliminate the need for devices altogether, an important economic consideration. A chapter on enabling acoustics completes the chapters on specific methods of prevention.

Preventing hearing loss has a monetary cost and health planners will need to consider this in order to make the best use of the health funds available. When evaluated, many preventative strategies are extremely cost effective. The chapter on economic analysis considers the cost of hearing loss and that of the failure to prevent it and provides a rational basis for intervening with preventative strategies.

To benefit from the methods of prevention outlined in earlier chapters, pregnant women and those who are hearing impaired need to be able to access health care. Two chapters are devoted to ways in which having or not having adequate access affects health in general and hearing care in particular, and includes examples of national programmes which have been set up in three large countries to prevent hearing impairment in all three aspects – detection, treatment and re/habilitation. The programmes show what can be accomplished.

The final chapter attempts to synthesize all of the endeavours to date, achievements as well as omissions and describes many areas where progress is needed and outlines some of the advances expected in the near future.

This book has drawn upon the knowledge and experience of contributors from various disciplines to demonstrate that in many instances prevention of deafness is feasible. The resulting benefits to individuals and to society described here show that in all instances it is desirable.

List of Contributors

Peter W Alberti, MB, BS, PhD, FRCS, Professor Emeritus, Department of Otolaryngology, University of Toronto, Canada.

Arum Kumar Agarwal, MB, BS, MS (ENT), Director-Professor of ENT & Dean, Maulana Azad Medical College, New Delhi, India.

Robert MP Baltussen, PhD. Department of Primary and Community Care, Radboud University, Nijmegen Medical Center, Nijmegen, Holland.

Maria Cecilia Bevilacqua, PhD, Professor of Audiology, University of São Paulo, Campus Bauru, Brazil.

Emma Brunskill, PhD, Professor, Computer Science Department, Carnegie Mellon University, Pittsburgh, PA, USA.

Xingkuan Bu, MD, Professor of Otolaryngology, WHO Collaborating Center for Preventing of Deafness and Hearing Impairment, Jiangsu Province Hospital, Nanjing Medical University, Nanjing, China.

Shelly Khanna Chadha, MB, BS, MS (ENT), Professor of ENT, Maulana Azad Medical College, New Delhi, India.

Adrian Davis, OBE, FFPH, FSS, PhD, MSc, BSc, Professor, Medical Research Council (MRC) Hearing and Communication Group, London, UK.

Katrina Davis, MB, BChir, MRCPsych, South London and Maudsley National Health Service (NHS) Trust, London, UK.

Seth M Flaxman BA, Computer Science Department, Carnegie Mellon University, Pittsburgh, PA, USA.

Andrew Forge, PhD, Professor of Auditory Cell Biology, Centre for Auditory Research, UCL Ear Institute, London WC1X 8EE

Howard J Hoffman, MA, Epidemiology and Statistics Program, National Institute on Deafness and Other Communication Disorders (NIDCD), National Institutes of Health (NIH), Bethesda, MD, USA.

Janet R Jamieson, PhD, Professor, Department of Educational and Counselling Psychology, and Special Education, Faculty of Education, University of British Columbia Canada.

A. Abraham Joseph, MBBS, DCH, MD MSc, Director, Christian Institute of Health Science and Research, Nagaland, India.

Amanda J. Leach MAgSci, PhD, Program Leader, Ear Health, Child Health Division, Menzies School of Health Research, Casuarina, NT. Australia.

Maya Mascarenhas MPH, Department of Epidemiology and Biostatistics, University of California, San Francisco, California, USA.

Colin D Mathers, PhD, Department of Health Statistics and Informatics, World Health Organization, Geneva, Switzerland.

Peter S. Morris, MBBS, FRACP, PhD, Deputy Leader, Child Health Division, Menzies School of Health Research, Casuarina, New Territories. Australia.

Valerie E Newton, MB, ChB, MSc, MD, FRCP, Professor Emerita, Department of Audiology, University of Manchester, UK.

John O'Keefe, BASc., MSc, PEng, FIOA, Aercoustics Engineering Limited, Toronto, Canada.

Bolajoko O Olusanya, MBBS, MSc, FRCP, Medical Officer, Institute of Child Health and Primary Care, University of Lagos, Lagos, Nigeria.

Kathleen Pichora-Fuller, PhD, RMPM, Professor, Department of Psychology, University of Toronto, Mississauga, Ontario, Canada.

Nathaniel H Robin, MD, Professor of Genetics and Pediatrics, University of Alabama at Birmingham, Department of Genetics, Birmingham, Alabama, USA.

Ulf Rosenhall, M.D., Ph.D. Professor, Department of Audiology and Neurotology, Karolinska University Hospital, Stockholm and Department of Clinical Science, Intervention and Technology, Karolinska Institutet, Stockholm, Sweden.

Katherine Dewer Rutledge, MS, CGC, Director of Genetic Counseling Services, University of Alabama at Birmingham, Department of Genetics, ,Birmingham, Alabama, USA.

Andrew W Smith, BSc, MB BS, MSc, MRCP, Honorary Professor, International Centre for Evidence on Disability , International Centre for Eye Health, London School of Hygiene and Tropical Health. London, UK.

Gretchen A Stevens, DSc, Department of Health Statistics and Informatics, World Health Organization, Geneva, Switzerland.

Dianne Toe, PhD, Senior Lecturer, Early Learning, Development and Inclusion, Melbourne Graduate School of Education, The University of Melbourne, Victoria, Australia.

In: Prevention of Hearing Loss
Editors: V. Newton, P. Alberti and A. Smith

ISBN: 978-1-61942-745-7
© 2012 Nova Science Publishers, Inc.

Chapter I

Hearing Loss: Definitions and Classification

*Andrew W. Smith**

Abstract

This chapter covers definitions and classifications of hearing loss in order to provide a foundation on which the main structure of the book is built.

After an introduction on some of the difficulties with terminology in this field, the next section of the chapter defines the different types of hearing loss, and attempts to bring clarity to the way that different terms are used to describe hearing difficulties. It includes causes of hearing loss along the auditory pathway as well as in the ear.

The third section provides a classification of hearing loss in terms of (1) its types, location and timing; (2) quantification of hearing loss, according to the different tests of hearing loss that are currently in use; (3) international systems of classification developed by the World Health Organization (WHO), and information on systems used or proposed by other bodies.

Introduction

On reading scientific papers and the media, there are many ways of describing and naming difficulties with hearing, and much confusion is generated by overlaps and alternative usages of terms and their different meanings. This chapter is an attempt to light up this area. Full illumination may not be possible, however, since ultimately we tend to behave like Humpty-Dumpty in *Through the Looking Glass* who said 'When I use a word, it means just what I choose it to mean — neither more nor less.' [1].

The title of this chapter illustrates the problem – "hearing loss" was selected out of several alternatives because it appears to be the most neutral term with the least "baggage".

---

* Corresponding author: andrew.smith@LSHTM.ac.uk.

The expression "hearing loss" is meant to include all types of hearing difficulty or problem. A few might criticize the word "loss" since individuals who have inherited their hearing problems could be said to have never had any hearing so cannot "lose" it. This boils down to a question of semantics again, and in this book, inherited hearing problems, whenever they occur, are included.

The next section of this chapter defines key terms in this field, as they are generally used and as they have been used in this book. The rest of the chapter classifies hearing loss according to different parameters: type and location in the auditory system, the different ways that hearing loss is measured and quantified, its age of onset, according to different international systems of classification developed by the World Health Organization, and some other relevant systems currently in use or proposed to grade severity of hearing loss. Only brief descriptions of each item are given and it is not intended that the description should be sufficient to enable a particular test of hearing to be conducted.

Definitions of Hearing Loss

Hearing Loss

This term can be used, as it has in this book, to designate all types and levels of hearing difficulty whenever they occur. However it is also used in a more specific way to indicate hearing that previously existed but has now been lost. Thus it has been defined in the on-line dictionary of audiology [2] as follows: "The amount in decibels by which an individual's hearing threshold level changes for the worse, commonly understood to refer to the combined loss from all causes. The term may also be applied to that part of the overall loss which is attributable to a known influence (for example, noise-induced hearing loss) or a combination of contributing causes (for example, age-associated hearing loss). The related term threshold shift implies before-and-after comparison whereas hearing loss commonly assumes a notional starting point such as audiometric zero." However, the starting point may be considered as anything less sensitive than 'normal', which would therefore include levels greater than audiometric zero.

Hearing Disorder

This is another generic term covering all types and levels of hearing difficulty which has been defined by the American Speech-Language-Hearing Association (ASHA) in 1993 as follows:

"A hearing disorder is the result of impaired auditory sensitivity of the physiological auditory system. A hearing disorder may limit the development, comprehension, production, and/or maintenance of speech and/or language. Hearing disorders are classified according to difficulties in detection, recognition, discrimination, comprehension, and perception of auditory information." [3].

Hearing Impairment

Hearing impairment is a generic descriptive term of hearing loss. It includes all persons whose hearing is outside the normal range. It covers those who are deaf and those who are hard of hearing, as defined below. It can refer to the whole range or only part of the auditory spectrum.[4]

The WHO International Classification of Functioning, Disability and Health (ICF) lists hearing impairment among Hearing Functions, which are a subgroup of group b: Bodily Functions:

"b230: Hearing functions. Sensory functions relating to sensing the presence of sounds and discriminating the location, pitch, loudness and quality of sounds. *Inclusions: functions of hearing, auditory discrimination, localization of sound source, lateralization of sound, speech discrimination; impairments such as deafness, hearing impairment and hearing loss."[5]*

A description of the overall structure and functioning of the ICF is given later in the chapter.

The terms "hearing impairment" or "hearing-impaired" may not be acceptable to all people with hearing loss, as the following statement on the website of the World Federation of the Deaf indicates:- "'hearing-impaired" is often viewed as negative. It focuses on what people cannot do. It establishes the standard as "hearing" and anything different as "impaired," or substandard, hindered, or damaged. It implies that something is not as it should be and ought to be fixed if possible. To be fair, this is probably not what people intended to convey by the term "hearing impaired."'[6]

Hearing Disability, and Hearing Handicap

These terms were used in the International Classification of Impairment, Disability and Handicap, ICIDH, 1980 [7] which has now been fully superceded by the ICF [8] (sometimes called ICIDH-2 to show that it is in effect a second edition of the ICIDH even though it has a different name). In the ICF the term "handicap" is no longer used and disability only appears under group e, environmental factors. Section 3.c) includes further information about the ICIDH. However, these terms remain in common usage, so the definitions of them used by the ICIDH are given in a box later in this chapter.

Hard of Hearing

The term hard of hearing is used for those with mild to severe hearing loss who can benefit from amplification [3]. As defined by the International Federation of Hard of Hearing People (IFHOH), the "definition of hard of hearing people, whose usual means of communication is by speech and appropriate technology, includes people with a hearing loss, late deafened adults, people who experience tinnitus or Menière's disease, people who have a cochlear implant, people who have hyperacusis" [9]. In this definition, tinnitus, Menière's

Disease and hyperacusis are some of the few conditions which are hearing impairments, but not hearing losses, although they may be associated with hearing loss. The IFHOH also includes people with prelingual hearing impairment who develop good speech and language following cochlear implantation [10].

ASHA has defined hard of hearing as "a hearing disorder, whether fluctuating or permanent, which adversely affects an individual's ability to communicate. The hard-of-hearing individual relies on the auditory channel as the primary sensory input for communication". [3].

Deafened and Late-Deafened

The UK National Association of Deafened People (NADP) states that "Deafened people are those who have used spoken language for communication but then have lost most or all of their natural hearing"[11].

The loss is generally severe or profound and is usually sudden but may have a more gradual onset. They distinguish themselves from hard of hearing people who, they state, have a gradual-onset, mild/moderate hearing loss, causing words or parts of conversations to be missed.

The term "late-deafened" generally refers to people who become deaf from any cause later in childhood, in young adulthood, during the working years, and sometimes later in life. For example, the Association for Late-Deafened Adults, ALDA, in the USA [12] caters for this group.

The term "adventitious deafness" has been used to mean a hearing loss that occurs sometime after birth [13], so that deafened and late-deafened are sub-groups of this.

Deaf, Deafness

The terms "deaf" and "deafness", with lower-case "d", are usually used to describe people with profound hearing loss, such that no benefit can be obtained from amplification. However in countries such as the UK and others in South Asia "deaf" and "deafness" are used by the media or in everyday usage to refer to any level of hearing loss. ASHA has defined "deaf" as "a hearing disorder that limits an individual's aural/oral communication performance to the extent that the primary sensory input for communication may be other than the auditory channel." [3].

However, it would perhaps be better to apply this definition to the noun "deafness" rather than the adjective "deaf". The word Deaf, written with an upper-case "D", is used to refer to someone who belongs to the Deaf Culture, which is seen by some as a distinctive cultural group with its own language. The World Federation of the Deaf (WFD) states:

"Deaf and hard of hearing people do not identify as having a disability or see themselves as experiencing a limitation. Instead, they identify as a member of a cultural and linguistic group" [14].

Deaf-Blind

This refers to both visual impairment and hearing impairment occurring in combination with each other in one person. Examples of causes are Usher's syndrome where hearing loss is combined with Retinitis pigmentosa, or congenital rubella which now mainly occurs in countries where there are no or inadequate immunization programmes (see Chapter 6). Frequently, other disabilities occur with visual and hearing impairment such as in congenital rubella. The combination of these disabilities causes significant challenges which need specific solutions that are often different from those for persons with either hearing loss or visual loss alone. This disability has not been specifically addressed in this book.

Auditory Processing Disorders

These are conditions which affect the auditory nerve or more central parts of the auditory pathway.

Auditory Neuropathy Spectrum Disorder (ANSD)

"Auditory neuropathy" is a relatively recent clinical diagnosis used to describe individuals with auditory temporal processing disorders due to dysfunction of the synapse between the inner hair cells and the auditory nerve, and/or dysfunction of the auditory nerve itself. Patients with auditory neuropathy show clinical evidence of normally functioning outer hair cells but typically demonstrate impaired speech understanding, and show normal to severely impaired speech detection and pure tone thresholds. Their ability to process rapidly changing acoustic signals, i.e. auditory temporal processing, is affected.

There are multiple designations for this disorder, so to simplify terminology a recent set of guidelines recommended using the term "Auditory Neuropathy Spectrum Disorder" (ANSD) [15]. The guideline authors stated that the term "auditory neuropathy" has gained wide-spread acceptance, and was retained in order to avoid confusion for patients and professionals. The expression of this disorder encompasses a spectrum ranging from limited or mild effects (complaints of difficulty "hearing" in noisy listening conditions) to profound effects (inability to "hear" in any listening condition, functionally "deaf"). In addition, the term "spectrum" was felt to expand the concept of this disorder to include sites of the lesion other than the auditory nerve.

Auditory Processing Disorder (APD)

The following description is taken from the Position Statement on Auditory Processing Disorder (APD) by the British Society of Audiology published on 31st March 2011 [16]

"APD is characterised by poor perception of both speech and non-speech sounds. Auditory 'perception' is the awareness of acoustic stimuli, forming the basis for subsequent action. Perception results from both sensory activation (via the ear) and neural processing that integrates this 'bottom-up' information with activity in other brain systems (e.g. vision, attention, memory). Insofar as difficulties in perceiving and understanding speech sounds could arise from other causes (e.g. language impairment, non-native experience of a particular language), poor perception of speech alone is not sufficient evidence of APD.

APD has its origins in impaired neural function. The mechanisms underlying APD can include both afferent and efferent pathways in the auditory system, as well as higher level processing that provides 'top-down' modulation of such pathways.

APD impacts on everyday life primarily through a reduced ability to listen, and so respond appropriately to sounds. The term 'listening' has been used to imply an active process while 'hearing' implies a more passive process; it is possible to hear without listening attentively". This condition is also called Central Auditory Processing Disorder (CAPD) [17, 18].

Classifications of Hearing Loss Types, Location and Timing of Hearing Loss

Conductive

Hearing loss caused by blockage of the external ear or by blockage or derangement of the middle ear, resulting in a reduction of transmission of sound energy reaching the cochlea in the inner ear.[2].

Sensorineural (Hair Cell or Neural Damage)

In descending order of frequency, this is hearing loss due to a lesion or disorder of the outer or inner hair cells of the inner ear (sensory hearing loss) or of the auditory nervous system (neural hearing loss) or of the auditory centres in the brain. Most authorities would consider the term sensorineural to include ANSD and APD above, though they would be regarded as not typical sensorineural hearing loss [15]. The causes of sensorineural hearing loss can be inherited, congenital or acquired. Formerly called perceptive loss or nerve loss; both these terms are now obsolete [2]. This is the most common type of permanent hearing loss [19].

Mixed

Sometimes a conductive hearing loss occurs in combination with a sensorineural hearing loss (SNHL). In other words, there may be damage in the outer or middle ear and in the inner ear (cochlea) or auditory nerve. When this occurs, the hearing loss is referred to as a mixed hearing loss [19].

Bilateral and Unilateral

Bilateral hearing loss occurs in both ears. Unilateral hearing loss (UHL) means that hearing is normal in one ear but there is hearing loss in the other ear. The hearing loss can be conductive or sensorineural affecting the outer, middle or inner ear, range from mild to very severe, occur in both adults and children and can be either peripheral or central [19].

Symmetrical and Asymmetrical Hearing Loss

Symmetrical means the degree and configuration of hearing loss are the same in each ear. Asymmetrical means degree and configuration of hearing loss are different in each ear [19]. The amount of difference for a hearing loss to be designated asymmetric has clinical importance, for example when deciding whether to conduct a Magnetic Resonance Imaging (MRI) scan for an asymmetric hearing loss to rule out acoustic neuroma. This is currently a matter of clinical opinion and beyond the scope of this book.

Progressive and Sudden Hearing Loss

Progressive hearing loss becomes worse over a prolonged period of time. Sudden hearing loss occurs suddenly over a maximum of 3 days. Sudden hearing loss requires immediate medical attention to determine its cause and treatment [19]. However, many people experience a 'slight' acute (sudden) hearing loss which usually resolves. The amount of hearing loss which would be therefore be deemed medically important is also a clinical decision and beyond the scope of this book.

Fluctuating Versus Stable Hearing Loss

Fluctuating hearing loss changes over time—thresholds sometimes improving, sometimes worsening, and may be due to conductive or sensorineural causes. It is frequently bilateral and may be associated with progressive hearing loss [20]. Stable hearing loss shows no change in degree of hearing loss over time.

Age of Onset: Pre-Lingual, Post-Lingual

Prelingual Hearing Loss

This type of hearing loss is sustained prior to the acquisition of language, and can thus occur as a result of a congenital condition or through hearing loss in early infancy. A recent US review stated that more than 50% of prelingual hearing loss is genetic, most often (>80%) autosomal recessive and non-syndromic, and a small percentage of prelingual deafness is syndromic or autosomal dominant non-syndromic [21,22]. These figures are not necessarily true in parts of the developing world where immunization has not been effective.

Congenital CMV infections and connexin mutations have been estimated to be the two major causes of hearing loss at birth, while enlarged vestibular aqueduct along with congenital CMV infection are the major causes of pre-lingual hearing loss that are expressed after birth [23].

Prelingual hearing loss can have a profound effect on the development of language unless there is early detection through neonatal hearing screening followed by early intervention.

Post-Lingual Hearing Loss

Post-lingual hearing loss occurs after the acquisition of language, and may be due to any of the acquired childhood causes, as well as delayed-onset genetic hearing loss such as otosclerosis, and other conditions acquired in adulthood.

Peripheral versus Central Hearing Loss

Peripheral hearing loss is any type of hearing loss where the lesion is in the outer, middle or inner ear or in the auditory or cochlear nerve, arbitrarily before it becomes the vestibulo-cochlear nerve. Most definitions of peripheral hearing loss include lesions of the auditory or cochlear nerve (the distal part of the VIIIth Cranial nerve) [24]

Peripheral hearing loss has also been defined as "abnormal encoding of the auditory system" [25].

Central hearing loss occurs somewhere along the pathway of the central auditory system i.e. vestibulo-cochlear nerve, cochlear nucleus, trapezoid body, superior olivary complex, lateral lemniscus, inferior colliculi, medial geniculate nucleus, primary auditory cortex.

Cortical deafness occurs when there is damage to the primary auditory cortex usually caused by bilateral embolic stroke. It is characterized by an inability to interpret either verbal or nonverbal sounds with preserved awareness of the occurrence of sound (as for instance by a startle reaction to a clap) [26]. This condition is very rare because most of the causes are incompatible with life. However one patient, studied over 20 years, had MRI-confirmed bilateral absence of considerable portions of her temporal lobes resulting in cortical deafness. Her speech characteristics were those usually associated with a person with profound peripheral hearing loss [27].

Quantification of Hearing Loss

The purpose of this section is to list current tests in general use with a very brief description of the type of test. It is not intended to enable the reader to conduct the test. In the ICF classification these measuring methods would be respectively at the level of the body (hearing) or at the level of the activity (listening).

Testing Hearing with No or Basic Equipment

Questionnaire to subject with hearing loss, or their care-giver. The questions record the subject's or the care-giver's observations of the subject's response to sound. If the subject is a baby, the respondent would usually be a parent, preferably the mother.

Response to voice. The tester uses his or her own voice to observe response to sound, generally in a more controlled environment (e.g. quiet part of a health centre).

Response to noise-maker(s). The tester uses one or more noisemakers such as a rattle to observe response to sound. Some noise makers can be made and calibrated to produce specific intensities and frequencies of sound (e.g. the Manchester Rattle [28]). This rattle is still used in some locations, as evidenced by its continuing availability from medical suppliers in the UK and Ireland [29].

Tuning fork – Rinne and Weber tests. The tuning fork tests ability to respond to the tone produced by the tuning fork transmitted via air conduction (AC) or bone conduction (BC). The Rinne test compares perception of sounds as transmitted by AC through the middle ear with sounds transmitted by BC through the mastoid in the same ear. The Weber test is a qualitative BC test that is used to assess if both ears hear equally [30]. Tuning forks are commonly used also to compare the hearing of the subject with that of the tester.

Distraction testing assesses the response to different frequencies and intensities of a noise-maker in an infant at the instant when a visual distraction is stopped.

Pure Tone Audiometry

This group of tests generally determines the threshold of audibility to pure tones at different sound frequencies, delivered through earphones or in a free field. The subject indicates the sound has been heard by raising a finger, or pressing a button, or saying "yes". The free field method may be used for a child that cannot cooperate and is conducted by presenting the sound from an audiometer held a certain distance from the ear, or via loudspeakers in a sound-proof booth. Other variants are (1) Visual Response Audiometry where a young child is rewarded by sight of a light or a toy when correctly responding by looking at a sound source; (2) conditioned play audiometry in a slightly older child (up to 4-5 years), where the child is trained to perform a simple activity such as putting a block in a box, whenever a sound is heard.

If the outer or middle ear is obstructed, the test can be done by pure-tone bone conduction, using a vibrator placed on the skin where a skull bone is near the skin surface. The skull bones transmit sound energy to the inner ear, by-passing the outer and middle ear. The 'air-bone gap' is a measure of conductive loss, since it is the difference between the hearing threshold measured by air conduction and the threshold measured by bone conduction.

Speech Audiometry

This tests the speech reception threshold in older children and adults, which is the faintest speech that can be heard half the time. Word recognition or the ability to correctly repeat back words at a comfortable loudness level may also be tested.

Telephone and Internet Screening

A development of the speech-in-noise test is telephone screening for hearing loss. This was originally developed in The Netherlands and is now available in the UK [31]. By telephone, a random series of digit triplets is generated automatically from pre-recordings and the subject responds using the telephone keypad. The test has been well validated with high sensitivity and specificity [32] and has been successfully implemented in fixed line telephones, computers, smartphones and tablets, such as the iPAD, via the internet.

The tests in the sections above are partially subjective since they require a conscious response to the presented sound.

Oto-Acoustic Emission (OAE) Testing

An OAE is vibrational energy originating from motile behaviour of the outer hair cells in the cochlea and observable as sound in the external ear canal. Such emissions may be spontaneous (SOAE) or evoked by an externally applied acoustic stimulus.

Oto-acoustic emissions evoked by a transient acoustic stimulus (e.g. a click) occur with a time delay of a few milliseconds and are termed transient-evoked oto-acoustic emissions (TEOAE). They can be evoked by a click or tone-burst stimulus [2]. Distortion-product oto-acoustic emissions (DPOAE) are evoked using a pair of primary tones f_1 and f_2 with particular intensity. OAEs disappear after the inner ear has been damaged, so OAEs are used as a measure of inner ear health [33]. They are the basis of a simple, non-invasive, test for hearing defects in newborn babies and in children who are too young to cooperate in conventional hearing tests. This test is the basis of most Universal Neonatal Hearing Screening Programmes that many countries are implementing around the world. (See Chapter 9: Screening and Surveillance). Oto-acoustic emissions can also assist in differential diagnosis of cochlear and higher level hearing losses such as Auditory Neuropathy Spectrum Disorder, (ANSD), although if used as the only screening tool will fail to identify ANSD. In other words, OAE tests, in the absence of a conductive block, are specifically tests for outer hair cell function.

Electric Response Audiometry

These tests measure auditory function by externally recording electrical potentials evoked by acoustic stimuli applied to the ear. Techniques are distinguished according to the site of origin of the potential.

Cortical ERA (CERA) records potentials from the auditory cortex; this is also known as slow vertex response (SVR). This is ineffective in infants because of an immature central nervous system.

Auditory brainstem response (ABR) records potentials from the brainstem; this was formerly also known as brainstem evoked response audiometry (BERA).

Electrocochleography (ECochG) records the potentials existing in and around the cochlea, using an electrode placed either externally or transtympanically [2].

Auditory Steady State Response (ASSR). This is an auditory evoked potential, elicited with modulated tones that can be used to predict hearing sensitivity in patients of all ages. It uses statistical measures to determine if and when a threshold is present and create a valid estimated audiogram. Both ABR and ASSR, and also CERA, can be used to estimate threshold for patients who cannot or will not participate in traditional behavioral measures.

Tests in the above two sections (OAE and Electric Response Audiometry) are objective tests and do not require any conscious response from the subject. However, their interpretation is subjective.

International Systems of Classification of Hearing Loss Developed by WHO

The family of International Classifications at WHO includes the following top-level Reference Classifications and several derived classifications. The 3 Reference Classifications are the main classifications on basic parameters of health, prepared by WHO and approved by the WHO's governing bodies for international use. They comprise:

- International Classification of Diseases (ICD)
- International Classification of Functioning, Disability and Health (ICF)
- International Classification of Health Interventions (ICHI)

The first two classifications will be covered in this section. The third is still in preparation. Further information about this family of classifications can be found on the WHO website [34].

International Classification of Diseases 10th Revision (ICD-10)

ICD-10 comprises 22 chapters covering all health and disease conditions. Each chapter is identified by a letter, and subsections of chapters are numerically coded, as shown against each item below. It can be fully accessed on-line [35].

Causes of hearing loss and the different aspects of hearing loss are found in the following sections of the ICD-10:-

1) Chapter VIII Diseases of the ear and mastoid process (H60-H95)
2) The 1st page of the on-line chapter gives links to various other sections that include conditions that cause hearing loss but are not part of Chapter VIII: Diseases of the ear and mastoid process (H60-H95).
3) There are also various other conditions which may cause hearing loss, but are not mentioned as being excluded from Chapter VIII, as follows:-
   - B05.3 Measles complicated by otitis media (H67.1)
   - G00 Bacterial meningitis, not included elsewhere (Haemophilus, Pneumococcal, Streptococcal)
   - A39 Meningococcal infection, Meningococcal meningitis
   - Q16 Congenital malformations of the ear causing impairment of hearing (excl: congenital deafness (H90.-)

International Classification of Functioning, Disability and Health (ICF)

The ICF classifies health and health-related domains from the perspective of the body, and individual and societal perspectives by means of two lists: a list of body functions and structure, and a list of domains of activity and participation. An individual's functioning and disability occur in a context, so the ICF includes a list of environmental factors [36].

The ICF acknowledges that every human being can experience a decrement in health and thereby experience some degree of disability. The ICF 'mainstreams' the experience of disability and recognises it as a universal human experience. It shifts the focus from cause to impact and therefore places all health conditions on an equal footing allowing them to be compared using a common metric. The ICF also takes into account the social and environmental aspects of disability so that their impact on the person's functioning can be recorded.

Locations of items in the ICF specifically relevant to hearing loss are listed as follows. More details can be found by searching the on-line version of the ICF, items being identified by the lettering and numbering system shown below [37].

b BODY FUNCTIONS and BODY STRUCTURES
Chapter 2 (in Functions) on sensory functions includes Hearing Function (b230)
Chapter 2 (in Structures) on The Eye, Ear and related structures.(s240-s299)

d ACTIVITIES AND PARTICIPATION
Chapter 1: Learning and applying knowledge (d110-d119),
Chapter 2: Communication (d310-d360)

e ENVIRONMENTAL FACTORS
Chapter 1: Products and Technology e125 - e155 (including devices for amplification, and building design)
Chapter 2: Natural Environment including Sound (e250)
Chapter 3: Support and Relationships including relevant Health Professionals (e355)
Chapter 5: Services, Systems and Policies including architecture and construction (e515), Education and training (e5851).

The International Classification of Impairments, Disabilities and Handicaps (ICIDH)

The development of the ICF built on the strengths of its predecessor, the International Classification of Impairments, Disabilities and Handicaps (ICIDH), and addressed its weaknesses.

The ICIDH, published in 1980, provided key definitions, for that time, of impairment, disability, and handicap (see box) but these have been superceded by the ICF.

The ability of the ICIDH not only to classify an individual's circumstances but to provide a theoretical framework to inter-relate impairment, disability and handicap made it a powerful tool for a range of applications including:

- clinical diagnosis and rehabilitation assessment,
- record keeping in health and rehabilitation settings,
- development of medical and rehabilitation monitoring systems,
- program evaluation.

Major improvements of the ICIDH by the ICF were the shift in focus from cause to impact of disabilities and the more specific recognition of the social construction of disability and the critical role played by environmental or contextual factors in restricting full participation [38] as described in the previous section.

Definitions of the ICIDH 1980

(now superceded by the International Classification of Functioning, Disability and Health)

The International Classification of Impairments, Disabilities and Handicaps (ICIDH), provides a conceptual framework for disability which is described in three dimensions-impairment, disability and handicap:

Impairment: In the context of health experience an impairment is any loss or abnormality of psychological, physiological or anatomical structure or function.

Disability: In the context of health experience a disability is any restriction or lack (resulting from an impairment) of ability to perform an activity in the manner or within the range considered normal for a human being.

Handicap: In the context of health experience a handicap is a disadvantage for a given individual, resulting from an impairment or a disability, that limits or prevents the fulfillment of a role that is normal (depending on age, sex, and social and cultural factors) for that individual.

Impairment is considered to occur at the level of organ or system function.

Disability is concerned with functional performance or activity, affecting the whole person.

The third dimension-'handicap'-focuses on the person as a social being and reflects the interaction with and adaptation to the person's surroundings. The classification system for handicap is not hierarchical, but is constructed of a group of dimensions, with each dimension having an associated scaling factor to indicate impact on the individual's life.

WHO Prevention of Deafness and Hearing Impairment (PDH) Definitions

WHO Prevention of Deafness and Hearing Impairment (PDH), part of the WHO Programme for Prevention of Blindness and Deafness (PBD), currently defines hearing impairment as any level of hearing loss from mild, through moderate and severe to profound. The levels or grades are given in a table on the WHO website [39] and in Figure 1.1.

WHO has also defined *disabling hearing impairment* in adults and children [40] as follows:

Disabling hearing impairment in adults should be defined as a permanent unaided hearing threshold level for the better ear of 41 dB HL or greater; for this purpose the hearing threshold level is to be taken as the better ear average hearing threshold level for the four frequencies 0.5, 1, 2, and 4 kHz.

Disabling hearing impairment in children under the age of 15 years should be defined as a permanent unaided hearing threshold level for the better ear of 31 dB HL or greater; for this purpose the hearing threshold level is to be taken as the better ear average hearing threshold level for the four frequencies 0.5, 1, 2, and 4 kHz.

Grades or levels of impairment	WHO Hearing threshold levels in decibels for the better ear taken as the average of the unaided pure-tone threshold levels for the frequencies of 0.5, 1, 2, 4 kHz	WHO definition of Disabling Hearing Impairment in children less than 15 years of age	WHO definition of Disabling Hearing Impairment in adults aged 15 years and older
No Impairment	<26 dB HL		
Slight or Mild impairment	26-40 dB HL		
Moderate Impairment	41-60 dB HL	**Average threshold levels 31 db HL or greater for the frequencies 0.5, 1, 2, 4 kHz**	**Average threshold levels 41 db HL or greater for the frequencies 0.5, 1, 2, 4 kHz**
Severe Impairment	61-80 dB HL		
Profound Impairment	≥81 dB HL		

Audiometric threshold measurements according to the international standard ISO 8253-1 .

Figure 1.1. WHO definitions of Hearing Impairment. (adapted from Pascolini D and Smith A [44] and used with permission from INFORMA HEALTH CARE).

However there is concern amongst some audiologists that the WHO hearing levels for adult-onset disabling hearing impairment and for any level of hearing loss were set too high, because of the recognition that significant moderate and mild disability respectively exists at thresholds below the current WHO levels. There is also disquiet about having different levels for adults and children for defining disabling hearing impairment.

There are a number of other classifications of hearing loss in use in different countries. Two examples are from American Speech-Language-Hearing Association ASHA in the USA [41], and the British Society of Audiology in the UK [42].

Having different scales of severity in different parts of the world makes it difficult to compare epidemiological surveys of prevalence accurately, since the different scales have a highly significant effect on the numbers of subjects discovered. A study in 1999 [43] showed that prevalence results varied from 6 to 30% in women and 10 to 49% in men, depending on which scale was used to group the subjects. Thus it is essential that all such studies adopt the same standard. The WHO scale shown in Fig. 1.1 was an attempt to do this, and a number of surveys have been conducted and analysed using this scale [44]. If the recommended scale were to change, the results of previous surveys using the current WHO levels should be re-calculated, by going back to the original datasets.

Recently, the expert group on hearing loss working for the new initiative on the Global Burden of Disease (GBD) [45] in which WHO is involved, addressed this issue. As stated in Chapter 2, the Global Burden of Disease (GBD) Expert Group on Hearing impairment "did not find the current categories, and particularly the different categorization for children and adults, compelling in understanding the needs of the hearing impaired population." The group has proposed a new classification which takes into account concerns that the lower bounds for any level of impairment or for disabling hearing impairment, as given above, are set too high, and that mild, unilateral and child-onset hearing losses have been ignored.

The new classification defines mild hearing loss as 20.0 to 34.9 dB HL, better ear average at 0.5, 1, 2, and 4 kHz, and disabling hearing loss as 35.0 dB HL or above in children and adults at the same average frequencies. It also defines seven levels of severity of hearing loss, from -10 dB HL to +94.9dB HL, each defined by a 14.9 dB HL range band in hearing level in the better ear; total impairment ("deaf") is defined as a hearing loss ≥95 dB HL in the better ear (see chapter 2, in particular the section "Defining Hearing Impairment" and table 2.1, for further information).

Use of this new classification could lead to a substantial increase in the numbers worldwide with "disabling hearing loss". Thus, recalculation using these new cut-offs of the data from 4 recent population-based surveys in 4 different provinces of China conducted using the WHO Ear and Hearing Disorders Survey Protocol [46] increases the overall prevalence of moderate or worse ("disabling") hearing loss from 4.7% using the current WHO cut-offs (31/41dB HL or greater in children and adults respectively) to 7.6% using the new GBD cut-off (35 dB HL or greater), and from 14.5% to 40.9% respectively for mild or worse hearing loss (using the new GBD cut-off of 20.0 dB HL or greater) [47].

It should be emphasised that these new levels have not so far been officially accepted yet by WHO or elsewhere.

Conclusion

As with any rapidly developing field, there are a large number of definitions and classify-cations which are often confusing, overlapping or even contradictory. They are also frequently changing, and this chapter is merely a snapshot of a particular moment, but which may be useful to locate and relate the more important contributions that form the rest of this book.

References

[1]   Carroll, Lewis. *Through the Looking Glass and What Alice Found There*. Macmillan, London, 1871.

[2]   Lawton, B.W., Robinson, D.W. (2003). A Concise Vocabulary of Audiology and allied topics. Part 1: Vocabulary. On-line version © 2003 Institute of Sound and Vibration Research. Available from: http://www.isvr.co.uk/reprints/vocab.htm (Accessed 6 August 2011).

[3]   American Speech-Language-Hearing Association. (1993). Definitions of Communication Disorders and Variations 1993. Available from: http://www.asha.org /docs/pdf/-RP1993-00208.pdf (Accessed 16 October 2011).

[4]   Industry Canada. (2011). Definition: Hearing Impairment, in Assistive Technology Links, Industry Canada. Available from: http://www.apt.gc.ca/wat/wb14200 e.asp?did =5 (Accessed 6 August 2011).

[5]   World Health Organisation. (2011). Hearing functions: hearing impairment. WHO International Classification of Functioning, Disability and Health (ICF) – online version. Available from: http://apps.who.int/classifications/icfbrowser/ (Accessed 25 October 2011).

[6]   World Federation of the Deaf. (2011). Statement on term "Hearing Impaired". Available from: http://www.wfdeaf.org/faq (Accessed 6 August 2011).

[7]   World Health Organisation. (1980). International Classification of Impairment, Disability and Handicap (ICIDH), Geneva: World Health Organisation.

[8]   World Health Organisation. (2011). World Health Organisation International Classification of Functioning, Disability and Health (ICF). Available from: http://www. who.int/classifications/icf/en/ (Accessed 25 October 2011).

[9]   The International Federation of Hard of Hearing People (IFHOH), Brochure. Available from: http://www.ifhoh.org/pdf/ifhohbrochure.pdf

[10]   Angelo TC, Bevilacqua MC, Moret AL. Speech perception in pre-lingual deaf users of cochlear implant. Pro Fono, 22, 275-279.

[11]   Definition of "Deafened" in Information Booklet, National Association of Deafened People. Available from: http://www.nadp.org.uk/intr.htm (Accessed 25 October 2011)

[12]   The Association of Late-Deafened Adults, ALDA. Available from: http://alda.org/ (Accessed 1 October 2011).

[13]   Glossary of Hearing Loss and Other Terms Related to Ears. Available from: http://www.hearinglosshelp.com/glossary.htm#AdventHL (Accessed 9 August 2011).

[14]   Deaf Culture. Page on the website of the World Federation of the Deaf. Available from: http://www.wfdeaf.org/our-work/focus-areas/deaf-culture-2. (Accessed 7 August 2011).

[15]   Guidelines for Identification and Management of Infants and Young Children with Auditory Neuropathy Spectrum Disorder. Hayes D, Sininger Y (Co-chairs for Guidelines Development Conference), The Children's Hospital, Colorado, USA 2008. Synopsis of guidelines available from: http:.childrenscolorado.org/ conditions/ speech/ danielscenter/ANSD-Guidelines.aspx. (Accessed 6 August 2011).

[16] British Society of Audiology, APD Special Interest Group, Position Statement on Auditory processing disorder (APD). (2011). *British Society of Audiology.* Available from:

http://www.thebsa.org.uk/images/stories/docs/BSA_APD_PositionPaper_31March11_F INAL.pdf (Accessed 9 August 2011).

[17] American Academy of Audiology (AAA). (2010). Diagnosis, treatment and management of children and adults with central auditory processing disorder. Available from: www.audiology.org/resources/documentlibrary/Documents/CAPD%20Guide lines%208-2010.pdf (Accessed 4 October 2011).

[18] Central Auditory processing disorders in Definitions of Communication Disorders and Variations. American Speech-Language-Hearing Association. (1993). Available from: http://www.asha.org/docs/pdf/RP1993-00208.pdf (Accessed 15 October 2011).

[19] Types of Hearing Loss. American Speech-Language-Hearing Association http://www. asha.org/public/hearing/Types-of-Hearing-Loss/ (Accessed 25 October 2011).

[20] Review of Progressive and Fluctuating Hearing Loss. Ross D. Paper on CDC Website at http://www.cdc.gov/ncbddd/hearingloss/documents/unilateral/DRossPkg04-Progressive & Fluctuating-cleared.pdf (Accessed 5 January 2012).

[21] Smith, R., Hildebrand, M., Van Camp, G.(2010). Deafness and Hereditary Hearing Loss Overview. Gene Reviews Bookshelf ID: NBK1434 PMID: 20301607 Initial Posting: February 14, 1999; Last Update: October 14, 2010.

[22] Denoyelle, F., Weil, D., Maw, M.A., Wilcox, S.A., Lench, N.J., Allen-Powell, D.R., Osborn, A.H., Dahl, H.H., Middleton, A., Houseman, M.J., Dodé, C., Marlin, S., Boulila-ElGaïed, A., Grati, M., Ayadi, H., BenArab, S., Bitoun, P., Lina-Granade, G., Godet, J., Mustapha, M., Loiselet, J., El-Zir, E., Aubois, A., Joannard, A., Petit, C. (1997). Prelingual deafness: high prevalence of a 30delG mutation in the connexin 26 gene. Human Molecular Genetics, 6, 2173-2177.

[23] Nance, W., Limb, G., Dodson, K. (2006). Importance of congenital cytomegalovirus infections as a cause for pre-lingual hearing loss. *Journal of Clinical Virology* 35, 221–225

[24] The Ears and Hearing. North Queensland Hearing Services. Available from: http://www.hearingservices.com.au/ears.php (Accessed 15 October 2011).

[25] Koravand, A., Jutras, B., Roumy, N.(2010). Peripheral hearing loss and auditory temporal ordering ability in children. *International Journal of Pediatric Otorhin olaryngology* 74,50–55

[26] Hain T. Central Hearing Loss. Paper on Website Dizziness-and-Balance.com, based on Hain TC, Micco A. "Cranial Nerve 8: Vestibulocochlear Nerve" in. Textbook of Neurology, Goetz and Pappert Eds, Saunders, 2003, (2nd Edn). Available from: http://www.dizziness-and-balance.com/disorders/hearing/cent_hearing.html. (Accessed 9 August 2011).

[27] Hood, L.J., Berlin, C.I., Allen, P. (1994).Cortical deafness: a longitudinal study. *Journal of the American Academy of Audiology,* 5, 330-342.

[28] Kettlety, A.(1987).The Manchester high pitch rattle. British Journal of Audiology, 21, 73-74.

[29] Manchester Rattle suppliers: Available from: http://www.wms. co.uk/ ENT/ENT InstrumentsandAccessories/Manchester_Rattle http://www. medstore. ie/ manchester-rattle-p-357.html

[30] Dickens, O. (2011). Tuning fork tests: a basic primary hearing assessment approach to improving clinical efficiency. *Journal of Community Ear and Hearing Health Issue 11.* To be available from: http://disabilitycentre.lshtm.ac.uk/key-publications/journal-of-community-ear-and-hearing-health/

[31] Action on Hearing (formerly the Royal National Institute for the Deaf) Telephone or internet test of Hearing see: http://www.actiononhearingloss.org.uk/your-hearing/look-after-your-hearing/check-your-hearing/take-the-check.aspx (Accessed on 6 August 2011).

[32] Smits, C., Kapteyn, T.S., Houtgast, T. (2004). Development and validation of an automatic speech-in-noise screening test by telephone. *International Journal of Audiology, 43,* 15-28.

[33] Otoacoustic Emission, Wikipedia. http://en.wikipedia.org/wiki/Otoacoustic_emission (Accessed 7 August 2011).

[34] Madden, R., Sykes, C., Ustun, T. (2007). World Health Organization Family of International Classifications: definition, scope and purpose. Geneva: World Health Organisation. Available from: http://www.who.int/classifications/en/Family Document 2007.pdf (Accessed 8 August 2011).

[35] World Health Organisation. (2007). International Classification of Diseases 10th Revision (ICD-10). Available from: http://apps.who.int/classifications/apps /icd/icd10 online/ (Accessed 8 August 2011).

[36] World Health Organisation. (2001). International Classification of Functioning, Disability and Health (ICF), overview. Available from: http://www.who.int /classifi-cations/icf/en/ (Accessed 8 August 2011).

[37] World Health Organisation. (2001). International Classification of Functioning, Disability and Health (ICF). Available from: http://apps.who.int/classifications /icfbrowser/ (Accessed 8 August 2011).

[38] What is disability? on Australian Indigenous Health Infonet. Available from:http:// www.healthinfonet.ecu.edu.au/related-issues/disability/reviews/background-information (Accessed 8 August 2011).

[39] World Health Organisation Programme for Prevention of Blindness and Deafness. Grades of Hearing Impairment. Available from: http://www.who.int/pbd/deafness/ hearing_impairment_grades/en/index.html (Accessed 6 August 2011).

[40] World Health Organisation. (1991,1997). Report of the informal working group on prevention of deafness and hearing impairment: programme planning. Geneva: World Health Organisation. 1991 at http://whqlibdoc.who.int/hq/1991/WHO_PDH_91.1.pdf . With adaptations from: Report of the first informal consultation on future programme developments for the prevention of deafness and hearing impairment, Geneva: World Health Organisation. 23-24 January 1997, WHO/PDH/97.3. Available from: http:// whqlibdoc.who.int/hq/1997/WHO_PDH_97.3.pdf .

[41] Degree of Hearing Loss: a page in section "Information for the Public" American Speech-Language-Hearing Association (ASHA). http://www.asha.org/public/hearing/ Degree-of-Hearing-Loss/ (Accessed 10 August 2011).

[42] British Society of Audiology Recommended Procedure: Pure-tone air-conduction and bone-conduction threshold audiometry with and without masking. 24th September 2011. http://www.thebsa.org.uk/docs/Guidelines/BSA_RP_PTA_FINAL_24Sept11.pdf (Accessed 23 October 2011).

[43] Duijvestijn, J.A., Anteunis, L.J., Hendriks, J.J., Manni, J.J. (1999). Definition of hearing impairment and its effect on prevalence figures. A survey among senior citizens. *Acta Otolaryngologica*, 119, 420-423.

[44] Pascolini, D. and Smith, A. (2009). Hearing impairment in 2008: a compilation of available epidemiological studies. *International Journal of Audiology*, 48, 1–13.

[45] Global Burden of Disease Study. (2010). Available from: www.globalburden.org (Accessed 1 October 2011).

[46] World Health Organization. (1999). WHO Ear and Hearing Disorders Survey: Protocol and Software Package. Document WHO/PBD/PDH/99.8. Geneva: World Health Organization.

[47] Mackenzie, I., Smith, A. (2009). Deafness – The Neglected And Hidden Disability. *Annals of Tropical Medicine and Parasitology*, 103, 565–571.

In: Prevention of Hearing Loss
Editors: V. Newton, P. Alberti and A. Smith

ISBN: 978-1-61942-745-7
© 2012 Nova Science Publishers, Inc.

Chapter II

Global and Regional Hearing Impairment Prevalence

Gretchen A. Stevens, *Seth M. Flaxman,*
Maya Mascarenhas, Katrina Davis, Emma Brunskill,
Adrian Davis, Andrew W. Smith,
Howard J. Hoffman and Colin D. Mathers

Abstract

Hearing impairment is a leading cause of disease burden, yet studies of its prevalence are rare. We present estimates of the global prevalence of hearing impairment generated for the Global Burden of Disease 2010 study. We estimated that 1.2% (0.8%-1.8%) of children under age 15, 9.8% (7.7%-13.2%) of females over age 15, and 12.2% (9.7%-16.2%) of males over age 15 experienced moderate or worse hearing impairment in 2008 (defined as a hearing level of 35 decibels or more). We found very high prevalences of adult hearing impairment in low-income regions, especially in sub-Saharan Africa and in South and Southeast Asia; childhood onset of hearing impairment was also higher in these regions that other regions. While hearing aid use reduces the burden of hearing impairment in high-income regions, there is little evidence of their use in the developing countries where the burden of hearing impairment is greatest.

Introduction

Hearing impairment is a leading cause of disability worldwide [1]. Childhood hearing impairment can result in reduced ability to communicate, inability to interpret speech sounds leading to poor language acquisition, economic and educational disadvantage, and social isolation. While childhood hearing impairment has more serious implications due to its potential for interfering with language acquisition, it is far less common than adult onset

* Corresponding author: stephensg@who.int.

hearing impairment. Most people will experience some hearing loss in their lives. Despite its high prevalence and burden, hearing impairment receives little attention. This fact, combined with the significant logistical hurdles involved in collection of hearing impairment data, such as the need for a quiet setting for the testing (preferably a soundproof booth), means that measured hearing impairment data are very sparse, and few studies are nationally representative.

The Global Burden of Disease (GBD) project aims to produce cause-specific estimates of global mortality, disease burden and risk factors for fatal and nonfatal conditions such as hearing impairment. A key principle of the GBD framework is to make the best possible estimates for every condition and population, producing estimates and corresponding uncertainty intervals even when data are sparse [2]. These estimates are updated periodically. The current update is the GBD 2010 study, which has generated estimates of burden of disease and risk factors in 1990, 2005, and 2010. In this chapter, we describe our estimates of the prevalence and causes of hearing impairment, which were carried out as part of the GBD 2010 study[2]. These estimates were carried out under the guidance of an international Expert Group on Hearing Loss convened for the GBD project.

To evaluate the prevalence of hearing impairment, we synthesized available data from population-based surveys of hearing impairment[3]. We accessed papers from a published literature review [4] and obtained additional detailed data tabulations from investigators. We fit a Bayesian hierarchical model, making estimates by region, sex, age and hearing level (severity of hearing impairment). We used Bayesian methods because they are well-suited to accurately reflect the uncertainty associated with estimates, particularly when data are sparse. We also estimated the proportion of individuals with hearing impairment who had access to a hearing aid.

An analytic challenge in this work is that hearing impairment is defined using different audiometric thresholds in the literature. Under the guidance of the Expert Group, we have used new hearing impairment categories which fully describe the range of hearing impairment, from mild to total. An important feature of our modeling approach is its inclusion of the level of hearing loss, in dB HL, as a term. As a result, we are able to model data reported using various definitions, and we are able to quantify the relationship we observed between hearing impairment prevalence and hearing loss threshold.

Defining Hearing Impairment

Many models of classification of hearing impairment based on the audiogram have been devised to suit the needs of researchers and clinicians. The classification published by the World Health Organization is one of the most commonly employed models to date, particularly by those publishing information about developing countries.[5,6] WHO guidelines suggest different categorizations for hearing impairment in children and adults. In the USA, UK and other parts of Europe different definitions and models have been used [7, 8].

The expert group convened to advise on estimates for the GBD project did not find the current categories, and particularly the different categorization for children and adults, compelling in understanding the needs of the hearing impaired population. The expert group has proposed a unified classification for adults and children. They proposed to use the average threshold in the better ear across the 0.5, 1, 2 and 4 kHz frequencies (as in the WHO classification). Additionally, the GBD classification uses the four frequency pure-tone hearing average, better ear thresholds in equally spaced (15 dB HL intervals) to classify hearing as "not impaired", *viz.*, excellent hearing (-10 to <5 dB HL) or good hearing (5 to <20 dB HL) in the better ear, to total impairment ("deaf") with hearing loss ≥95 dB HL in the better ear (see Table 2.1). A category for unilateral hearing impairment was also included, resulting in 7 categories of hearing impairment. Some studies have shown that there is higher compliance, better use and greater benefit from managing hearing impairment with hearing aids as a major component of the clinical management plan at ≥35 dB HL.[9-11] In addition, prevalence estimates in some studies are more robust for ≥35 dB HL because not all studies used ISO standard audiometric booths for measurement of hearing level. We have therefore used this cut-off point as a major definition of need (being able to be met by appropriate provision of hearing aids), whilst maintaining a category of 'mild' hearing impairment for those with unilateral hearing impairment or bilateral hearing impairment between 20-34 dB HL. Those with mild or unilateral hearing impairment (children as well as adults) still have substantial disability in terms of hearing in noisy environments and will become an increasing burden with a growing elderly population, but there are problems in compliance in the use of hearing aids for this group as well as lack of evidence on what other treatments may substantially reduce the burden [12].

Table 2.1. Hearing impairment categories used in this analysis

Hearing impairment category	Better ear hearing level (dB HL)	Hearing in a quiet environment	Hearing in a noisy environment
Unilateral	<20 in the better ear; ≥35 in the worse ear	Does not have problems unless sound is near poorer hearing ear	May have real difficulty following / taking part in a conversation
Mild	20-34	Does not have problems hearing what is said	May have real difficulty following / taking part in a conversation
Moderate	35-49	May have difficulty hearing a normal voice	Has difficulty hearing and taking part in conversation
Moderately Severe	50-64	Can hear loud speech	Has great difficulty hearing and taking part in conversation
Severe	65-79	Can hear loud speech directly in one's ear	Has very great difficulty hearing and taking part in conversation
Profound	80-94	Has great difficult hearing	Cannot hear any speech
Total	≥95	Cannot hear any speech	Cannot hear any speech

Global and Regional
Prevalence of Hearing Impairment

We estimated hearing impairment prevalence, for 8 world regions (Table 2.2 and Figure 2.1). We used all available data to estimate age-specific prevalence of hearing impairment, and used 2008 population data to calculate the prevalence of hearing impairment. Our analysis was carried out in the following steps: 1) collection of hearing impairment data from population-based surveys; 2) use of a statistical model to estimate hearing impairment levels by country, age, sex, and hearing threshold, for ages greater than 5 years; 3) compilation of cross-sectional analyses of hearing impairment aetiology among school-aged children; and 4) estimation of the rate of congenital hearing impairment using estimates of hearing impairment prevalence among school-aged children and aetiological data.

Data Sources: School-Aged Children and Adults

We considered measured hearing loss data from population-based studies of hearing impairment identified in a systematic review by Pascolini and Smith.(4) Pascolini and Smith identified 50 studies carried out in 31 countries, of which we excluded 12 for methodological reasons, including non-random sampling, inclusion of only ethnic minorities; no reporting of hearing loss for the better ear; and insufficiently described sampling methods.

We also excluded 6 surveys, because data were not reported by age, and 2 school studies because we considered that it is not possible to accurately measure hearing impairment below 40 dB HL in school settings, which tend to be noisy. We sent requests to investigators identified in Pascolini and Smith's review for tabulations of the study data using the detailed hearing impairment categories developed for the GBD study. We also asked these investigators to provide information on hearing aid use by hearing level, and to refer us to other unpublished data sources. Detailed tabulations were collected from 11 studies, representing 10 countries. In addition, 12 new studies, representing 7 countries, were personally communicated to us.

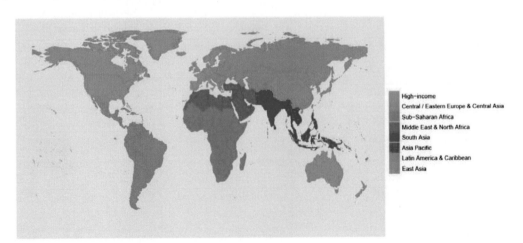

High-income
Central / Eastern Europe & Central Asia
Sub-Saharan Africa
Middle East & North Africa
South Asia
Asia Pacific
Latin America & Caribbean
East Asia

Figure 2.1. Map of analysis regions.

Table 2.2. Hearing impairment prevalence, for 8 world regions.

Subregion	Countries
East Asia region	
East Asia	China, Hong Kong SAR (China), Macau SAR (China), Democratic People's Republic of Korea, Taiwan
Asia Pacific region	
Southeast Asia	Cambodia, Indonesia, Lao People's Democratic Republic, Malaysia, Maldives, Myanmar, Philippines, Sri Lanka, Thailand, Timor-Leste, Viet Nam
Oceania	Cook Islands, Fiji, French Polynesia, Kiribati, Marshall Islands, Micronesia (Federated States of), Nauru, Palau, Papua New Guinea, Samoa, Solomon Islands, Tonga, Vanuatu
South Asia region	
South Asia	Afghanistan, Bangladesh, Bhutan, India, Nepal, Pakistan
Central / Eastern Europe and Central Asia region	
Central Asia	Armenia, Azerbaijan, Georgia, Kazakhstan, Kyrgyzstan, Mongolia, Tajikistan, Turkmenistan, Uzbekistan
Central Europe	Albania, Bosnia and Herzegovina, Bulgaria, Croatia, Czech Republic, Hungary, Montenegro, Poland, Romania, Serbia, Slovakia, Slovenia, Macedonia (Former Yugoslav Republic of)
Eastern Europe	Belarus, Estonia, Latvia, Lithuania, Moldova, Russian Federation, Ukraine
Middle East and North Africa region	
North Africa and Middle East	Algeria, Bahrain, Egypt, Iran (Islamic Republic of), Iraq, Jordan, Kuwait, Lebanon, Libyan Arab Jamahiriya, Morocco, Occupied Palestinian Territory, Oman, Qatar, Saudi Arabia, Syrian Arab Republic, Tunisia, Turkey, United Arab Emirates, Yemen
Sub-Saharan Africa region	
Central Africa	Angola, Central African Republic, Congo, Democratic Republic of the Congo, Equatorial Guinea, Gabon
East Africa	Burundi, Comoros, Djibouti, Eritrea, Ethiopia, Kenya, Madagascar, Malawi, Mauritius, Mozambique, Rwanda, Seychelles, Somalia, Sudan, Uganda, United Republic of Tanzania, Zambia
Southern Africa	Botswana, Lesotho, Namibia, South Africa, Swaziland, Zimbabwe
West Africa	Benin, Burkina Faso, Cameroon, Cape Verde, Chad, Côte d'Ivoire, Gambia, Ghana, Guinea, Guinea-Bissau, Liberia, Mali, Mauritania, Niger, Nigeria, Senegal, Sierra Leone, São Tomé and Príncipe, Togo
Latin America and Caribbean region	
Andean Latin America	Bolivia, Ecuador, Peru
Central Latin America	Colombia, Costa Rica, El Salvador, Guatemala, Honduras, Mexico, Nicaragua, Panama, Venezuela (Bolivarian Republic of)
Southern Latin America	Argentina, Chile, Uruguay
Tropical Latin America	Brazil, Paraguay
Caribbean	Antigua and Barbuda, Bahamas, Barbados, Belize, Bermuda, British Virgin Islands, Cuba, Dominica, Dominican Republic, Grenada, Guyana, Haiti, Jamaica, Netherlands Antilles, Puerto Rico, Saint Kitts and Nevis, Saint Lucia, Saint Vincent and the Grenadines, Suriname, Trinidad and Tobago
High-income region	
Asia-Pacific, high-income	Brunei Darussalam, Japan, Republic of Korea, Singapore
Australasia	Australia, New Zealand
North America, high-income	Canada, United States of America
Western Europe	Andorra, Austria, Belgium, Cyprus, Denmark, Finland, France, Germany, Greece, Greenland, Iceland, Ireland, Israel, Italy, Luxembourg, Malta, Netherlands, Norway, Portugal, Spain, Sweden, Switzerland, United Kingdom

In our final analysis dataset, we included 42 studies carried out between 1973 and 2010 in 29 countries (Table 2.3). 18 studies were in high-income countries and 24 in low- or middle-income countries. 13 studies only considered children and adolescents under age 20, while 12 tested only adults and 17 reported data for subjects of all ages. Age-specific data on adults in low- and middle- income countries were particularly sparse: only 12 studies reported this type of information. These studies were carried out in Brazil, China, Ecuador, India, Indonesia, Madagascar, Myanmar, Nigeria, Oman, Sri Lanka and Vietnam; study years ranged from 1995-2010. No data were located from the Central / Eastern Europe and Central Asian region. We identified more than one data source from a few countries. Two studies on children were available for one high-income (United States) and three developing countries (Nigeria, Tanzania, and Brazil). For adults, more than one data source was available for seven countries (Australia, Brazil, Finland, Norway, Sweden, the United Kingdom, and the US). When more than one data source was available from a country, they were often not directly comparable because they considered different subnational populations.

Statistical Methods: School-Aged Children and Adults

We used Bayesian hierarchical logistic regression to estimate hearing impairment prevalence for each country-age-severity group [13,14]. Prevalence data is geographically nested: a single survey is conducted in a specific subregion; subregions are part of a wider geographical region; and several regions make up the globe. We built our model hierarchically to reflect this nesting: a hierarchical model allows regional estimates to be informed both by survey data from that region and by survey data from other regions. The relative weight given to the data from the same region *vs.* from other regions is informed by the availability and consistency of the within-region data compared to the availability and consistency of data from other regions. In this way, a hierarchical Bayesian model allows us to "borrow strength" where appropriate as informed by the data, while quantifying our uncertainty.

Different studies in our dataset have different sample sizes. We incorporate the different degrees of uncertainty implied by different sample sizes into our model using a binomial probability distribution. For each study, the sample size and the number of subjects experiencing hearing loss at a certain threshold tell us the likelihood of a given prevalence estimate (given the binomial probability distribution). This information is used to fit the various coefficients of our regression in a Bayesian framework as follows: the current values of the parameters are used to make an estimate of the prevalence, and the binomial probability distribution tells us the likelihood of this estimate, with smaller sample sizes implying less certainty and larger sample sizes more certainty. Then, the parameters are updated using a Markov chain Monte Carlo (MCMC) algorithm, moving us towards values which give estimates that are more likely. Once the model has converged, the MCMC algorithm will iterate through different sets of parameters with similar likelihoods. These sets of parameter values are used to calculate a distribution of hearing impairment prevalences for each region, age, and sex, which is called the posterior distribution. The median hearing impairment from the posterior distribution is our central estimate, and we estimate the 95% uncertainty interval around our estimate with the 2.5-97.5 percentiles of the posterior distribution.

Table 2.3. Characteristics of data sources used in the analysis

Country	Year	Sample size	Ages	Location	Hearing aid coverage data	Reference
Sub-Saharan Africa region						
Angola	1982	1030	5-15	Two districts in Luanda, one middle-class one slum, school based	no	Bastos, I., et al. (1993).Chronic otitis media and hearing loss in urban schoolchildren in Angola - a prevalence study. *Journal of Audiological Medicine, 2,* 129-140.
Dem. Rep. Of the Congo	1995	2286	5-16	Several locations in Kinshasa, school based	no	Tshiswaka, M.T., et al. (1995). Etudes basees sur la population pour evaluer la prevalence des alterations de l'ouue chez les ecolier de 5 a 16 ans dans la ville de Kinshasa (Zaire). Report from the service ORL Cliniques Universitaires de Kinshasa.
Kenya	1996	2869	1-14	8 districts	no	Chege, J.M., et al. (1998). A survey on prevention of deafness in children in Kenya. Report of a project of the Kenya Society for Deaf Children Nairobi, Kenya.
Madagascar	2003	5572	All ages	Province of Antananarivo	no	Randrianarisoa, T., et al. (2008). Resultat de l'enquete sur defience auditive dans la province d'Anatananarivo, Madagascar. Unpublished report, Antananarivo, Madagascar. Re-analysed by author.
Nigeria	1995	359	4-10	Mushin Local Government Area of Lagos State, 8 urban schools	no	Olusanya, B.O., et al. (2000). The hearing profile of Nigerian school children. *International Journal of Pediatric Otorhinolaryngology,55,* 73-79. Re-analysed by author.
Nigeria	2000	8975	All ages	Akwa Ibom, Benue, Katsina states	no	Nwawolo, C.C. (2003).Presentation: The WHO Ear and Hearing Disorders Survey Protocol: Practical Challenges in its use in a Developing Country(Nigeria). Informal Consultation on Epidemiology of Deafness.
Sierra Leone	1992	2015	5-15	Eastern province around the town of Panguma, rural	no	Seely, D.R., et al. (1995). Hearing loss prevalence and risk factors among Sierra Leonean children. *Archives of Otolaryngology - Head and Neck Surgery,121,* 853-858.

Table 2.3. (Continued)

Country	Year	Sample size	Ages	Location	Hearing aid coverage data	Reference
South Africa	1990	401	6-13	Western Cape, rural, school based	no	Prescott, C.A., et al. (1991). Ear and hearing disorders in rural grade 2 (Sub B) schoolchildren in the western Cape. *South African Medical Journal, 79*, 90-93.
Tanzania	1995	802	5-20	Dar es Salaam, urban/rural	no	Minja, B.,and Machemba, A. (1996). Prevalence of otitis media, hearing impairment and cerumen impaction among school children in rural and urban Dar es Salaam, Tanzania. *International Journal of Pediatric Otorhinolaryngology, 37*, 29-34.
Tanzania	1993	854	6-16	Mohi and Monduli districts, urban and rural	no	Bastos, I., et al. (1995). Middle ear disease and hearing impairment in northern Tanzania. A prevalence study of schoolchildren in the Moshi and Monduli districts. *International Journal of Pediatric Otorhinolaryngology, 32*, 1-12.
Zimbabwe	1998	5528	5-12	Manicaland province, eastern Zimbabwe, mostly rural, school based	no	Westerberg, B.D., et al.(2005). Prevalence of hearing loss in primary school children in Zimbabwe. *International Journal of Pediatric Otorhinolaryngology, 69*, 517-525.
Latin America and Caribbean region						
Brazil	2003	2427	4+	Canoas, metropolitan Porto Allegre	yes	Beria, J., et al. (2007).Hearing impairment and socioeconomic factors: a population-based survey of an urban locality in southern Brazil. *Revista Panamericana de Salud Pública 2007; 21*, 381-387. Re-analysed by author.
Brazil	2006	577	All ages	urban Monte Negro, Rondonia, Northern Brazil	no	Bevilacqua, C., et al.(2009). A survey of hearing disorders in an urban population in Montenegro, Rondonia, Brazil. Unpublished paper. Re-analysed by author.
Ecuador	2010	7067	All ages	National	no	Ullauri, A., et al. (2010).WHO

Country	Year	Sample size	Ages	Location	Hearing aid coverage data	Reference
Middle East and North Africa region						
Oman	1997	11402	All ages	Whole country	no	Al Khabori, M., et al. (2004).The prevalence and causes of hearing impairment in Oman: a community-based cross-sectional study. *International Journal of Audiology, 43,*486-492.
High-income region						
Australia	1993, 2007	1530, 154	70+, 75+	Adelaide metropolitan area	yes	Sanchez, L. and Luszcz, M. (2009).The Australian Longitudinal Study of Ageing: 1992-continuing, Flinders Centre for Ageing Studies, Flinders University, South Australia. 2009. Re-analysed by author.
Australia	1997-2004	2956	55-99	Blue Mountains Hearing Study, west of Sydney	yes	Gopinath, B., et al. (2009). Prevalence of age-related hearing loss in older adults: Blue Mountains Study. *Archives of Internal Medicine,169,* 15-6. Re-analysed by author.
Denmark	1991, 2006	905, 1315	31-51, 46-66	Ebeltoft, Jutland, rural district	yes	Karlsmose, B., et al. (1999).Prevalence of hearing impairment and subjective hearing problems in a rural Danish population aged 31-50 years. *British Journal of Audiology, 33,* 395-402. Reanalysed by author.
Finland	1997	5400	5-75	Northern Ostrobothnia	no	Uimonen, S., et al. (1999).Do we know the real need for hearing rehabilitation at the population level? Hearing impairments in the 5- to 75-year-old cross-sectional Finnish population. *British Journal of Audiology, 33,* 3-9.
Finland	1990, 2000	202, 42	80, 90	City of Jyvaskyla	no	Hietanen, A. et al. (2004).Changes in hearing in 80-year-old people: a 10-year follow-up study. *International Journal of Audiology, 43,*126-135.
Italy	1989	2170	18+	5 representative cities of North, South and Center	no	Quaranta, A., et al.(1996). Epidemiology of hearing problems among adults in Italy. *Scandinavian Audiology Supplementum, 42,* 9-13.
Norway	1977	1449	20+	Norwegian Sor-Trondelag	no	Molvær, O.I., et al.(1983). Hearing Acuity in a Norwegian Standard Population, *Scandinavian Audiology,12,* 29-236. Re-analysed by author.

Table 2.3. (Continued)

Country	Year	Sample size	Ages	Location	Hearing aid coverage data	Reference
Norway	1996	50273	18-101	Nord Trondelag County	yes	Tambs, K., et al. (2003).Hearing loss induced by noise, ear infections, and head injuries: results from the Nord-Trondelga Hearing Loss Study. *International Journal of Audiology*, *42*, 89-105. Re-analysed by author.
Sweden	1998	590	20-80	Ostergotland province	no	Johansson, M.S.K., et al. (2003). Prevalence of hearing impairment in a population in Sweden. *International Journal of Audiology*, *42*, 8-28. Re-analysed by author.
Sweden	1986, 1990, 1991, 1992	223, 197, 249, 133	70, 75, 85, 90	City of Gothenburg	yes	Jönsson, R., et al.(1998). Auditory function in 70 and 75-year-olds of four age cohorts. A cross-sectional and time-lag study of presbyacusis. *Scandinavian Audiology*, *27*, 81-93. Jönsson, R., Rosenhall, U. (1998). Hearing in advanced age. A study of presbyacusis in **85-, 88-, and 90-year-old people.** *Audiology*, *37*,207-218. Re-analysed by author. Karlsson, A.K., et al. (1998).Aural Rehabilitation in the Elderly: Supply of Hearing Aids Related to Measured Need and Self-Assessed Hearing Problems. *Scandinavian Audiology*, *27*,153-160.
United Kingdom	1983	2910	17-80	Cardiff, Glasgow, Nottingham, Southhampton	yes	Davis, A.C. (1989). The Prevalence of Hearing Impairment and Reported Hearing Disability among Adults in Great Britain. *International Journal of Epidemiology*, *18*, 911–917. Re-analysed by author.
United Kingdom	1994	346	15-29	Nottingham	no	Smith, P., et al. (1999). Hearing in young adults: Report to ISO/TC43/WG1. *Noise and Health*,*1*, 1-10. Re-analysed by author.
United Kingdom	2000	351	55-79	Nottingham and Southampton	no	Davis, A., et al. (2007).Acceptability, benefit and costs of early screening for hearing disability: a study of potential screening tests and models. *Health Technology Assessment*, 11, Re-analysed by author.

Country	Year	Sample size	Ages	Location	Hearing aid coverage data	Reference
USA	1973	6827	25-74	US NHANES I, 1971-75	yes	Centers for Disease Control and Prevention (CDC). National Center for Health Statistics (NCHS).(2010). National Health and Nutrition Examination Survey Data. Hyattsville, MD: U.S. Department of Health and Human Services, Centers for Disease Control and Prevention, 1971-1975. Reuben, D.B. et al. (1998).Hearing loss in community-dwelling older persons: National prevalence data and identification using simple questions. *Journal of the American Geriatrics Society, 46*,1008-1011. Re-analysed by author.
USA	1978	5725	1-19	US NHANES II 1976-80	no	Centers for Disease Control and Prevention (CDC). National Center for Health Statistics (NCHS).(2010). National Health and Nutrition Examination Survey Data. Hyattsville, MD: U.S. Department of Health and Human Services, Centers for Disease Control and Prevention, 1976-1980. Re-analysed by author.
USA	2001	5346	20-74	US NHANES 1999-2004	yes	Centers for Disease Control and Prevention (CDC). National Center for Health Statistics (NCHS). (2010). National Health and Nutrition Examination Survey Data. Hyattsville, MD: U.S. Department of Health and Human Services, Centers for Disease Control and Prevention, 1999-2004. Re-analysed by author.
USA	2005	2745	10-19, 65-85+	US NHANES 2005-2006	yes	Centers for Disease Control and Prevention (CDC). National Center for Health Statistics (NCHS). (2010). National Health and Nutrition Examination Survey Data. Hyattsville, MD: U.S. Department of Health and Human Services, Centers for Disease Control and Prevention, 2005-2006. Re-analysed by author.
South Asia						
India	1997	5428	6 mo+	Vellore District, Tami Nadu, rural and semi-urban setting	no	Mackenzie, I. (2003).Hearing Impairment in Asia - Final report of 4 country survey. Unpublished. Re-analysed by author.

Table 2.3. (Continued)

Country	Year	Sample size	Ages	Location	Hearing aid coverage data	Reference
Nepal	1990	15845	5+	Mid Western and Eastern	no	Little, P., et al. (1992).Hearing Impairment and ear pathology in Nepal. *The Journal of Laryngology and Otology,107,* 395-400.
Pakistan	1997	607	5-15	Sialkot District, Punjab, rural	no	Elahi, M.M., et al. (1998). Paediatric hearing loss in rural Pakistan. *Journal of Otolaryngology, 27,*348-353.
Asia Pacific region						
Indonesia	1998	5604	6 mo+	Bandung, urban to rural areas in West Java	no	Mackenzie, I. (2003). Hearing Impairment in Asia - Final report of 4 country survey. Unpublished.
Myanmar	2001	6340	6 mo+	Hlaing Thar Yar township, Yangoon	no	Mackenzie, I. (2003). Hearing Impairment in Asia - Final report of 4 country survey. Unpublished.
Sri Lanka	2001	4858	All ages	Kandy District	no	Mackenzie, I. (2003).Hearing Impairment in Asia - Final report of 4 country survey. Unpublished.
Thailand	1989	12395	6-15	Bangkok and 9 rural provinces, school based	no	Prasansuk, S. (2000).Incidence/prevalence of sensorineural hearing impairment in Thailand and Southeast Asia. *Audiology, 39,*207-211.
Viet Nam	2001	13120	All ages	3 northern and 3 southern provinces	no	Dung, T.T. et al. (2003). Preliminary result of survey "Ear and Hearing disorder" in Vietnam. Informal Consultation on Epidemiology of Deafness and Hearing Impairment in Developing Countries and Update of the WHO Protocol. 2003. World Health Organization, Geneva
East Asia region						
China	2006	29246	4 mo+	Jiangsu, Guizhou, Sichuan, Jilin provinces	no	Bu, X. (2002). Results from WHO Ear and Hearing Disorders Survey in 4 Provinces (Jiangsu, Sichuan, Guizhou, and Jilin) China. Unpublished report. Ear and Hearing Research Unit. Dept. of Otolaryngology. Jiangsu Province Hospital. Nanjing Medical University. Nanjing, China

Our final model had the following elements (see Appendix for more details): 1) a sub-region-specific offset parameter for each of the 21 GBD subregions, modeled hierarchically to be nested in eight world regions, which in turn shared a global prior; 2) age as a two-knot linear spline to flexibly model age patterns; 3) linear and quadratic terms for hearing impairment level (dB HL), allowing for modeling of hearing impairment at any threshold; and 4) a sex ratio, *i.e.*, the percent of the sample population that was female. The prevalence of adult hearing impairment may vary due to differences in a region's age structure (that is, a higher proportion of older adults in Europe vs. in developing regions) or due to differences in age-specific hearing impairment prevalence. For comparability, we present age-standardized prevalences using the WHO reference population [15]. We also calculate unadjusted prevalences, which reflect the proportion of each region's population with a hearing impairment.

Hearing Impairment among Pre-Lingual Children

Hearing loss among pre-lingual children is difficult to measure in household-based surveys. In order to determine the proportion of childhood hearing loss that is present at birth vs. acquired during childhood, we carried out a systematic review of studies of hearing impairment among school-aged children. We identified 38 studies that reported the timing of hearing impairment onset in the broadly defined categories of congenital, perinatal, postnatal, and unidentified. We included data regardless of the definition of hearing impairment used, but excluded 10 of those studies because the time of onset was unidentified for more than 40% of children in the study. The 28 studies we finally used are listed in Table 2.4. To calculate the rate of congenital hearing loss, we modelled data on congenital onset of childhood hearing loss using a logistic regression. We first redistributed unknown time of onset pro-rata to the congenital/perinatal and postnatal groups in each data source. The percent of childhood hearing impairment that was congenital was strongly related to development level, thus our final model had as its independent variable log of GDP per capita (see Appendix). We then calculated congenital hearing impairment rates by multiplying the estimated percent of childhood hearing impairment that is congenital by the prevalence of hearing loss among school-age children (ages 5-14 years), estimated with the Bayesian hierarchical model described above.

Estimates of Hearing Impairment Prevalence

Hearing impairment prevalence increased with age (Figure 2.2) and was higher among males than females. Globally, the prevalence of hearing impairment ≥ 35 dB HL for males aged 15 years or over was 12.2% (9.7%-16.2%) while for females aged 15 years or older it was 9.8% (7.7%-13.2%). (Figure 2.3). Our results suggest that adult-onset hearing impairment has substantially higher prevalence in low- and middle-income countries than in high-income countries, demonstrating the need for attention to hearing impairment globally. After adjusting for differences in age structure, the prevalence of hearing impairment was highest in developing regions and lowest in high-income regions (Figure 2.4 and Table 2.5).

Table 2.4. Studies reporting onset or timing of hearing impairment among school-aged children

Country	Year	Better ear hearing threshold (dBHL)	Sample Size	Proportion of childhood HI with congenital onset (%)	Proportion of childhood HI with postnatal onset (%)	Proportion of childhood HI with unknown onset (%)	Reference
Oman	2004	60	1400	58	8	34	Al Khabori, M. (2004). Causes of severe to profound deafness in Omani paediatric population. *International Journal of Pediatric Otorhinolaryngology, 68*, 1307-1313.
USA	1999	35	211	61	7	32	Billings, K. R. and M. A. Kenna (1999). Causes of pediatric sensorineural hearing loss: yesterday and today. *Archives of Otolaryngology Head and Neck Surgery, 125*, 517-521.
UK	1996	30	339	55	7	38	Das, V. K. (1996). Aetiology of bilateral sensorineural hearing impairment in children: a 10 year study. *Archives of Diseases in Childhood, 74*, 8-12.
Belgium	2003	Deaf school	190	61	6	33	Deben, K., et al. (2003). Epidemiology of hearing impairment at three Flemish Institutes for Deaf and Speech Defective Children. *International Journal of Pediatric Otorhinolaryngology, 67*, 969-975.

Country	Year	Better ear hearing threshold (dBHL)	Sample Size	Proportion of childhood HI with congenital onset (%)	Proportion of childhood HI with postnatal onset (%)	Proportion of childhood HI with unknown onset (%)	Reference
Turkey	2000	Deaf school	130	28	46	26	Derekoy, F. S. (2000). Etiology of deafness in Afyon school for the deaf in Turkey. *International Journal of Pediatric Otorhinolaryngology, 55,* 125-131.
Nigeria	2007	71	115	11	54	35	Dunmade, A. D., et al. (2007). Profound bilateral sensorineural hearing loss in Nigerian children: any shift in etiology? *Journal of Deaf Studies and Deaf Education, 12,* 112-118.
Turkey	2003	Deaf school	162	46	34	20	Egeli, E., et al. (2003). Etiology of deafness at the Yeditepe School for the deaf in Istanbul. *International Journal of Pediatric Otorhinolaryngology,67,* 467-471.
Turkey	2000	Deaf school	130	24	43	33	Derekoy, F. S. (2000). Etiology of deafness in Afyon school for the deaf in Turkey. *International Journal of Pediatric Otorhinolaryngology, 55,*125-131.
UK	1997	40	653	70	16	14	Fortnum, H. and Davis A. (1997). Epidemiology of permanent childhood hearing impairment in Trent Region, 1985-1993. *British Journal of Audiology, 31,* 409-46.

Table 2.4. (Continued)

Country	Year	Better ear hearing threshold (dBHL)	Sample Size	Proportion of childhood HI with congenital onset (%)	Proportion of childhood HI with postnatal onset (%)	Proportion of childhood HI with unknown onset (%)	Reference
China	2010	25	813	29	69	2	Fu, S., et al. (2010). Prevalence and etiology of hearing loss in primary and middle school students in the Hubei Province of China. *Audiology and Neurootology, 15*, 394-398.
Cyprus	2000	50	100	75	25	0	Hadjikakou, K. and Bamford, J. (2000). Prevalence and age of identification of permanent childhood hearing impairment in Cyprus. *Audiology 39*,198-201.
UK	2003	40	130	76	7	17	MacAndie, C., et al. (2003). Epidemiology of permanent childhood hearing loss in Glasgow, 1985-1994. *Scottish Medical Journal, 48*, 117-119.
Finland	1998	40	112	61	2	38	Maki-Torkko, E.M., et al. (1998). Epidemiology of moderate to profound childhood hearing impairments in northern Finland. Any changes in ten years? *Scandinavian Audiology, 27*, 95-103.

Country	Year	Better ear hearing threshold (dBHL)	Sample Size	Proportion of childhood HI with congenital onset (%)	Proportion of childhood HI with postnatal onset (%)	Proportion of childhood HI with unknown onset (%)	Reference
Tanzania	1998	Deaf school	354	10	68	22	Minja, B. M. (1998). Aetiology of deafness among children at the Buguruni School for the Deaf in Dar es Salaam, Tanzania. *International Journal of Pediatric Otorhinolaryngology, 42*, 225-231.
Pakistan	2011	NR	300	50	33	17	Musani, .A., et al. (2011). Frequency and causes of hearing impairment in tertiary care center. *Journal of the Pakistan 61*,141-144.
Austria	2001	40	165	54	10	36	Nekahm D, et al. (2001). Epidemiology of permanent childhood hearing impairment in the Tyrol, 1980-94. *Scandinavian Audiology, 30*,197-202.
Nigeria	1987	Profound	267	20	49	31	Obiako, M.N. (1987). Profound childhood deafness in Nigeria: a three year survey. *Ear and Hearing 8*, 74-77.
Turkey	2005	Deaf school	840	55	34	11	Ozturk, O., et al. (2005). Evaluation of deaf children in a large series in Turkey. *International Journal of Pediatric Otorhinolaryngology, 69*, 367-373.

Table 2.4. (Continued)

Country	Year	Better ear hearing threshold (dBHL)	Sample Size	Proportion of childhood HI with congenital onset (%)	Proportion of childhood HI with postnatal onset (%)	Proportion of childhood HI with unknown onset (%)	Reference
Denmark	2001	20	214	45	45	10	Parving, A. and A.-M. Hauch (2001). Permanent Childhood Hearing Impairment - Some Cross-Sectional Characteristics from a Surveillance Program. *International Pediatrics, 16*, 1-5.
Greece	2005	NR	94	82	3	15	Riga, M., et al. (2005). Etiological diagnosis of bilateral, sensorineural hearing impairment in a pediatric Greek population. *International Journal of Pediatric Otorhinolaryngology 69*, 449-455.
Australia	2003	NR	134	95	5	0	Russ S.A., et al. (2003). Epidemiology of congenital hearing loss in Victoria, Australia. *International Journal of Audiology, 42*, 385-90.
Nicaragua	2007	30	96	72	11	17	Saunders, J. E., et al. (2007). Prevalence and etiology of hearing loss in rural Nicaraguan children. *Laryngoscope, 117*, 387-398.
Turkey	2004	Deaf school	550	66	16	18	Silan, F., et al. (2004). Syndromic etiology in children at schools for the deaf in Turkey. *International Journal of Pediatric Otorhinolaryngology 68*, 1399-406.

Country	Year	Better ear hearing threshold (dBHL)	Sample Size	Proportion of childhood HI with congenital onset (%)	Proportion of childhood HI with postnatal onset (%)	Proportion of childhood HI with unknown onset (%)	Reference
Germany	1998	Deaf school	314	55	14	31	Streppel, M., et al. (1998). Epidemiology and etiology of acquired hearing disorders in childhood in the Cologne area. *International Journal of Pediatric Otorhinolaryngology,44*, 235-243.
Egypt	1998	Deaf school	223	60	20	20	Tantawy, A.Z., et al. (1998). Studying the etiology of deafness in the "deaf" schools of Alexandria. *Journal of the Egyptian Public Health Association 73*, 125-136.
Estonia	2000	40	172	88	12	0	Uus, K. and Davis, A.C. (2000). Epidemiology of permanent childhood hearing impairment in Estonia, 1985-1990. *Audiology 39*,192-197.
UK	2010	40	54	67	17	16	Watkin, P. M. and Baldwin, M. (2011). Identifying deafness in early childhood: requirements after the newborn hearing screen. *Archives of Diseases in Childhood, 96*, 62-6.

Table 2.4. (Continued)

Country	Year	Better ear hearing threshold (dBHL)	Sample Size	Proportion of childhood HI with congenital onset (%)	Proportion of childhood HI with postnatal onset (%)	Proportion of childhood HI with unknown onset (%)	Reference
Saudi Arabia	2002	76	302	80	10	10	Zakzouk, S. M. and Al-Anazy F. (2002). Sensorineural hearing impaired children with unknown causes: a comprehensive etiological study. *International Journal of Pediatric Otorhinolaryngology 64*, 17-21.

Notes: NR = not reported.

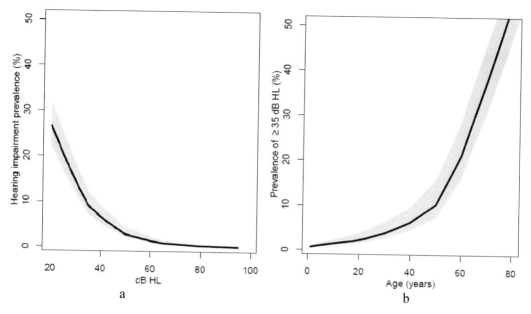

Figure 2.2. Global pattern of hearing impairment (A) by hearing threshold and (B) by age. Panel A displays cumulative prevalence, that is, prevalence of hearing impairment at each threshold and at higher thresholds.

Age-standardized hearing impairment ≥35 dB HL ranged from 3.7% in high-income countries (3.0%-4.8%) to 11.9% in Sub Saharan Africa region (8.7%-15.5%) and 13.0% in the South Asian region (8.3%-20.2%). Adult males in South Asia had the highest prevalence of impairment: 15.0% (9.6%-22.9%). Mild, moderate, severe, profound, and total hearing impairment were modeled to have the same geographic pattern. We estimated that the age-standardized prevalence of hearing impairment ≥35 dB HL was 4 (2.3-6.6) times higher in South Asia than in high-income regions.

We found that time of onset of childhood hearing impairment is strongly related to level of development, with the percent of childhood hearing impairment occurring in the congenital period ranging from 86% (85%-87%) in high-income countries to 37% (34%-39%) in South Asia and 28% (25%-30%) in sub-Saharan Africa (Figure 2.4). The global prevalence of hearing impairment ≥35 dB HL among children under 15 years of age was 1.2% (95% uncertainty interval 0.8%-1.8%).

The prevalence of mild hearing impairment was 18.1% (15.6%-20.8%) for males and 15.1% (12.9%-17.5%) for females (Table 2.5). The corresponding prevalences of moderate hearing impairment were 6.4% for males (5.1%-8.1%) and 5.2% for females (4.2%-6.6%), and of moderately severe hearing impairment were 1.9% (1.5%-2.8%) for males and 1.5% (1.2%-2.2%) for females. The prevalence of severe hearing impairment was 0.6% (0.4%-0.9%) for males and 0.4% (0.3%-0.8%) for females. Profound and total hearing impairment have a global prevalence of 0.5% (0.4%-1.0%) for males and 0.3% (0.2%-0.7%) for females. Globally, we estimate that 93.6% (90.7%-95.2%) of children and 68.3% (62.2%-73.2%) of adults have a hearing threshold <20 dB HL in the better ear.

We estimate 21 million children (15-34 million), 299 million men (237-396 million), and 239 million women (189-324 million) have hearing impairment ≥35 dB HL. Calculating prevalence as the number impaired over the total population, the lowest prevalence of hearing impairment ≥35 dB HL among adults 15 years and over was in the Middle East and North Africa region (5.9%, 3.0%-11.5%) and the high-income regions (7.7%, 6.4%-9.8%). The greatest percentage of adults with hearing impairment ≥35 dB HL was in the South Asian region (13.2%, 8.1%-21.4%) and Central / Eastern Europe and Central Asian region (13.9%, 2.9%-51.0%).

Ageing has likely caused a large increase in the prevalence of hearing impairment in recent years, and the trend is expected to continue. Assuming that the prevalence of hearing impairment at specific ages did not change, the worldwide prevalence of hearing impairment ≥35 dB HL increased from 6.9% (5.4%-9.8%) in 1990 to 8.3% (6.6%-11.1%) in 2008.

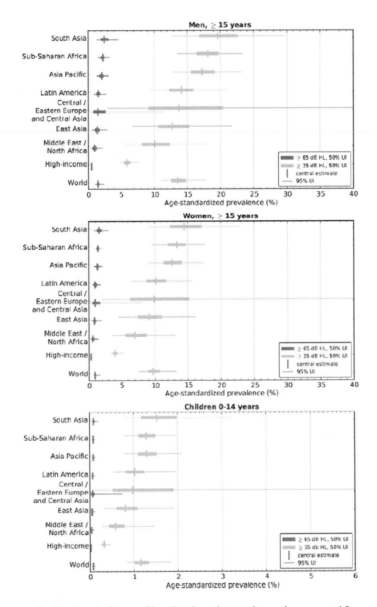

Figure 2.3. Age-standardized prevalence of hearing impairment by region, men ≥15 years, women ≥15 years, and children under 15 years of age. UI = uncertainty interval.

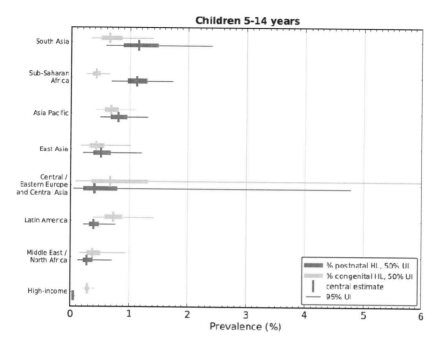

Figure 2.4. Prevalence of hearing impairment ≥ 35 dB HL among children aged 5-14 years, disaggregated by time of onset.

As people are living longer in all regions of the world, [16] it is likely that the prevalence of hearing impairment will continue to increase, primarily driven by demographic trends. This trend can be attenuated by preventing of hearing impairment and by correcting hearing impairment.

Use of Hearing Aids

We obtained data from 8 studies that recorded hearing aid coverage by hearing level, of which one was from Brazil and the remainder were from high-income countries. We modelled data on current hearing aid use, by hearing impairment level, from high-income countries using a logistic regression. Our final model accounted for improvements in coverage over time (see Appendix).

In high-income countries, use of a hearing aid was most common among those with profound hearing loss and increased over time (Figure 2.5). Coverage was estimated to increase from 6% (5%-7%) among those with mild hearing impairment to 89% (83%-93%) among those with profound hearing impairment. Among those with total hearing impairment, for whom a hearing aid is unlikely to be effective, 62% (49%-74%) had a hearing aid. In the high-income region, 40 million (35-49 million) people use a hearing aid, of whom 26 million have hearing impairment ≥35 dB HL (22-34 million, corresponding to 43% of those with hearing impairment ≥35 dB HL).

We did not have sufficient data to estimate hearing aid use in developing countries, but suspect that coverage is small to negligible: one study in Brazil did not identify anyone who used a hearing aid, and combining our data with data on hearing aid production indicates that few hearing aids are sold in developing countries [17,18].

Table 2.5. Prevalence of hearing impairment by region, impairment category, and demographic group (estimates for 2008). Percentages are reported for adult males and females; rates per 1,000 are reported for children

Region	Population ('000s)	Mild (20-34 dB HL)	Moderate (35-49 dB HL)	Moderately severe (50-64 dB HL)	Severe (65-79 dB HL)	Profound (80-94 dB HL)	Deaf (≥95 dB HL)
Males, 15+ years (per cent)							
High-income region	387,609	16.8 (14.9-19.3)	5.8 (4.9-7.2)	1.6 (1.3-2.2)	0.4 (0.3-0.6)	0.1 (0.1-0.2)	0.1 (0.1-0.2)
Central / Eastern Europe and Central Asia region	155,901	23.8 (8.7-33.5)	9.6 (2.2-26.6)	3.1 (0.5-14.3)	0.9 (0.1-6.4)	0.3 (0.0-2.7)	0.2 (0.0-2.8)
Sub-Saharan Africa region	232,208	24.1 (19.3-28.8)	8.3 (6.0-10.9)	2.5 (1.7-3.5)	0.7 (0.5-1.1)	0.2 (0.1-0.3)	0.2 (0.1-0.3)
Middle East and North Africa region	154,985	16.4 (10.1-25.3)	4.9 (2.6-9.0)	1.3 (0.6-2.8)	0.4 (0.2-0.8)	0.1 (0.0-0.3)	0.1 (0.0-0.2)
South Asia region	543,896	26.9 (20.1-33.4)	10.2 (6.6-15.6)	3.2 (1.8-5.5)	1.0 (0.5-1.9)	0.3 (0.2-0.6)	0.3 (0.1-0.6)
Asia Pacific region	212,693	25.5 (20.8-30.1)	9.4 (7.0-12.6)	2.9 (2.0-4.3)	0.9 (0.6-1.4)	0.3 (0.2-0.4)	0.2 (0.1-0.4)
Latin America and Caribbean region	200,837	22.5 (16.9-28.1)	8.2 (5.6-11.8)	2.6 (1.6-4.1)	0.8 (0.4-1.4)	0.2 (0.1-0.5)	0.2 (0.1-0.4)
East Asia region	556,140	22.7 (14.9-30)	8.2 (4.4-13.5)	2.5 (1.1-4.8)	0.7 (0.3-1.6)	0.2 (0.1-0.5)	0.2 (0.1-0.4)
World	2,444,268	22.7 (19.8-25.7)	8.4 (6.8-10.6)	2.6 (2.0-3.7)	0.8 (0.6-1.2)	0.2 (0.2-0.4)	0.2 (0.1-0.4)
Females, 15+ years (per cent)							
High-income region	408,794	15 (13.3-17.2)	5.3 (4.4-6.6)	1.4 (1.1-2.0)	0.4 (0.3-0.5)	0.1 (0.1-0.2)	0.1 (0.1-0.1)
Central / Eastern Europe and Central Asia region	178,626	21.6 (8.7-31.4)	9.2 (2.2-23.7)	3.0 (0.5-13.2)	0.9 (0.1-6.1)	0.3 (0.0-2.6)	0.2 (0.0-2.8)
Sub-Saharan Africa region	238,564	19.6 (15.3-23.9)	6.4 (4.6-8.5)	1.8 (1.2-2.6)	0.5 (0.3-0.8)	0.2 (0.1-0.2)	0.1 (0.1-0.2)
Middle East and North Africa region	148,927	12.8 (7.7-20.4)	3.7 (1.9-6.9)	0.9 (0.4-2.0)	0.2 (0.1-0.6)	0.1 (0.0-0.2)	0.1 (0.0-0.1)
South Asia region	515,635	22.3 (16.2-29.4)	7.8 (5.0-12.2)	2.4 (1.3-4.2)	0.7 (0.4-1.3)	0.2 (0.1-0.4)	0.2 (0.1-0.4)
Asia Pacific region	219,241	21.2 (16.9-25.8)	7.5 (5.5-10.2)	2.3 (1.5-3.3)	0.7 (0.4-1.0)	0.2 (0.1-0.3)	0.2 (0.1-0.3)
Latin America and Caribbean region	210,768	18.5 (13.7-24.1)	6.6 (4.4-9.6)	2.0 (1.2-3.3)	0.6 (0.3-1.1)	0.2 (0.1-0.4)	0.2 (0.1-0.3)

Region	Population ('000s)	Mild (20-34 dB HL)	Moderate (35-49 dB HL)	Moderately severe (50-64 dB HL)	Severe (65-79 dB HL)	Profound (80-94 dB HL)	Deaf (≥95 dB HL)
East Asia region	531,769	18.6 (12.1-26.1)	6.4 (3.4-10.7)	1.9 (0.8-3.7)	0.5 (0.2-1.2)	0.2 (0.1-0.4)	0.1 (0.1-0.3)
World	2,452,325	19 (16.4-21.8)	6.8 (5.5-8.6)	2.0 (1.5-3.0)	0.6 (0.4-1.0)	0.2 (0.1-0.4)	0.2 (0.1-0.3)
Children, 0-14 years (per 1,000)							
High-income region	155,818	16.1 (11.8, 23.7)	2.5 (1.9, 3.8)	0.5 (0.4, 0.7)	0.1 (0.1, 0.2)	0.0 (0.0, 0.1)	0.0 (0.0, 0.0)
Central / Eastern Europe and Central Asia region	65,496	46.8 (6.1, 291)	7.8 (1.0, 87.1)	1.5 (0.2, 19.5)	0.4 (0.0, 4.9)	0.1 (0.0, 1.4)	0.1 (0.0, 1.2)
Sub-Saharan Africa region	322,090	56.5 (37, 82.6)	9.7 (6.1, 15)	1.9 (1.2, 3.0)	0.5 (0.3, 0.7)	0.1 (0.1, 0.2)	0.1 (0.1, 0.2)
Middle East and North Africa region	124,201	28.7 (12.9, 67.3)	4.6 (2.0, 11.5)	0.9 (0.4, 2.3)	0.2 (0.1, 0.5)	0.1 (0.0, 0.2)	0.1 (0.0, 0.1)
South Asia region	480,060	69.3 (38, 127.5)	12 (6.2, 25)	2.4 (1.2, 5.0)	0.6 (0.3, 1.2)	0.2 (0.1, 0.4)	0.1 (0.1, 0.3)
Asia Pacific region	157,568	60.1 (39, 92.2)	10.2 (6.3, 16.5)	2.0 (1.2, 3.3)	0.5 (0.3, 0.8)	0.1 (0.1, 0.2)	0.1 (0.1, 0.2)
Latin America and Caribbean region	153,566	49.3 (27, 87.2)	8.1 (4.3, 15.5)	1.6 (0.8, 3.1)	0.4 (0.2, 0.7)	0.1 (0.1, 0.2)	0.1 (0.0, 0.2)
East Asia region	262,960	39.9 (16.8, 86.1)	6.5 (2.7, 15.2)	1.3 (0.5, 3.0)	0.3 (0.1, 0.7)	0.1 (0.0, 0.2)	0.1 (0.0, 0.2)
World	1,721,759	53 (39.4, 75.2)	9.1 (6.6, 14.4)	1.8 (1.3, 2.9)	0.4 (0.3, 0.7)	0.1 (0.1, 0.2)	0.1 (0.1, 0.2)

A primary obstacle to hearing aid provision in developing countries is their high cost [18]. There is likely a large unmet need for innovative interventions including low-cost hearing aids in developing countries.

While hearing aids provide an important improvement in hearing acuity, current technology does not eliminate most hearing impairments.

The GBD Expert Group has suggested that hearing aid use improves hearing by one hearing impairment category, that is, a person with a moderately severe hearing impairment and a hearing aid may achieve the level of hearing functioning of a person with a moderate hearing impairment, and a person with a mild hearing impairment and a hearing aid may function like a person with no hearing impairment.

Using this assumption, and additionally assuming that countries in Eastern Europe have hearing aid coverage 50% of that in the high-income regions, we estimated the prevalence of hearing impairment ≥35 dB HL to be 4.9% (4.1%-6.4%) in the high-income regions (*vs.* 6.4%, 5.3%-8.2% without adjusting for hearing aid use) and 8.0% (6.4%-10.7%) in the world (*vs.* 8.3%, 6.6%-11.1% without hearing aids; Figure 2.6).

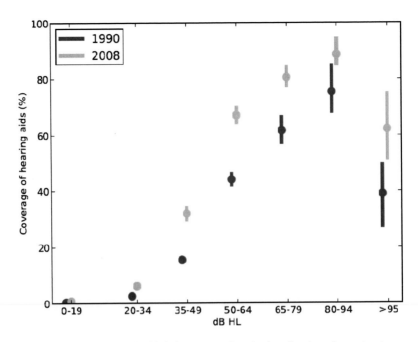

Figure 2.5. Hearing aid coverage in the high-income region, by hearing impairment category and year.

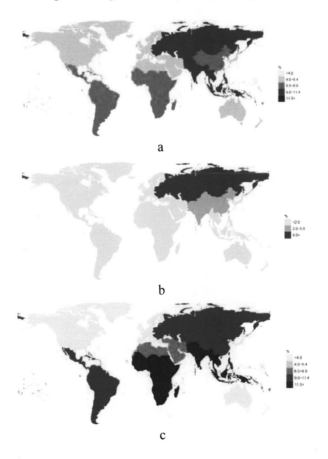

Figure 2.6. (Continued).

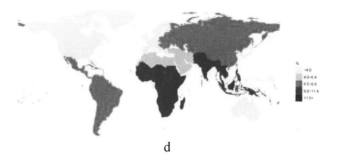

d

Figure 2.6. Hearing impairment ≥35 dB HL adjusted for use of a hearing aid in 8 world regions, A) prevalence in 2008, B) standard error of prevalence in 2008, C) age-standardized male prevalence; and D) age-standardized female prevalence.

Challenges in Describing the Epidemiology of Hearing Impairment

The main limitation in describing the prevalence of hearing impairment is the scarcity of data. As a result of this scarcity, we were unable to estimate time trends in hearing impairment prevalence.

Data on adults were available for high-income regions from 1973 to 2005, including several countries with more than one data source, but for developing regions data were only available from 1995 or later, and no repeated national surveys were available from any developing country.

While we expect that age-specific hearing impairment prevalences may have changed over time, our data were not sufficient to quantify those changes for all world regions. We suspect the sparsity of population-based data is a result of the low position of hearing impairment on the global health agenda, and the logistic hurdles involved in measuring hearing impairment in the field.

Conclusion

Hearing impairment is positively related to age, male sex, and low- and middle-income regions.

The prevalence of adult hearing impairment is very high n low-income regions, especially in sub-Saharan Africa and in South and Southeast Asia. While hearing aid use reduces the burden of hearing impairment in high-income regions, there is little evidence of hearing aid use in developing countries. There is a clear unmet need for treatment of conditions that cause hearing impairment and for low-cost interventions that reduce the disability associated with hearing impairments.

In addition, repeated cross-sectional and longitudinal studies of hearing impairment prevalence are needed, particularly in the regions where this disabling condition is highly prevalent, in order to generate more accurate estimates of trends.

Acknowledgments

This work was undertaken as a part of the Global Burden of Diseases, Injuries, and Risk Factors study. The results in this paper are prepared independently of the final estimates of the Global Burden of Diseases, Injuries, and Risk Factors study. Bill and Melinda Gates Foundation provided funding for this analysis. We thank Richard White for assistance preparing figures, Catherine Michaud for research coordination, Donatella Pascolini of the WHO Prevention of Blindness and Deafness program for assistance with data sources. We also wish to thank the GBD Expert Group on Hearing Loss, Jose M. Acuin (Philippines), Peter Alberti (Canada), Mazin Al-Khabori (Oman), Jorge Umberto Beria (Brazil), Maria Cecilia Bevilacqua (Brazil), Xingkuan Bu (China), Adrian Davis (UK), Luciana Petrucci Gigante (Brazil), Howard J. Hoffman (USA), Abraham Joseph (India), Young-Ah Ku (South Korea and WHO), Ian Mackenzie (UK), Thais C. Morata (Brazil and USA), Katrin Newmann (Germany), Valerie E. Newton (UK), Bolajoko Olusanya (Nigeria), Agneta Parving (Denmark), and Andrew W. Smith (UK, formerly WHO; Expert Group Leader).

We are indebted to many others who supplied new tabular data for the analysis (by country): *Australia* Blue Mountains: Dr. Bamini Gopinath (Dr. Catherine McMahon, Professor Paul Mitchell); ALSA: Dr. Linnett Sanchez, Dr. Mary Luszcz; *Brazil*: Dr. Cecilia Bevilacqua; *Brazil*: Dr. Beatriz Raymann, Dr. Luciana Gigante; *Denmark*: Dr. Bo Karlsmose (Dr. Torsten Lauritzen, Dr. Janus Laust Thomsen); *Ecuador*: Dr. Alejandra Ullauri, Carlos Jimenez; *India:* Dr. Abraham Joseph, (Dr Anand Job); Madagascar: Dr. Theodore Randrianarisoa (Dr. Rinasoa Andriamampianina); *Nigeria*: Dr. Bola Olusanya; *Norway*: Dr. Kristian Tambs, Dr. Bo Engdahl, Dr. Otto Inge Molvær; Sweden: Dr. Ulf Rosenhall; *United States* NHANES I, II, III, 1999–2004, and 2005–2006: Dr. Chia-Wen Ko.

References

[1]   World Health Organization. The global burden of disease: 2004 update. Geneva: World Health Organization; 2008.

[2]   Murray, C. J. L., Lopez, A. D., Black, R. E., Mathers, C. D., Shibuya, K., Ezzati, M, Salomon, J. A., Michaud, C. M., Walker, N., Vos, T. (2007). Global Burden of Disease 2005: call for collaborators. *Lancet,* 370,109-110.

[3]   Stevens, G. A., Flaxman, S., Brunskill, E., Mascarenhas, M., Mathers, C. D., Finucane, M. M. Global and regional hearing impairment prevalence: an analysis of 42 studies in 29 countries. *European Journal of Public Health.* In press.

[4]   Pascolini, D., Smith, A. (2009). Hearing Impairment in 2008: A compilation of available epidemiological studies. *International Journal of Audiology,* 48, 473-485.

[5]   World Health Organization. (1991).Report of the Informal Working Group on Prevention of Deafness and Hearing Impairment Programme Planning. Geneva: World Health Organization; 1991. Report No.: WHO/PDH/91.1.

[6]   World Health Organization.(1997) Future programme developments for prevention of deafness and hearing impairment. Report No.: WHO/PDH/97.3. Geneva: World Health Organization.

[7]   British Society of Audiology. (2004). Pure tone air and bone conduction threshold audiometry with and without masking and determination of uncomfortable loudness levels: Reading: *British Society of Audiology.*

[8]   American Speech-Language-Hearing Association. (2001).Type, degree, and configuration of hearing loss. Rockville, Maryland: American Speech-Language-Hearing Association.

[9]   Davis, A., Smith, P., Ferguson, M., Stephens, D., Gianopoulos, I.(2007). Acceptability, benefit and costs of early screening for hearing disability: a study of potential screening tests and models. *Health Technology Assessment,* 11,1-294.

[10]   Gianopoulos, I., Stephens, D., Davis, A. (2002).Follow up of people fitted with hearing aids after adult hearing screening: the need for support after fitting. *British Medical Journal,* 31, 325-471.

[11]   Stephens, D., Lewis, P., Davis, A., Gianopoulos, I., Vetter, N.(2001). Hearing aid possession in the population: lessons from a small country. *Audiology,* 40,104-111.

[12]   Pronk, M., Kramer, S. E., Davis, A. C., Stephens, D., Smith, P. A., Thodi, C., Anteunis, L. J., Parrazzini, M., Grandori, F. 920110. Interventions following hearing screening in adults: A systematic descriptive review. *International Journal of Audiology,* 50, 594-609.

[13]   Gelman, A., Hill, J. (2007). Data analysis using regression and multilevel/hierarchical models. In: R. M. Alvarez, N. L. Beck, L. L. Wu, (Eds.), (pp 207). New York, NY: Cambridge University Press.

[14]   Gelman, A. (2006). Multilevel (hierarchical) modeling: what it can and cannot do. *Technometrics,* 48, 432-434.

[15]   Ahmad, O., Boschi-Pinto, C., Lopez, A. D., Murray, C. J. L., Lozano, R., Inoue, M. (2001). Age standardization of rates: a new WHO standard. *GPE Discussion Paper No* 31. Geneva: WHO.

[16]   United Nations Population Division. (2011). World Population Prospects: 2010 revision. New York: United Nations Population Division.

[17]   Sorensen, T. W. (2005). Time to concentrate: 7th annual hearing aid industry report. Copenhagen: Carnegie Securities Research.

[18]   Hearing aids and services for developing countries. *Revisa Panamericana Salud Publica.* 2001, 10, 139- 142.

In: Prevention of Hearing Loss
Editors: V. Newton, P. Alberti and A. Smith

ISBN: 978-1-61942-745-7
© 2012 Nova Science Publishers, Inc.

Chapter III

Mechanisms of Hearing Loss of Cochlear Origin

Andrew Forge[*]

Abstract

Normal auditory function depends upon the activity of the sensory "hair" cells of the organ of Corti in the cochlea, the nerves that innervate them and the maintenance of the physiological environment in which they operate. Damage or functional disruption of any of these elements will lead to hearing impairment. There are two types of hair cell arranged in rows along the cochlear spiral. Inner hair cells (IHC) are innervated exclusively by afferent nerves and are the primary receptor cells. Outer hair cells (OHC) actively enhance sound-induced vibrations in the cochlea providing amplification of the signal detected by the inner hair cells. Death of hair cells is the most common cause of sensorineural deafness. Ageing, noise and certain chemical agents with "ototoxic" effects are the primary causes of hair cell death and acquired hearing loss. Ototoxic chemicals include aminoglycoside antibiotics, cis-platinum and certain organic solvents. In almost all cases of acquired deafness and most genetically-related deafness, loss of hair cells is usually progressive and occurs in a distinct pattern. OHC at the basal end of the cochlear spiral, where high frequencies are normally detected, die first. Damage then spreads progressively apically to cause threshold shifts at successively lower frequencies. (Organic solvents are an exception: hair cells in the mid-frequency range are first affected). Loss of IHC, and subsequently of their afferent innervation, follows loss of OHC, usually after some delay. OHC loss will correspond to an auditory threshold shift of around 60dB, the degree of amplification those cells provide, with greater threshold shifts as IHC die. The effects of almost all conditions that cause hair cell loss result in activation of a biochemical "programmed cell death pathway" leading to apoptosis. A common activating trigger is the generation of excess free radicals. Potential means to protect hair cells from lethal damage either by targeting the stress-activated cell death pathways or through suppression of excess free-radical generation ("anti-oxidant" therapy) are being devised. While the effects of damaging agents maybe upon the hair cells directly, other cochlear tissues that are involved in maintaining their physiological

---

[*] Corresponding author: a.forge@ucl.ac.uk.

environment (homeostasis) may be affected either as well as or preceding hair cell loss. OHC in particular appear vulnerable to adverse physiological conditions, and disruption of homeostasis may therefore be a direct cause of, or exacerbate direct effectson, hair cells. In addition, interactions between the effects of different agents may cause greater damage than that resulting from one agent alone, and underlying genetic background may influence the sensitivity of hair cells to damage. For these reasons the clinical signature of auditory dysfunction sometimes may not be simply related to a specific lesion site.

Anatomy and Physiology of the Cochlea

The cochlea is formed of a membranous canal enclosed in a bony channel [1]. The canal and the surrounding bony channel coil in a spiral around a central axis, the modiolus, which contains the nerve and blood supply. The number of turns of the spiral from base to apex varies with species; there are approximately two and a half turns in the human cochlea. The membranous cochlear canal is triangular in cross-section (Figure 3.1) and creates three compartments (scalae). The lumen of the canal forms the scala media with the scala vestibuli above and scala tympani below. Scala vestibuli and scala tympani contain perilymph, a fluid in which there is a high concentration sodium ions (Na^+), similar in composition to other extracellular fluids. The fluid within scala media is endolymph, which, unusually for an extracellular fluid, has a high potassium ion (K^+) (and low Na^+) concentration. Cochlear endolymph also has a high positive resting electrical potential of ca. +80mV, the endocochlear potential (EP).

The cochlear tissues form the walls of the scala media. The partition between the scala tympani and the scala media is formed of the acellular basilar membrane and the organ of Corti, the sensory epithelium of the cochlea,that sits upon it (Figure 3.1). The basilar membrane is freely permeable to perilymph so that the cell bodies and nerves of the sensory epithelium are exposed to perilymph. The border between perilymph and endolymph is created by ionic barriers formed by tight junctional sealing at the apical (luminal) end of the epithelial cells. Consequently the apical surfaces of the cells of the organ of Corti are bathed in K^+-rich endolymph, while the cell bodies are bathed in Na^+-rich perilymph. Scala media is separated from scala vestibuli by the Reissner's membrane.

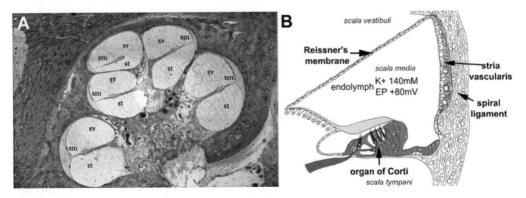

Figure 3.1. A. Cross-section of cochlea in human temporal bone: sm=scala media, st=scala tympani, sv=scala vestibuli. B. Diagrammatic cross section of single cochlear turn.

Along the lateral wall of the scala media is the stria vascularis an ion transporting epithelium that is responsible for the production and maintenance of endolymph. The stria vascularis rests on the spiral ligament that sits upon the lateral bony wall of the cochlea. The extracellular spaces of the ligament are filled with perilymph, so that the stria vascularis forms a border between the two cochlear fluids.

The Organ of Corti and Transduction of Sound Signals

The organ of Corti [1] (Figure 3.2) is composed of sensory "hair" cells and various types of supporting cells. Hair cells, various forms of which are the mechano-sensory cells of hearing and balance organs in all vertebrate classes, are characterised by and derive their name from, the organised bundle of erect projections at their apical end. Each hair cell is separated from its neighbours by intervening supporting cells so no two hair cells contact each other. This arrangement creates a regular mosaic of cells at the apical surface of the organ of Corti that is called the reticular lamina (Figure 3.2). Overlying the organ of Corti and the hair cells is another acellular, fibrous structure, the tectorial membrane (Figure 3.1).

In the organ of Corti there are two types of hair cells that are arranged in parallel rows along the length of the cochlear spiral (Figure 3.2). There is a single row of inner hair cells (IHC) and three to five rows (depending on the species) of outer hair cells (OHC). In humans there are about 3000 IHC and 9000 OHC along the length of the organ of Corti [2]; in mice (a commonly used animal model for studies of the cochlea) about 725 IHC and 2300 [3] and in guinea pigs, another good animal model, approximately 2000 IHC and 7000 OHC[4].

The hair bundle at the apical end of the hair cell is formed of rows of "stereocilia" that increase in height in one particular direction across the cell apex (Figure 3.2). The apical surfaces of the hair cells are bathed in endolymph, into which the stereocilia project, whilst the body of the cell is surrounded with perilymph (Figure 3.1).

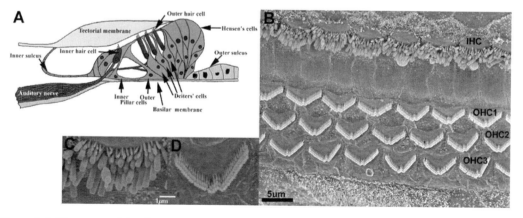

Figure 3.2. The organ of Corti. A. Diagram of a cross-section of the organ of Corti. B. Scanning electron micrograph of the apical (luminal, endolymphatic) surface of the organ of Corti, (the reticular lamina) of a mouse. There is a single row of inner hair cells (IHC) and three rows of outer hair cells (OHC1, OHC2, OHC3). Each hair cell is separated from its neighbour by intervening supporting cells. Single inner (C) and outer (D) hair cell to show the apical hair bundle of each. Each hair bundle is formed of rows of stereocilia. The stereocilia increase in height from the innermost row to the outermost row.

Deflection of the stereocilia stimulates the hair cell. Deflection towards the longest row of stereocilia, opens non-selective cation channels (the "transducer channels); deflection in the opposite direction closes them [5]. During sound stimulation, vibration of the stapes footplate displaces fluid along the scala vestibuli and scala tympani resulting in up and down displacement of the basilar membrane and the organ of Corti. Relative motion between the tectorial membrane and the reticular lamina is thereby produced and leads to deflection of the stereocilia alternately towards and away from the longest row of stereocilia. The consequent opening and closing of the transducer channels modulates a K^+ current flowing through the hair cells from the K^+ rich endolymph at the apical surface to the Na^+-rich perilymph around the hair cell body. The opening of the transducer channels leads to increased K^+ entry resulting in depolarisation of the hair cell; deflection in the opposite direction closes the channels and the hair cell becomes hyperpolarized. The changes in electrical potential stimulate hair cell activity. The high positive EP coupled with a negative resting potential inside the HC, provides a driving force for the current flow from endolymph into the hair cell increasing the sensitivity of the system [6].

There are a number of systematic dimensional variations of the basilar membrane and organ of Corti along the length of the spiral which affect the mechanical properties of the system such that for different frequencies of the sound stimuli, maximal vibration of the basilar membrane occurs at different locations: sounds of particular frequency cause maximal stimulation at a particular place; a place-frequency relationship or tonotopic organisation along the organ of Corti. High frequency (high pitched) sounds cause maximum displace-ment, and thus stimulation of the hair cells, at the base of the cochlea and low frequencies are detected at the apical end. This means that differential damage to the organ of Corti along its length will be reflected in differential loss of frequency perception; if hair cells at the basal end of the cochlea are affected a high frequency hearing loss results but the ability to detect low frequencies may be unimpaired.

The two hair cell types in the cochlea have different roles. IHC are the primary receptor cells. They are directly innervated exclusively by afferent nerve fibres (that is nerves that carry information to the brain). Each IHC synapses with several different fibres, and around. 90-95% of the total afferent innervation to the cochlea terminates on IHC [7]. The changes in electrical potential of IHC upon stereociliary deflection lead to neural excitation. OHC on the other hand have a modulatory role. They have an extensive direct efferent innervation (i.e. nerves carrying information sent from the brain) [7]. Recording of the neural activity of individual cochlear afferent nerves in response to sound, which represents output from a single IHC, shows that each nerve is extremely sensitive to one particular frequency, its "characteristic frequency". This "tuning" of the nerve to a particular frequency is physiologically vulnerable. When OHC are lost but IHC remain intact there is a loss of sharp neural tuning, and thus, in the ability to discriminate between sounds of different frequency, and in the ability to detect sounds lower than 60dB in sound pressure level (i.e. there is a severe hearing impairment but loud sounds can be heard)[8]. It is believed that, *in vivo*, OHC actively influence the movement of the basilar membrane in response to sound in a way that amplifies the signal reaching the IHC. This increases sensitivity to sound (by around 60dB) [9,10]. Thus, if OHC are damaged or lost, there will be decrease or loss in cochlear amplification and hearing impairment. The power for the "cochlear amplifier" function of the OHC is thought to derive from the EP [10,11]. Consequently loss of EP results in hearing impairment because of a loss of amplification.

The Stria Vascularis and Spiral Ligament

The maintenance of cochlear endolymphatic K^+ and the generation and maintenance of the EP derives from the activity of the stria vascularis, the ion transporting epithelium that lines the lateral wall of the endolymphatic space (Figure 3.1). Damage to the stria vascularis will result in a loss of EP. The stria vascularis is composed of three cell types and encloses its own capillary blood supply

The marginal cells line the endolymphatic compartment and actively transport K^+ into endolymph. The intermediate cells are enclosed entirely within the stria and are melanocytic cells. The basal cells separate the stria vascularis from the underlying spiral ligament, which is freely permeable to perilymph. There is no direct diffusion pathway between the stria and either perilymph or endolymph, entry of oxygen and nutrients to the stria deriving from the enclosed vasculature. Numerous large gap junctions, sites of direct cell-to-cell communication, provide conduits for the passage of ions and small molecules between cells of the cochlear lateral wall [12,13,14].

The generation of EP is dependent upon the recycling of K^+ passing through the hair cells from endolymph to perilymph and from perilymph back to endolymph via the stria vascularis [15]. Beneath the stria is the spiral ligament which is part of the perilymphatic compartment. The ligament is formed of several sub-populations of fibrocytes. These cells take up K^+ from the perilymph in the extracellular spaces of the ligament. K^+ is then passed through cells of the ligament via gap junctions between fibrocytes, and then into the basal cells of the stria vascularis via the gap junctions between strial basal cells and ligament fibrocytes. Basal cells are connected to strial intermediate cells also by gap junctions [12,13]. EP is generated by electrogenic K^+ passage across the membrane of the intermediate cells.

As well as a role in K^+ re-cycling the various sub-populations of spiral ligament fibrocytes are involved in other aspects of cochlear homeostasis, including pH balance[16]. Damage to the spiral ligament can therefore be detrimental to cochlear function more generally. Death of certain sub-populations of spiral ligament fibrocytes, along with death of OHC and permanent hearing deficits, has been noted both following exposure to excess noise and with ageing [17,18]. Death of OHC in particular can be triggered by failures to maintain the physiological environment within the cochlea. Mutations in genes which encode proteins whose activity is necessary for maintenance of the characteristics of endolymph that are localised in cells of the lateral wall can cause deafness and progressive loss of hair cells is often apparent [19,20,21,22].

Physiological Tests of Auditory Function

The alternating changes in hair cell potentials in phase with the sound vibrations that are generated as transduction channels open and close can be recorded extracellularly from electrodes close to the round window as the cochlear microphonic potential (CM). CM recorded extracellularly is dominated by the responses of the OHC. There are three times as many OHCs as IHCs, and the resting intracellular potential of OHC is much lower (-70mV) than that of IHCs (-40mV), so that CM potentials are much greater in OHC than IHC.

The activity of the OHC that produces amplification in response to stimulating input sounds results in the emission of sound signals from the ear (otoacoustic emissions, OAE) [10,23]. Recording OAE involves merely the insertion of a small probe consisting of a microphone and loudspeaker assembly into the external ear canal. It provides a non-invasive, sensitive, objective measure of cochlear sensitivity; a decrease in OAE amplitude indicates an impairment of OHC activity and thus indicates hearing impairment. Because of the non-invasive nature of the test and because OAEs are a direct, objective measure of the cochlea's response to sound that does not require the participation of the subject under test, OAE recording has become not only a routine clinical audiological procedure, but it also enables assessment of hearing in new born babies thereby providing the basis for new born hearing screening programmes.

The activity of the auditory nerve upon sound stimulation recorded from extracellular electrodes as the compound action potential (CAP) is a measure of the neural output from the cochlea that derives primarily from IHC stimulation. The neural output from the cochlea can also be recorded non-invasively from the auditory brain stem response (ABR), which is the electrical activity associated with successive stimulations of a number of centres along the auditory neural pathway in the brainstem to the auditory cortex following reception of a sound in the cochlea. The test involves presentations of sounds of different intensities at a variety of frequencies and estimation of the lowest sound pressure level that provokes a just detectable response, the threshold, at each tested frequency. Permanent increases in the frequency thresholds of the ABRs ("threshold shifts" where louder sounds are necessary to elicit the response) indicate hearing impairment, and correlate with loss of hair cells at the particular appropriate locations in the cochlea.

Damaging Agents:
Some General Considerations

The most common type of hearing loss is sensorineural; that is, it results from malfunction of the cochlea. In the majority of cases, this is due to damage to or death of the hair cells and accompanying degeneration of afferent innervation, although there are some agents which produce temporary hearing impairment and do not cause hair cell death. Hair cell death may be the result of direct effects upon the hair cells themselves, but some agents affect the tissues of the lateral wall, the stria vascularis and/or spiral ligament, with consequent adverse effects on cochlear homeostasis that compromise hair cell survival. In non-mammalian vertebrates, such as birds, reptiles, amphibians and fish, lost hair cells are spontaneously replaced by new ones. This leads to functional restoration and recovery from any hearing impairment. Mammals, including humans, have no similar regenerative capacity so that once lost, hair cells are not replaced and the consequent hearing impairment is permanent.

Sensorineural hearing loss may be congenital, as a result of certain developmental defects or specific genetic conditions. About 1 in 1000-2000 babies are born with impaired hearing, approximately 50% of which is accounted for by genetic defects. There is a growing list of the genetic mutations which lead to permanent hearing impairment. Further information can be accessed via the internet through the Hereditary Hearing Loss web site (http://hereditary

hearingloss.org). Hereditary hearing loss will not be considered specifically in this chapter, although fundamentally at the cellular level the ultimate conditions and biochemical mechanisms that lead to hair cell death may be the same as those which are triggered in acquired hearing loss.

In the majority of cases sensorineural hearing loss is acquired after birth. Ageing, noise, and certain chemical agents with toxic effects on cells of the inner ear, so called ototoxins, are the major causes of acquired hearing impairment [24]. Otherwise valuable therapeutic agents such as aminoglycoside antibiotics [25] and the antitumour agent cis-platinum [26] as well as a number of industrial chemicals, most notably organic solvents [27,28,29], are ototoxic and cause hair cell death and permanent hearing impairment.

Patterns of Hair Cell Loss

The effects of ototoxins (with the exception of organic solvents, see later) as well as those of ageing are first apparent in the cochlea's basal turn, with damage spreading toward the apex with age or time post-exposure [2,17]. This corresponds functionally to hearing impairment that initially affects the high frequencies and then spreads progressively to involve successively lower frequencies. After acoustic overexposure, the loss of hair cells occurs at a location along the organ of Corti that is related to the frequency(ies) of the damaging sound(s) [30,31,32], but it also occurs in the basal turn with the extent of this hair cell loss increasing and spreading toward the apex of the cochlea with time post-exposure and with increases in sound intensity [32]. It is also generally found with ageing, exposure to ototoxins and noise that the extent of OHC loss is much greater than that of IHC and studies following the progression of hair cell loss over time have shown that after most insults OHC die before the IHC (Figure 3.3).

Thus, there is a pattern of hair cell loss in which OHC in the basal coil die first with a corresponding loss of cochlear amplification of the highest sound frequencies, with OHC loss then progressing apicalwards along the organ of Corti producing threshold shifts at ever lower frequenciesDeath of IHC follows later but its initiation maybe considerably delayed such that there can be extensive loss of OHC with relatively little loss of IHC. The death of IHC may, in fact, be a secondary consequence of the damage to the organ of Corti resulting from loss of OHC and the tissue repair processes that follow from it. Since IHC are the sensory cells that send information on the reception of sound signals to the brain, whereas OHC primarily are involved in amplification of the signal that reaches the IHC, the initiation of IHC loss will lead to progression to more severe or profound hearing loss than that which results from loss of only OHC and the amplification they provide.

The general pattern of hair cell loss that is found with acquired hearing loss is also observed as a consequence of the effects of many of the genetic mutations that cause deafness. This is the case not only for genes that are expressed in hair cells but also for many genes that are normally expressed in other cells in the organ of Corti or in the lateral wall tissues but not in hair cells. The adverse effects of these mutations are mostly upon maintenance of cochlear homeostasis (the physiological environment which maintains hair cell functioning and survival). That the differential loss of hair cells that is seen with environmental factors that produce acquired hearing loss is also apparent with genetic factors indicates the likelihood that OHC in the basal coil are intrinsically more vulnerable to stress than those at the apex, and that OHC are more sensitive to adverse physiological conditions than are IHC.

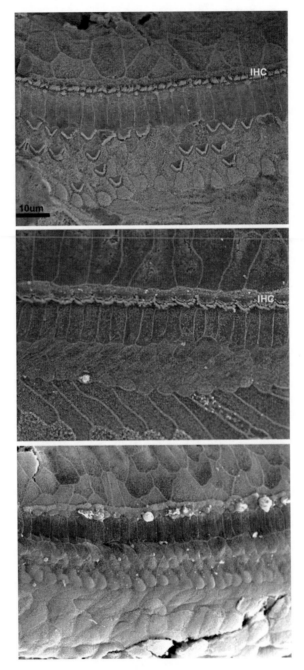

Figure 3.3. Progression of hair cell loss following aminoglycoside treatment. Outer hair cells die before inner hair cells (IHC).

This conclusion is supported by studies of the immature organ of Corti isolated from the cochlea and maintained *in vitro* as organotypic culture (i.e. maintained "in a dish") [33].

When the tissue in culture is incubated with ototoxins such that both apical and basal coils are exposed to identical conditions, there is the same differential basal coil-to-apical coil effect on OHC that is seen *in vivo*

Effects on Afferent Innervation

In regions where all of the OHCs are lost, and where IHCs are absent, afferent innervation is found to have degenerated. This is manifested as a decrease in the number of neuronal cell bodies within the spiral ganglion. It has generally been held that loss of IHC is the trigger for loss of innervation. The IHC produce neurotrophic factors that are crucial for neuronal survival and thus loss of IHC together with the loss of stimulation that IHC provide to neurons lead to neuronal death. However, some very recent work has suggested that loss of a sub-population of the afferent neurons that innervate IHC may be a primary consequence of the effects of noise and possibly aminoglycosides. If such is the case, then the initial degree of hearing impairment would be greater than that which would accrue from loss of only OHC. On the other hand, other recent work has suggested that the neurotrophins which are essential for survival of afferent innervation may be produced not only by the IHC but also by those supporting cells (the inner phalangeal and inner border cells) that surround them. This could enable survival of some afferent innervation in the absence of IHC and could be one factor underlying the prolonged survival of afferent innervation in the human cochlea which provides for the effectiveness of cochlear implants.

Mechanisms of Hair Cell Death

There is now considerable evidence that in most situations where hair cell loss occurs the majority of OHC show characteristics of apoptosis, the end stage of a programmed cell death pathway [34]. Programmed cell death (sometimes known colloquially as "cell suicide") occurs following activation of a cascade of biochemical reactions that result in the enzymatic self-destruction of the cell. The classical programmed cell death pathway is mediated by enzymes known as caspases (*c*ysteine proteases with *asp*artate specificity). Caspases are normally present in cells in inactive forms. When the cell death pathway is triggered there is a regulated activation of "initiator" caspases which in turn activate "effector" caspases (most notably caspase 3). The effector caspases activate proteases that destroy cell proteins, and nucleases that fragment DNA. Apoptosis is characterized by distinctive morphological features including condensation of nuclear chromatin accompanied by shrinkage of the nucleus ("pyknotic" nuclei); nuclear fragmentation; cell shrinkage; membrane blebbing; and breakdown of the cell into fragments, so-called "apoptotic bodies." Cells undergoing apoptosis retain an intact cell membrane, so they do not provoke an inflammatory response, the membrane enclosed apoptotic bodies eventually becoming phagocytosed by circulating macrophages or by neighbouring cells. Thus, because inflammation is not stimulated, cells dying by apoptosis can be removed without disrupting tissue integrity.

Different stimulators of apoptosis activate differing sets of caspases and/or different pathways depending on the cellular environment and cell type. Apoptosis occurs naturally in many tissues to control cell numbers and in the processes that shape tissues and organs during their development, for example in the formation of the semi-circular canals in the inner ear. Extracellular signaling molecules can induce programmed cell death on binding to "cell death receptors" on the surface of the cell thereby activating an "extrinsic" cell death pathway. However, apoptosis is also triggered when cells are damaged enabling removal of such cells without disrupting tissue integrity. When cells are under physiological stress or when DNA is damaged several biochemical pathways that constitute the "intrinsic" cell death programme, which involves proteins associated with mitochondria, are activated. Pyknotic nuclei, markers of the DNA fragmentation characteristic of apoptosis, and activated caspase-3 have all been observed in OHC during the progression of the hair cell loss that follows exposure of animals to noise, after treatment with aminoglycoside antibiotics or cis-platinum, and from the effects of many genetic mutations that are associated with hearing loss. Thus, the OHC death that results from all these conditions is thought to result from stress-activation of programmed cell death pathways.

One factor that induces cellular stress leading to apoptosis is the generation of excess free radicals [35,36]. Free radicals, most commonly singlet oxygen (superoxide), nitrogen, and hydroxyl radicals, are molecules that contain an unpaired electron and consequently are highly unstable. They regain stability by losing or gaining an electron (oxidation or reduction - redox activity) through interaction with nearby molecules. Such redox activity can disrupt cellular components, leading to damage that triggers apoptosis [35,36]. Free radicals are produced during normal cellular metabolism [37]. They can have crucial roles as signaling molecules within the cell, but excessive production is usually contained by endogenous free-radical scavenger systems that inactivate them.

Glutathione is the most ubiquitous free-radical scavenger in most cells along with the enzyme superoxide dismutase (SOD), which catalyzes the inactivation of reactive oxygen species (ROS). Cell damage occurs when free-radical production exceeds the capacity of these endogenous scavenger systems to neutralize them [35]. In preparations of isolated mature organ of Corti maintained in short-term culture, OHC in the basal coil die relatively rapidly whereas those in the apical coil survive for much longer. This differential vulnerability of basal coil OHC relative to those from the apical coil can be overcome by incubating the preparations in the presence of free-radical scavengers [38]. This suggests that OHC along the length of the organ of Corti are differentially vulnerable to free-radical activity.

The levels of glutathione in OHC also vary along the cochlear spiral with higher levels estimated for OHC in the apical coil than in those at the base [38] indicating differential free-radical scavenging activity may underlie differential susceptibility to free-radical attack. Mice in which SOD has been ablated by genetic manipulation show much greater hair cell loss and hearing impairment following noise exposure than do normal litter mates [39], and there is more rapid and more extensive hair cell loss with ageing in these animals [40]. In contrast, genetic manipulation that leads to greater production of SOD than normal (over expression of SOD) has the opposite effect: less hair cell loss and a lesser degree of hearing impairment following aminoglycoside treatment [41]. It is also possible to identify the products of free-radical attack (i.e. those molecules that result from the alterations caused by the free radicals) using immunohistochemistry, and free-radical products have been observed in cochleae after noise trauma, ototoxic injury and with ageing [42,43].

From these observations taken together it is thought that one common mechanism at the cellular level causing death at least of OHC in a variety of different conditions is stress-induced excess free radical production triggering apoptosis. This has provided a basis for attempts to ameliorate or prevent the hair cell loss by protecting hair cells from damage or by inhibiting the biochemical pathways that are activated by stress (see below).

Modes of Action of Some Specific Damaging Agents

Aminoglycoside Antibiotics

All commonly used aminoglycoside antibiotics, including amikacin, gentamcin, kanamycin neomycin and streptomycin, are ototoxic causing death of hair cells [25]. They affect both the cochlea and the vestibular system, but it has been recognized that some aminoglycosides appear to be more cochleotoxic than vestibulotoxic. In humans neomycin is predominantly cochleotoxic whereas streptomycin is vestibulotoxic but these differences between the aminoglycosides in preferential sites of action are to some extent species dependent [25], for reasons that are not yet entirely clear. Damage to the vestibular sensory epithelia is not covered specifically in this chapter but many of the features of aminoglycoside activity in the cochlea, including mechanisms of hair cell death, apply to the vestibular system.

The effects of aminoglycoside – a progressive hearing loss that begins with loss of the highest frequencies- are usually manifest only after chronic, repeated treatment regimes, and may not become apparent for some time after the initiation of treatment, indeed may not be recognized until after treatment has ended. Single doses of aminoglycoside administered systemically are not normally damaging, but application of a single dose at the round window can lead to extensive hair loss, a procedure that has been used to ablate vestibular hair cells in some cases of profound unilateral vestibular dysfunction such as that associated with Meniere's disease, although loss of cochlear hair cells can also occur with this procedure [44]. Patients who receive aminoglycosides over long periods, such as those with cystic fibrosis or tuberculosis, have been identified as "at risk" groups in whom there is a higher incidence of aminoglycoside-induced ototoxicity than in the general population [25]. A predisposition to aminoglycoside-induced hearing loss (but not vestibulotoxicity) has also been linked to mutations in a mitochondrial gene. Maternally inherited hypersensitivity to aminoglycoside-induced deafness has been found to be associated with development of hearing loss after exposure to aminoglycoside at doses that do not normally cause hearing impairment [45]. Affected individuals carry a mutation in the mitochondrial gene for 12S ribosomal RNA [46].

Pharmacokinetic studies have shown that following systemic administration aminoglycosides enter perilymph from the blood relatively rapidly but the levels reached in perilymph are always far less than the peak level in serum [47], so that accumulation in perilymph is not a reason for their specific ototoxic effects. They do, however, persist in perilymph for prolonged periods.

Aminoglycosides also enter endolymph after a delay [47], indicating that their appearance in endolymph follows entry to perilymph, and the persistence of the drug in perilymph can lead to increasing concentrations in endolymph. Aminoglycosides then gain entry specifically into hair cells, with greater amounts in basal coil OHC than in those at the apex [48] and it is now thought that the entry into hair cells is via the transduction channels at the apical (endolymphatic) end of the hair cells [49]. Agents that can block the transduction channel, and mutations that inhibit channel opening prevent entry of aminoglycosides into OHC and prevent hair cell death [49].

Aminoglycosides kill hair cells in both the vestibular and auditory sensory epithelia in all vertebrate classes as well as those of the lateral line systems of fish and amphibian and also in nematocysts [25]–mechanosensitive cells in aquatic and marine invertebrates – suggesting that the specific effects of aminoglycosides on hair cells is due to their ability to pass through the transduction channel. In the mammalian cochlea the probability that the transduction channel is open is greater for OHC in the basal coil than for those at the apex (i.e. at rest there are more transduction channels open in basal coil hair cells) and the open probability is greater in OHC than IHC [50]. This could be another factor underlying differential vulnerability of hair cells along the cochlea. It has also been found that exposure to loud, but non-damaging, sounds concomitant with aminoglycoside treatment enhances the amino-glycoside-induced hair cell loss [51].

This could result from increased transduction channel opening in response to the sound enabling greater entry of aminoglycoside into hair cells and may underlie the enhanced hearing impairment that is observed in patients exposed to noise and aminoglycoside together in comparison to those exposed to one or other agent alone. It would also suggest that hair cell death follows only after a "critical level" of aminoglycoside has entered the hair cell. Thus, the delay before effects are manifest and the progression of effects over a prolonged period may result from first the delay in entry into endolymph, then the accumulation of drug in endolymph such that with continued entry into hair cells the critical levels at which the cells are no longer able to accommodate the toxic effects are reached.

However, entry into the hair cells, by itself, does not account for the hair cell death. It has been found that aminoglycosides chelate (bind to) ferric iron ions (Fe^{3+}) and it has been proposed that inside the cell redox reactions involving transitions between the ferric and ferrous ionic states (Fe^{3+} - Fe^{2+}) generates free radicals (see [25] for review of details). In an animal model, co-administration of a powerful iron chelator (1,2 dihydroxybenzoate) with aminoglycoside significantly reduced both the hair cell loss and the threshold shifts that normally follow from aminoglycoside administration, providing some support for the hypothesis that the gentamicin-iron complex maybe the ultimate toxic entity, though whether this complex, which would have a different electrical charge and a larger molecular size than the native aminoglycoside molecule, can enter the transduction channel has not been demonstrated.

In addition to causing death of hair cells, chronic administration of aminoglycosides also leads to a progressive thinning (atrophy) of the stria vascularis [52]. This seems to be due mainly to progressive apoptotic death of the marginal cells. At least initially this does not appear to cause significant reductions in the level of EP and there is evidence that the stria has a considerable degree of structural "redundancy" such that function can be maintained even with quite extensive cellular losses [53]. However, when the stria has been compromised by the effects of one damaging agent it may be less able to accommodate subsequent challenges, and adverse conditions that normally would not cause significant functional impairment may then have significant consequences on the ability of the stria to maintain EP.

Cis-Platinum

The features of cis-platinum induced hair cell loss are very similar to those of aminoglycosides: hair cell death occurs progressively from base to apex only after chronic treatment regimes. It has also been found that cis-platinum enters endolymph after a delay and effects on hair cells can be identified only after entry to endolymph [54]. However, how the drug enters the cell is not clear and thus the basis of its specific activity on hair cells is not known.

There is evidence that once inside the cell cis-platinum may inhibit endogenous free-radical scavenging systems [55]. Its ototoxicity correlates with a decrease in cochlear glutathione and significant decrease in the activity of enzymes involved in its recycling - glutathione peroxidise and glutathione reductase – as well as in superoxide dismutase [56]. How this is achieved is not clear but interference with anti-oxidant systems may lead to accumulation of free-radicals. Cis-platinum may also cause increases in the generation of free radicals themselves through stimulation of certain enzymes system associated with oxidative metabolism that naturally produce free radicals. In support of the conclusion that generation of excessive free radicals follows from the effects of cis-platinum in the cochlea, agents which enable maintenance of glutathione levels (such as d-methionine and 4-methylbenzoic acid), have been claimed to be effective in preventing the ototoxic effects of cis-platinum *in vivo* [57] (discussed further below).

In addition to effects on hair cells, cis-platinum appears be directly toxic to the neural elements in the cochlea [58]. The amplitudes of the CAP and ABR, measures of neural output from the cochlea, are reduced to a greater extent than are CM or OAE, measures of OHC activity. Exposure to cis-platinum also can cause atrophy of the stria vascularis in association with a reduced endocochlear potential [59] and it can cause apoptosis of marginal along the entire length of the cochlea [60] even when hair cell loss is confined to the basal cochlear coil. This has suggested that there are potentially multiple sites of direct action of cis-platinum in the cochlea but which site is primarily affected may be altered by manipulating the dosing regime [61].

Noise

As discussed in detail elsewhere, excessive noise induces both temporary hearing loss (temporary threshold shifts TTS) where there is a some or complete recovery from the initial loss of auditory sensitivity, and permanent hearing loss (PTS) which results from death of hair cells. Several different factors have been suggested to underlie TTS. Following exposure to noise under conditions that induce only TTS, rupture of the tip links that gate the transduction channels has been reported [62] but it has been found from studies conducted *in vitro* that following tip link disruption and concomitant loss of transduction upon stimulation of the hair bundle, the tip-links can be reformed and transduction thereby restored [49,63]. Thus, *in vivo*, the mechanical effects of excessive stimulation of the hair bundle could lead to tip-link breakage, reduced transduction and then functional recovery as tip-links are regenerated.

There is also evidence for disruption of the organization of the hair bundle and damage to the stereocilia themselves following noise trauma, but it has been suggested that there is normally constant turnover the actin filaments that form the stereocilia and this turnover could allow repair of damaged stereocilia and thus functional recovery [64]. Excessive noise has also been found to produce swelling of the afferent nerve terminals at the base of IHC, so called excitotoxic injury,that is reversible and may resolve over the approximate time scale of a TTS [65].

Normally upon stimulation, IHC release a neurotransmitter chemical into the synapses with the afferent nerves which causes the opening of ion channels in the synaptic membrane of the nerve leading to neural stimulation. With over stimulation of the IHC due to high sound levels there may be excessive release of neurotransmitter leading to the opening of excessive numbers of ion channels and excessive entry of ions that disrupts osmotic balance such that water flows into the nerve ending and it swells. This would impede neural activity and result in hearing loss, but would be potentially reversible as neurotransmitter release ceases. All, any or some of these mechanisms may underlie TTS.

With PTS, the initial hair cell death occurs at a location along the cochlea that is related to the frequency place of the damaging sound, some of which may be due to significant mechanical injury directly rupturing cells and inducing necrosis [66]. Necrosis is acute cell death in which plasma membrane integrity is compromised, the cell itself and its nucleus swell, presumably due to the influx of water across the compromised plasma membrane, and eventually the cell bursts. OHC showing swollen nuclei characteristic of necrosis have been observed in the traumatised regions of the cochlea soon (minutes to hours) after noise exposure.

Damage then progressively spreads outwards both apically (into lower frequency regions) but more prominently basally (into higher frequency regions). This progression may occur over a prolonged time period so that the final stabilized level of PTS may not be established for several days after the initial insult. Furthermore, in addition to damage at the frequency place, there is a progressive hair cell loss initiated at the basal end of the cochlea, similar to that observed with ototoxins.

This progressive loss seems to occur through apoptosis; pyknotic nuclei and activated caspase 3 have been identified in OHC during the progressive hair cell loss that follows the initial trauma [39,43,66]. It is thought that this progressive hair cell loss results from the effects of excessive free-radicals generated due to the high levels of oxidative metabolism concomitant with overstimulation of the hair cells. The generation of free radicals in the cochlea following acoustic trauma has been demonstrated directly and the products of free radical activity have been identified in noise-damaged ears [43].

This latter procedure has also shown that free-radical generation may continue for some time after the initial trauma, which may underlie the prolonged period before the PTS stabilizes, and that there is change in the species of free radical that is generated with time. This has implications for procedure aimed at protecting the cochlea from free radical injury after noise exposure (see below).

Effects on hair cells may not be either the only or the initial consequence of acoustic trauma. Studies in animals have shown effects in a several different regions of the cochlea. In particular a loss of certain fibrocytes in the spiral ligament has been observed as an early effect of noise trauma, and strial atrophy resulting from loss of marginal cells and inhibition of EP maintenance have been demonstrated as occurring after more prolonged periods [17].

Ageing

As described above, hair cell loss with ageing follows the general pattern progressing from base to apex along the cochlea, concomitant with progression of hearing loss from high to lower frequencies, and more extensive loss of OHC than IHC. It is not easy to identify the mechanisms of hair cell death with age because the number of cells dying at any one time point during the life time of an animal is small, even in mouse strains where a "natural" loss of hair cells occurs early in life and which are increasingly being used as models to study age related hearing loss (ARHL). Nevertheless, there is some evidence that excessive free radical production may be one cause. The products of free radical attack have been identified in the cochleae of ageing mice [42]; some evidence of the stress-activated pathways that lead to apoptosis have also been identified in the OHC in such animals [67]; and as described above, animals with defective free radical scavenging systems in the cochlea show much earlier, more rapid and more extensive age-related hair cell loss than normal [40]. However, it is clear that genetic background affects the rate and extent of hair cell loss with age. While ca. 50-60% of elderly people have a significant hearing loss, there are many very old people with good hearing. Likewise there are some mouse strains in which the onset of hearing loss in the absence of any damaging agents occurs relatively early in life, at about 6-8 months of age, whereas other strains maintain good hearing across the frequency range for at least two years, almost the complete life span of the animals. Studies to identify the genetic factors that underlie susceptibility to ARHL are underway in several laboratories in order to determine likely mechanisms of hair cell death with age.

However, hair cell loss may not be the only or primary cause of ARHL. Studies of human temporal bones by Schuknecht [68] classified the causes of presbyacusis into four categories: hair cell loss; neural loss more extensive than hair cell loss; strial atrophy without extensive hair cell loss; and "mixed" pathologies in which all or some of the other abnormalities existed. Certainly studies of ageing in animals have shown effects in various cell types and tissues in the cochlea. Loss of a certain population of fibrocytes preceding hair cell loss has been reported in a strain of mouse [17]. In aged gerbils there is primarily atrophy of the stria that leads eventually to loss of EP without extensive hair cell loss [53]. Strial atrophy also occurs in some mouse models of ageing [69]. Consequently currently there is no definitive understanding of mechanisms underlying ARHL and it is likely that that there may be multiple potential pathologies and variations between individuals in the underlying cause.

Organic Solvents

A number of different aromatic solvents and industrial chemical including toluene, p-xylene, ethylbenzene, styrene, trichloroethylene have been implicated in ototoxicity [28,29]. These cause auditory deficits after prolonged exposure to high concentrations (but concentrations not high enough to induce the narcosis and neurotoxicity that these chemicals can also induce). The effects of solvents may be exacerbated by concurrent exposure to high noise levels, or noise induced hearing loss may become more pronounced with concomitant exposure to certain solvents [70]. This can present a significant occupational hazard.

While solvents can cause OHC death, the pattern of damage differs from that of the agents discussed heretofore. OHC loss occurs first and most extensively in the middle and apical turns of the organ of Corti, rather than in the basal coil, and this coincides with effects on the mid-frequency ranges of hearing rather than the high frequencies [71,72]. Damage may then progress along the cochlea with time, primarily in the apical, low frequency direction. Also there is a distinct spread of damage in the radial direction across the organ of Corti from the third (outermost) row of OHC inwards to involve subsequently the second and maybe the first row of OHC [71]. Additionally the supporting cells, especially the third (outermost) row of Deiters' cells, are affected. Supporting cells are usually unaffected by the other agents that cause hair cell loss discussed above. Since organic solvents are minimally water soluble their distribution in the inner ear is unlikely to be determined by entry into the fluid spaces. The pattern of damage across the organ of Corti, from outside to in, has suggested that the solvents reach the inner ear from the vasculature of the stria vascularis or the spiral prominence region just below it and then pass through the tissues to the organ of Corti [29]. Upon reaching the organ of Corti, the supporting cells of the organ of Corti may then become injured before the damage spreads to the OHC. The effects of the solvents may be upon the membranes of the cells. Loss of membrane integrity and cell swelling, perhaps as a consequence of membrane damage, have been described as early events in the progression of solvent-induced damage in the organ of Corti and it has been contended that the principle mode of cell death in the organ of Corti is necrosis [29]. However, why damage is initiated in the middle frequency region of the cochlea is not clear. In this regard it is perhaps of note that the stria vascularis in the middle and apical cochlear turns is affected by the industrial chemical trimethyltin [73] which might suggest some characteristic of the vascular pathways and blood flow that influences solvent distribution.

Agents and Procedure That Protect Hair Cells from Lethal Damage and Loss

The discovery that hair cell loss occurs through defined biochemical pathways that may be activated by generation of excess free radicals offers potential pharmaceutical interventions to prevent hair cell death [34]. There are a number of different approaches. These include interventions to inhibit the apoptotic pathway or the stress activated pathways that lead to it; enhancement the natural stress response pathways that are activated in cells in response to changes in their physiological environment; use of "anti-oxidants" to scavenge excess free radicals; or enhancement of the natural free radical scavenging systems.

Inhibition of caspases is one target for intervention to prevent caspase-dependent programmed cell death. A number of specific caspase inhibitors that target the active sites of these enzymes are available. Studies in vitro using organotypic cultures of isolated inner ear sensory epithelia showed caspase inhibition can rescue hair cells from the lethal effects of aminoglycosides or cis-platinum when present continuously from slightly before, during and for some time after exposure to the drug [74,75,76]. These studies confirmed apoptosis as a major and universal mechanism of hair cell death following an ototoxin challenge. Subsequent *in vivo* studies also established the potential of caspase inhibition as a means to preserve hair cell function. Since activation of caspases occurs following the initial effects of aminoglycoside and cis-platinum, the preservation of hearing when caspases are inhibited indicates that the initial effects of these ototoxins may not of themselves significantly affect hair cell function. The most effective means for *in vivo* delivery of the caspase inhibitors was by local perfusion of the drug; systemic administration was much less effective. Furthermore, a potential difficulty with the use of caspase inhibitors is the possibility of inappropriate inhibition of apoptosis in tissues where it is occurring normally as part of cell turnover and tissue maintenance. Unwanted side effects are less likely when inhibitors are perfused into inner ear fluids (i.e., local therapy), but the requirement for a local delivery device and the necessity for a surgical procedure to position it may restrict clinical application of caspase inhibition.

An alternative means to inhibit a cell death pathway is to target those biochemical pathway(s) activated in response to the induced stress that subsequently triggers apoptosis. Such inhibition should target only cells which have suffered stress through exposure to a damaging agent or trauma and thus would be relatively specific. Certain small, cell-permeable molecules that interfere with activation of certain stress pathways, in particular the "c-Jun stress-activated pathway" (the JNK pathway), can inhibit programmed cell death. Inhibition of this cell pathway can enhance survival of hair cells after aminoglycoside- and noise-induced injury [77,78]. However, blocking JNK signaling does not protect against cis-platinum ototoxicity [79], illustrating that different damaging agents trigger different pathways and that one particular therapeutic agent may not be universally effective. On the other hand there is evidence that small molecule inhibitors of stress-activated pathways can be delivered to the cochlea relatively easily either by application to the round window membrane or even after systemic administration via sub-cutaneous injection, although they are less effective following administration by this latter route.

Cells can also activate systems to protect themselves against stresses, in particular physical stress. Heat shock proteins (HSP) are expressed when cells are exposed to raised temperatures (hyperthermia). They interact with cellular proteins to protect them from heat-induced disruption, but HSP can also afford protection from free radical damage, and some may have direct anti-apoptotic activity [80]. Several different HSPs are expressed in the cochlea [81,82]. One of them, HSP 70, is up-regulated in the cochlea after exposure to damaging sound and warming animals to about 41°C for 6–24 hours, to induce HSP expression, before exposure to a traumatizing level of noise has been shown to reduce the level of the PTS that develops post-noise exposure [81,82]. HSP 70 has also been found to be expressed in hair cells exposed to cis-platinum or aminoglycoside and induction of HSP, by warming or pharmacologically with geranylgeranylacetone, reduces the extent of hair cell loss that would otherwise have occurred [83,84].

Exposure to noise at non-damaging levels has also been found to be a physical stress that affords some protection from subsequent exposure to loud noise, so-called "sound conditioning" [85]. In a number of animal studies, protection from the damage normally caused by loud noise has been obtained with a variety of different non-damaging pre-exposure sound conditions varying from 81 dB to 95 dB SPL for exposure periods of several days to 15 minutes [86,87]. The protective effects may last for up to at least 60 days after the end of the conditioning period before exposure to the traumatizing noise. The protection most likely results from local enhancement of stress-activated protective mechanisms, in particular pathways activated by glucocorticoids [88]. Glucocorticoids can regulate expression of genes that are involved in cell survival pathways including those that enhance free radical scavenging [89], and glucocorticoid receptors have been localized in the cochlea [90,91].

Various stresses induce a rise in an animal's level of circulating glucocorticoid [89] and increases in circulating glucocorticoid levels have been observed in animals after exposure to moderate noise levels [90]. Local application of corticosteroids or dexamethasone to the cochlea, either by absorption from the middle ear via the round window or by direct infusion, has also been reported to reduce the extent of noise-induced or aminoglycoside-induced hair cell loss [92,93]. These observations indicate the potential value of steroid therapies in protecting hair cells from stress-induced injury, which has led to the suggestion that direct application of corticosteroid to the cochlea at the time of surgery may be effective in enhancing hair cell survival after implantation of a cochlear prosthesis [94].

Protection of hair cells from the lethal effects of exposure to noise or ototoxins has also been shown to be afforded by agents that scavenge free radicals directly or enhance the production of natural scavenger systems within a cell. Many molecules with such antioxidant activity, as well as being essentially nontoxic, are relatively small so are able to gain access to the inner ear fluids readily either from the bloodstream, and thus after systemic administration, or by crossing the round window membrane. Salicylate, for example, is, amongst its other activities, a scavenger of reactive oxygen species (ROS) and hydroxyl radicals (OH) and is able to enter perilymph rapidly from the blood. Co-administration of salicylate with aminoglycoside or with cis-platinum to animals has been shown to prevent hair cell loss almost completely and preserve auditory thresholds [95,96] and the clinical effectiveness of salicylate as an "otoprotective" agent against aminoglycoside-induced hearing loss has been tested [97]. In a small double blind clinical trial carried out in China, salicylate at doses not much higher than those used for routine analgesia and taken by patients during and for some weeks following a course of the antibiotic treatment for common infections, was shown to significantly reduce the incidence of hearing loss in comparison with patients taking a placebo. However, this result has not been replicated in other small trials.

Salicylate on its own however, is not effective against noise-induced hearing loss but, in an animal model a combination of salicylate with a vitamin E derivative (trolox) did afford some protection even when administered shortly after noise exposure [98]. After noise exposure an initial production of ROS is followed by the generation of reactive nitrogen species (RNS) and the continuation of damage for several days after noise exposure may be because of this delayed secondary generation of RNS [98]. Vitamin-E and its derivatives scavenge RNS, whereas salicylate acts only upon ROS. This highlights the fact that several different reactive free radicals may be produced by a particular insult and that combinations of therapeutic agents may be required to suppress their effects. A particular combination that is currently being tested for its potential to protect against noise-induced hearing loss is composed of vitamins A, C and E together with magnesium [99]. While the vitamins act to scavenge different free radical species, the role of magnesium is not clear although it has been reported to afford some protection against noise-induced hearing loss on its own. Oral administration of this combination has been reported to provide significant protection against noise-induced hearing loss even when administered sometime after the traumatizing event, and it has also been suggested to be effective against ototoxic damage, though this has not been thoroughly tested.

Other agents with anti-oxidant activity that have been reported to afford protection to hair cells include L-N-acetylcysteine [100], d-methionine [101], and a synthetic product "ebselen" (2-phenyl-1,2-benzisoselenazol-3[2H]-one) [102]. D-methionine has been said to be particularly effective against cis-platinum induced hair cell loss and hearing impairment.

Although all of these agents have some anti-oxidant activity they all can also enhance the activity of the glutathione, the principal natural free radical scavenger in most cells of the body. Glutathione is formed of three amino acids (glutamic acid, cysteine and glycine.) Cysteine contains sulphur (contains a "thiol" group). Oxidation of glutathione by ROS, in particular peroxides through the action of glutathione peroxidase (GPX), generates glutathione disulfide through the formation of sulphur–sulphur bonds between the cysteines of two glutathione molecules. This acts to "scavenge" the free radicals. Both L-NAC and D-methionine contain active thiol groups and can act as precursors of glutathione through being cysteine donors. Ebselen is a mimetic for glutathione peroxidase (GPx) and may also act to induce the production of GPx [102].

It should be noted that glutathione is normally synthesized naturally in the body from its constituent amino acids that are derived from the proteins in food. The maintenance of glutathione levels is, thus, dependent on an organism's proper protein nutrition. Animals maintained on a low-protein diet have greater susceptibility to aminoglycoside and cis-platinum–induced hearing impairment and hair cell loss but dietary supplementation with glutathione will reduce the extent of the ototoxic damage [103,104]. The vitamins and minerals that are reported to help protect hair cells against the effects of damaging agents are also obtained from food and are maintained in the body at optimal levels when nutrition is adequate. This emphasizes the need for proper nutrition in maintaining resistance to stress-induced hearing loss and that a poor diet may be a contributing factor to susceptibility to acquired hearing loss.

Agents Producing Temporary Hearing Loss

As pointed out above, noise may cause only a temporary threshold shift from which there may be complete recovery, and there are other agents that cause only temporary hearing loss. A single dose of a loop diuretic – furosemide, bumetanide or ethacrynic acid – can cause hearing loss that affects all frequencies within minutes of administration, but the functional deficit is quite rapidly reversible; hearing returns to normal within a few hours [105,106]. Experimental studies have shown that loop diuretics act upon the stria vascularis and cause a rapid reversible decline in EP, and thus inhibition of cochlear amplification [11,107,108]. The diuretic-affected stria vascularis shows extensive intercellular oedema indicating inhibition of ion transport mechanisms [107,108] and the target for diuretic has been identified as a sodium-potassium co-transporter protein that is required for the rapid uptake of potassium into marginal cells and whose action is crucial to the physiological process underlying generation of EP [109]. The macrolide antibiotics such as erythromycin produce similar audiological and pathological effects [110] although whether their molecular target is the same as that of diuretics is not clear. The consequences of effects of these agents upon the cochlea, coupled with observations of strial atrophy upon examination of the temporal bones from patients whose audiological deficits were known, has led to the general conclusion that functional impairment of the stria vascularis will result in threshold shifts at all testable frequencies (that is affecting the almost the entire length of the cochlea) of up to ca. 60dB (the level of cochlear amplification).

However, while single doses of diuretic do not cause permanent hearing loss, co-administration of a diuretic with a single systemic dose of aminoglycoside, which by itself would not be expected to cause damage, results in very rapid (within 24-48 hours) and extensive death of hair cells and profound permanent hearing loss [111]. This is probably a consequence of greatly enhanced uptake of positively charged (anionic) aminoglycoside into endolymph, and thereby into hair cells, as a result of the rapid decline in EP from the normal high positive levels (+80mV) to negative values (ca. -40mV) that is caused by the effects of the diuretic on the stria vascularis [112] (Taylor and Forge, 2007). From a clinical view point, however, this drug combination may be the only possible therapy in certain life-threatening conditions.

Temporary hearing impairment also results from the effects of salicylate at high doses and of quinine [113,114]. Both drugs induce rises in auditory thresholds across the whole detectable sound frequency range that are rapid in onset, within minutes of administration, persist at a constant raised level for as long as the medication is given, with rapid return to normal auditory sensitivity when treatment ends. Both drugs enter perilymph rapidly from the blood capillaries in the connective tissue that surrounds scala tympani and scala vestibule, and thus can distribute throughout the cochlea [114,115]. This can explain effects at all frequency regions. Entry into perilymph potentially provides access to the bodies of the hair cells, to the synapses with nerves at the basal end of the hair cells and to the nerves themselves. Salicylate has been shown to affect cochlear amplification: there is a loss of the sharp neural tuning that is characteristic of normal hearing, which manifests audiologically as a decrement in the ability to discriminate speech in noise; and the cochlear responses to sounds of low intensity, 60dB and lower, are affected, whereas responses to sounds of higher intensity are not [116]. This identifies the amplification mechanism in the outer hair cell as the site of action of salicylate. There is evidence that salicylate interacts with the specialised "motor" protein ("prestin") in the lateral plasma membrane of the outer hair cell that is thought to be the molecular element associated with cochlear amplification [117,118]. Quinine, however, affects cochlear responses across all intensities and thus does not target the amplifier specifically [119]. Effects of quinine upon outer hair cell morphology have been reported and these cells are thought to be one target of quinine action but the molecular target(s) are as yet unconfirmed.

Conclusion

While the incidence of permanent hearing loss is often the result of direct effects upon hair cells that lead to their death, as has been alluded to above, exposure to a combination of factors, either simultaneously or sequentially, may cause more extensive damage than would be the case from exposure to those individual agents alone. Indeed hearing loss may result from combined exposures when the conditions of exposure to any of the individual factors alone would not have been expected to cause any significant hair cell loss at all. Exposure to noise and organic solvents together leads to greater hair cell loss than the noise exposure level alone or the solvent alone would have produced, illustrating the synergistic effect of these agents upon the cochlea. Noise levels below those that cause any traumatic effects in the cochlea enhance the ototoxic effects of aminoglycosides. It has also been demonstrated in studies with animals, that exposure to damaging noise early in life can exacerbate age-related hearing loss [120]; the extent of hair cell loss with age was greater in animals exposed to noise when young in comparison with those that were not so exposed. Perhaps most devastating is the interactive effect of a loop diuretic with aminoglycoside described above. These interactions suggest the possibility that in some cases a hearing loss may result from multiple challenges delivered simultaneously or sequentially to the cochlea, any one of which individually may have no or only sub-clinical effects, but render the cochlea vulnerable when additional or further challenges, perhaps even from agents that are not recognised normally as damaging to the cochlea, are delivered. It is also the case that hair cells may not be the only or the primary site of damage. As described earlier there may be damage to the stria vascularis and potential inhibition of EP generation, to fibrocytes affecting cochlear homeostasis, or direct primary effects on the afferent neurons. Hair cell loss may be a secondary consequence of damage elsewhere and may not be the primary cause of the permanent auditory deficit. Furthermore, the extent and even the onset of a hearing loss is likely influenced by genetic factors –different alleles of genes that encode key proteins - that affect the ability of cells in the cochlea to mount a defence against a stress (either positively or negatively) or the execution of cell death programmes. Taken together, these considerations indicate that in a clinical situation there may well be multiple factors contributing to a particular case of permanent hearing loss and its audiological signature and identifying the underlying sites and mechanisms of damage may not be straightforward.

References

[1]   Forge, A., and Wright, A. (2002). The molecular architecture of the inner ear. *British Medical Bulletin 63*, 5-24.

[2]   Wright, A., Davis, A., Bredberg, G., Ulehlova, L., Spencer, H. (1987). Hair cell distributions in the normal human cochlea. *Acta Otolaryngologica Suppl., 444*: 1-48.

[3]   Ding, D., McFadden, S.L., Salvi, R. (2001). Cochlear hair cell densities and inner-ear staining techniques. In: J.F. Willott, (Ed.) *Handbook of Mouse Auditory Research: From Behavior to Molecular Biology.* (pp. 189-204) Boca Raton: CRC Press. .

[4]   Thorne, P.R., and Gavin, J.B. (1984). The accuracy of hair cell counts in determining distance and position along the organ of Corti. *Journal of the Acoustical Society of America, 76*, 440-442.

[5]   Hudspeth, A.J. (1989). How the ear's works work. *Nature, 341*, 397-404.

[6]   Davis, H. (1965). A model for transducer action in the cochlea. *Cold Spring Harbor Symposia on Quantitative Biology, 30*, 181-190.

[7]   Spoendlin, H. (1975). Neuroanatomical basis of cochlear coding mechanisms. *Audiology, 14*, 383-407.

[8]   Harrison, R.V., and Evans, E.F. (1982). Reverse correlation study of cochlear filtering in normal and pathological guinea pig ears. *Hearing Research, 6*, 303-314.

[9]   Ashmore, J.F., and Kolston, P.J. (1994). Hair cell based amplification in the cochlea. *Current Opinion in Neurobiology, 4*, 503-508.

[10]   Dallos, P. (1996). The cochlear amplifier. Progress in Biophysics and Molecular Biology 65: Sg201-Sg201.

[11] Ruggero, M.A., and Rich, N.C. (1991). Furosemide alters organ of corti mechanics: evidence for feedback of outer hair cells upon the basilar membrane. *Journal of Neuroscience, 11*, 1057-1067.

[12] Forge, A. (1984). Gap junctions in the stria vascularis and effects of ethacrynic acid. *Hearing Research, 13*,189-200.

[13] Forge, A., Becker, D., Casalotti, S., Edwards, J., Marziano, N., Nevill, G. (2003). Gap junctions in the inner ear: comparison of distribution patterns in different vertebrates and assessement of connexin composition in mammals. *Journal of Comparative Neurology, 467*, 207-231.

[14] Kikuchi, T., Kimura, R.S., Paul, D.L., Takasaka, T., Adams, J.C. (2000). Gap junction systems in the mammalian cochlea. *Brain Research and Brain Research Reviews, 32*, 163-166.

[15] Wangemann, P. (2002). K(+) cycling and the endocochlear potential. *Hearing Research, 165*, 1-9.

[16] Spicer, S.S., and Schulte, B.A. (1996). The fine structure of spiral ligament cells relates to ion return to the stria and varies with place-frequency. *Hearing Research, 100*, 80-100.

[17] Hequembourg, S., and Liberman, M.C. (2001). Spiral ligament pathology: a major aspect of age-related cochlear degeneration in C57BL/6 mice. *Journal of the Association for Research in Otolaryngology, 2*, 118-129.

[18] Wang, Y., Hirose, K., Liberman, M.C. (2002). Dynamics of noise-induced cellular injury and repair in the mouse cochlea. *Journal of Associated Research in Otolaryngology, 3*, 248-268.

[19] Boettger, T., Hubner, C.A., Maier, H., Rust, M.B., Beck, F.X., Jentsch, T.J. (2002) Deafness and renal tubular acidosis in mice lacking the K-Cl co-transporter Kcc4. *Nature, 416*, 874-878.

[20] Cohen-Salmon, M., Ott, T., Michel, V., Hardelin, J.P., Perfettini. I., Eybalin, M., Wu, T., Marcus, D.C., Wangemann, P., Willecke, K., Petit, C. (2002). Targeted ablation of connexin26 in the inner ear epithelial gap junction network causes hearing impairment and cell death. *Current Biology, 12*, 1106-1111.

[21] Rozengurt, N., Lopez, I., Chiu, C.S., Kofuji, P., Lester, H.A., Neusch, C. (2003) Time course of inner ear degeneration and deafness in mice lacking the Kir4.1 potassium channel subunit. *Hearing Research, 177*, 71-80.

[22] Steel, K.P., and Kros, C.J. (2001). A genetic approach to understanding auditory function. *Nature Genetics, 27*, 143-149.

[23] Kemp, D.T. (1978) Stimulated acoustic emissions from within the human auditory system. *Journal of the Acoustical Society of America, 64*, 1386-1391.

[24] Hawkins, J.E., Jr. (1973). Comparative otopathology: aging, noise, and ototoxic drugs. *Advances in Otorhinolaryngology, 20*, 125-141.

[25] Forge, A., and Schacht, J. (2000). Aminoglycoside antibiotics. *Audiology and Neurootology, 5*, 3-22.

[26] Rybak, L.P., and Kelly, T. (2003). Ototoxicity: bioprotective mechanisms. *Current Opinion in Otolaryngology Head and Neck Surgery, 11*, 328-333.

[27] Fuente, A., Slade, M.D., Taylor, T., Morata, T.C., Keith, R.W., Sparer J, Rabinowitz PM. (2009) Peripheral and central auditory dysfunction induced by occupational exposure to organic solvents. *Journal of Occupational and Environmental Medicine, 5,* 1202-1211.

[28] Morata, T.C., Dunn, D.E., Sieber, W.K. (1994). Occupational exposure to noise and ototoxic organic solvents. *Archives of Environmental Health, 49,* 359-365.

[29] Campo, P., and Maguin, K. (2007). Solvent-induced hearing loss: mechanisms and prevention strategy. *International Journal of Occupational and Medical Environmental Health, 20,* 265-270.

[30] Saunders, J.C., Dear, S.P, Schneider, M.E. (1985). The anatomical consequences of acoustic injury: A review and tutorial. *Journal of the Acoustical Society of America, 78,* 833-860.

[31] Slepecky, N. (1986). Overview of mechanical damage to the inner ear: noise as a tool to probe cochlear function. *Hearing Research, 22,* 307-321.

[32] Yoshida, N., Hequembourg, S.J., Atencio, C.A., Rosowski, J.J., Liberman, M.C. (2000). Acoustic injury in mice: 129/SvEv is exceptionally resistant to noise-induced hearing loss. *Hearing Research, 141,* 97-106.

[33] Richardson, G.P., and Russell, I.J. (1991). Cochlear cultures as a model system for studying aminoglycoside induced ototoxicity. *Hearing Research, 53,* 293-311.

[34] Forge, A., Van de Water, T.R. (2008) Protection and repair of inner ear sensory cells. In: R.J.Salvi, A.N.Popper, R. Fay (Eds.). Hair cell regeneration, repair and protection. (pp.141-198). New York: Springer.

[35] Evans, P., and Halliwell, B. (1999). Free radicals and hearing. Cause, consequence, and criteria. *Annals of the New York Academy of Science, 884,* 19-40.

[36] Halliwell, B. (2011). Free radicals and antioxidants - quo vadis? *Trends in Pharmacological Science, 32,* 125-130.

[37] Murphy, M.P., Holmgren, A., Larsson, N.G., Halliwell, B., Chang, C.J., Kalyanaraman, B., Rhee, S.G., Thornalley, P.J., Partridge, L., Gems, D., Nyström, T., Belousov, V., Schumacker, P.T., Winterbourn, C.C. (2011). Unraveling the biological roles of reactive oxygen species. *Cell Metabolism, 13,* 361-366.

[38] Sha, S.H., Taylor, R., Forge, A., Schacht, J. (2001). Differential vulnerability of basal and apical hair cells is based on intrinsic susceptibility to free radicals. *Hearing Research, 155,* 1-8.

[39] Ohlemiller, K.K., McFadden, S.L., Ding, D.L., Flood, D.G., Reaume, A.G., Hoffman, E.K., Scott, R.W., Wright, J.S., Putcha, G.V., Salvi, R.J. (1999). Targeted deletion of the cytosolic Cu/Zn-superoxide dismutase gene (Sod1) increases susceptibility to noise-induced hearing loss. *Audiology and Neurootology, 4,* 237-246.

[40] Keithley, E.M., Canto, C., Zheng, Q.Y., Wang, X., Fischel-Ghodsian, N., Johnson, K.R. (2005) Cu/Zn superoxide dismutase and age-related hearing loss. *Hearing Research, 209,* 76-85.

[41] Sha, S.H., Zajic, G., Epstein, C.J., Schacht, J. (2001). Overexpression of copper/zinc-superoxide dismutase protects from kanamycin-induced hearing loss. *Audiology and Neurootology, 6,* 117-123.

[42] Jiang, H., Talaska, A.E., Schacht, J., Sha, S.H. (2007). Oxidative imbalance in the aging inner ear., *Neurobiology of Aging, 28,* 1605-1612.

[43] Yamashita, D., Jiang, H.Y., Schacht, J., Miller, J.M. (2004). Delayed production of free radicals following noise exposure. *Brain Research, 1019*, 201-209.

[44] Forge, A., Li, L., Nevill, G. (1998). Hair cell recovery in the vestibular sensory epithelia of mature guinea pigs. *Journal of Comparative Neurology, 397*, 69-88.

[45] Prezant, T.R., Agapian, J.V., Bohlman, M.C., Bu, X., Oztas, S., Qiu, W.Q., Arnos, K.S., Cortopassi, G.A., Jaber, L., Rotter, J.I. (1993). Mitochondrial ribosomal RNA mutation associated with both antibiotic-induced and non-syndromic deafness. *Nature Genetics, 4*, 289-294.

[46] Hutchin, T., Haworth, I., Higashi, K., Fischel-Ghodsian, N., Stoneking, M., Saha, N., Amos., Cortopassi, G. (1993). A molecular basis for human hypersensitivity to aminoglycoside antibiotics. *Nucleic Acids Research, 21*, 4174-4179.

[47] Tran Ba Huy, P., Manuel, C., Meulemans, A., Sterkers, O., Amiel, C. (1981). Pharmacokinetics of gentamicin in perilymph and endolymph of the rat as determined by radioimmunoassay. *Journal of Infectious Diseases, 143*, 476-486.

[48] Hiel, H., Schamel, A., Erre, J.P., Hayashida, T., Dulon, D., Aran, J.M. (1992) Cellular and subcellular localization of tritiated gentamicin in the guinea pig cochlea following combined treatment with ethacrynic acid. *Hearing Research, 57*, 157-165.

[49] Gale, J.E., Marcotti, W., Kennedy, H.J., Kros, C.J., Richardson, G.P. (2001). FM1-43 dye behaves as a permeant blocker of the hair-cell mechanotransducer channel. *Journal of Neuroscience, 21*, 7013-7025.

[50] Russell, I.J., and Kossl, M. (1992). Sensory transduction and frequency selectivity in the basal turn of the guinea-pig cochlea. *Philosophical Transactions of the Royal Society of London Series B, Biological Sciences, 336*, 317-324.

[51] Decory, L., Hiel, H., Aran, J.M. (1991). In vivo noise exposure alters the in vitro motility and viability of outer hair cells. *Hearing Research, 52*, 81-88.

[52] Forge, A., Wright, A., Davies, S.J. (1987). Analysis of structural changes in the stria vascularis following chronic gentamicin treatment. *Hearing Research, 31*, 253-265.

[53] Spicer, S.S., Gratton, M.A., Schulte, B.A. (1997). Expression patterns of ion transport enzymes in spiral ligament fibrocytes change in relation to strial atrophy in the aged gerbil cochlea. *Hearing Research, 111*, 93-102.

[54] McAlpine, D., and Johnstone, B.M. (1990). The ototoxic mechanism of cisplatin. *Hearing Research, 47*, 191-203.

[55] Minami, S.B., Sha, S.H., Schacht, J. (2004). Antioxidant protection in a new animal model of cisplatin-induced ototoxicity. *Hearing Research, 198*, 137-143.

[56] Ravi, R., Somani, S.M., Rybak, L.P. (1995). Mechanism of cisplatin ototoxicity: antioxidant system. *Pharmacology and Toxicology, 76*, 386-394.

[57] Rybak, L.P, and Whitworth, C.A. (2005). Ototoxity: therapeutic opportunities. *Drug Discovery Today, 10*, 1313-1321.

[58] van Ruijven, M.W., de Groot, J.C., Klis, S.F., Smoorenburg, G.F. (2005). The cochlear targets of cisplatin: an electrophysiological and morphological time-sequence study. *Hearing Research, 205*, 241-248.

[59] Klis, S.F., O'Leary, S.J., Hamers, F.P., De Groot, J.C., Smoorenburg, G.F. (2000). Reversible cisplatin ototoxicity in the albino guinea pig. *Neuroreport,11*, 623-626.

[60] Alam, S.A., Ikeda, K., Oshima, T., Suzuki, M., Kawase, T., Kituchi T., Takasaka, T. (2000). Cisplatin-induced apoptotic cell death in Mongolian gerbil cochlea. *Hearing Research, 141*, 28-38.

[61] Rybak, L.P., Whitworth, C.A., Mukherjea, D., Ramkumar, V. (2007). Mechanisms of cisplatin-induced ototoxicity and prevention. *Hearing Research, 226,* 157-167.

[62] Clark, J.A., and Pickles, J.O. (1996). The effects of moderate and low levels of acoustic overstimulation on stereocilia and their tip links in the guinea pig. *Hearing Research, 99,* 119-128.

[63] Zhao, Y., Yamoah, E.N., Gillespie, P.G. (1996). Regeneration of broken tip links and restoration of mechanical transduction in hair cells. *Proceedings of the National Academy of Sciences, USA,* 93, 15469-15474.

[64] Schneider, M.E., Belyantseva, I.A., Azevedo, R.B., Kachar, B. (2002). Rapid renewal of auditory hair bundles. *Nature, 418,* 837-838.

[65] Ruel, J., Wang, J., Rebillard, G., Eybalin, M., Lloyd, R., Pujol, R., Puel, JL. (2007). Physiology, pharmacology and plasticity at the inner hair cell synaptic complex. *Hearing Research, 227,* 19-27.

[66] Henderson, D., McFadden, S.L., Liu, C.C., Hight, N., Zheng, X.Y. (1999). The role of antioxidants in protection from impulse noise. *Annals of the New York Academy of Sciences, 884,* 368-380.

[67] Sha, S.H., Chen, F.Q., Schacht, J. (2009). Activation of cell death pathways in the inner ear of the aging CBA/J mouse. *Hearing Research, 254,* 92-99.

[68] Schuknecht, H.F., and Gacek, M.R. (1993). Cochlear pathology in presbycusis. *Annals of Otology, Rhinology and Laryngology, 102,* 1-16.

[69] Ohlemiller, K.K. (2009). Mechanisms and genes in human strial presbycusis from animal models. *Brain Research, 1277,* 70-83.

[70] Morata, T.C. (1998). Assessing occupational hearing loss: beyond noise exposures. *Scandinavian Audiology Suppl., 48,* 111-116.

[71] Campo, P., Lataye, R., Cossec, B., Placidi, V. (1997). Toluene-induced hearing loss: a mid-frequency location of the cochlear lesions. *Neurotoxicology and Teratology, 19,* 129-140.

[72] Johnson, A.C., and Canlon, B. (1994). Progressive hair cell loss induced by toluene exposure. *Hearing Research, 75,* 201-208.

[73] Fechter, L.D., and Carlisle L. (1990). Auditory dysfunction and cochlear vascular injury following trimethyltin exposure in the guinea pig. *Toxicology and Applied Pharmacology, 105,* 133-143.

[74] Forge, A, Li, L. (2000). Apoptotic death of hair cells in mammalian vestibular sensory epithelia. *Hearing Research, 139,* 97-115.

[75] Matsui, J.I., Ogilvie, J.M., Warchol, M.E. (2002). Inhibition of caspases prevents ototoxic and ongoing hair cell death. *Journal of Neuroscience, 22,* 1218-1227.

[76] Cunningham, L.L., Cheng, A.G., Rubel, E.W. (2002). Caspase activation in hair cells of the mouse utricle exposed to neomycin. *Journal of Neuroscience, 22,* 8532-8540.

[77] Pirvola, U., Xing-Qun, L., Virkkala, J., Saarma, M., Murakata, C., Camoratto, A.M., Walton, K.M., Ylikoski, J. (2000). Rescue of hearing, auditory hair cells, and neurons by CEP-1347/KT7515, an inhibitor of c-Jun N-terminal kinase activation. *Journal of Neuroscience, 20,* 43-50.

[78] Wang, J., Van De Water, T.R., Bonny, C., de Ribaupierre, F., Puel, J.L., Zine, A. (2003) A peptide inhibitor of c-Jun N-terminal kinase protects against both amino-glycoside and acoustic trauma-induced auditory hair cell death and hearing loss. *Journal of Neuroscience, 23,* 8596-8607.

[79] Wang J, Ladrech, S., Pujol, R., Brabet, P., Van De Water, T.R, Puel, J.L. (2004) Caspase inhibitors, but not c-Jun NH2-terminal kinase inhibitor treatment, prevent cisplatin-induced hearing loss. *Cancer Research, 64*, 9217-9224.

[80] Richter, K., Haslbeck, M., Buchner, J. (2010). The heat shock response: life on the verge of death. *Molecular Cell, 40,* 253-266.

[81] Altschuler, R.A., Fairfield, D., Cho, Y., Leonova, E., Benjamin, I.J., Miller, J.M., Lomax, M.L. (2002). Stress pathways in the rat cochlea and potential for protection from acquired deafness. *Audiology and Neurootology, 7*, 152-156.

[82] Yoshida, N., Kristiansen, A., Liberman, M.C. (1999) Heat stress and protection from permanent acoustic injury in mice. *Journal of Neuroscience, 19*, 10116-10124.

[83] Takumida, M., Anniko, M. (2005). Heat shock protein 70 delays gentamicin-induced vestibular hair cell death. *Acta Otolaryngologica, 125,* 23-28.

[84] Taleb, M., Brandon, C.S., Lee, F.S., Harris, K.C., Dillmann, W.H., Cunningham, L.L. (2009) Hsp70 inhibits aminoglycoside-induced hearing loss and cochlear hair cell death. *Cell Stress Chaperones 14*, 427-437.

[85] Canlon, B., and Fransson, A. (1995). Morphological and functional preservation of the outer hair cells from noise trauma by sound conditioning. *Hearing Research, 84*, 112-124.

[86] Kujawa, S.G., and Liberman, M.C. (1999). Long-term sound conditioning enhances cochlear sensitivity. *Journal of Neurophysiology, 82*, 863-873.

[87] Yoshida, N., and Liberman, M.C. (2000). Sound conditioning reduces noise-induced permanent threshold shift in mice. *Hearing Research, 148*, 213-219.

[88] Tahera, Y., Meltser, I., Johansson, P., Salman, H., Canlon, B. (2007). Sound conditioning protects hearing by activating the hypothalamic-pituitary-adrenal axis. *Neurobiology of Disease, 25*, 189-197.

[89] Wang, Y., and Liberman, M.C. (2002). Restraint stress and protection from acoustic injury in mice. *Hearing Research, 165*, 96-102.

[90] Rarey, K.E., Curtis, L.M., ten Cate WJ (1993) Tissue specific levels of glucocorticoid receptor within the rat inner ear. *Hearing Research, 64*, 205-210.

[91] Terunuma, T., Hara, A., Senarita, M., Motohashi, H., Kusakari, J. (2001). Effect of acoustic overstimulation on regulation of glucocorticoid receptor mRNA in the cochlea of the guinea pig. *Hearing Research, 15*, 121-124.

[92] Himeno, C., Komeda, M., Izumikawa, M., Takemura, K., Yagi, M., Weiping, Y., Doi, T., Kuriyama, H., Miller, J.M., Yamashita, T. (2002) Intra-cochlear administration of dexamethasone attenuates aminoglycoside ototoxicity in the guinea pig. *Hearing Research, 167*, 61-70.

[93] Takemura, K., Komeda, M., Yagi, M., Himeno, C., Izumikawa, M., Doi, T., Kuriyama, H., Miller, J.M., Yamashita, T. (2004). Direct inner ear infusion of dexamethasone attenuates noise-induced trauma in guinea pig. *Hearing Research, 196,* 58-68.

[94] Eshraghi, A.A. (2006). Prevention of cochlear implant electrode damage. *Current Opinion in Otolaryngology Head and Neck Surgery, 14,* 323-328.

[95] Li, G., Sha, S.H., Zotova, E., Arezzo, J., Van de Water, T., Schacht, J. (2002). Salicylate protects hearing and kidney function from cisplatin toxicity without compromising its oncolytic action. *Laboratory Investigation, 82*, 585-596.

[96] Sha, S.H., and Schacht, J. (1999). Salicylate attenuates gentamicin-induced ototoxicity. *Laboratory Investigation, 79*, 807-813.

[97] Chen, Y., Huang, W.G., Zha, D.J., Qiu, J.H., Wang, J.L., Sha, S.H., Schacht, J. (2007). Aspirin attenuates gentamicin ototoxicity: from the laboratory to the clinic. *Hearing Research, 226*, 178-182.

[98] Yamashita, D., Jiang, H.Y., Le Prell, C.G., Schacht, J., Miller, J.M. (2005). Post-exposure treatment attenuates noise-induced hearing loss. *Neuroscience, 134*, 633-642.

[99] Le Prell, C.G., Hughes, L.F., Miller, J.M. (2007). Free radical scavengers vitamins A, C, and E plus magnesium reduce noise trauma. *Free Radical Biology and Medicine, 42*, 1454-1463.

[100] Kopke, R.D., Jackson, R.L., Coleman, J.K., Liu, J., Bielefeld, E.C., Balough, B.J. (2007). NAC for noise: from the bench top to the clinic. *Hearing Research, 226*, 114-125.

[101] Campbell, K.C., Meech, R.P., Klemens, J.J., Gerberi, M.T., Dyrstad, S.S., Larsen, D.L., Mitchell, D.L., El-Azizi, M., Verhulst, S.J., Hughes, L.F. (2007). Prevention of noise- and drug-induced hearing loss with D-methionine. *Hearing Research, 226*, 92-103.

[102] Lynch, E.D., and Kil, J. (2005). Compounds for the prevention and treatment of noise-induced hearing loss. *Drug Discovery Today, 10*, 1291-1298.

[103] Garetz, S.L., Altschuler, R.A., Schacht, J. (1994). Attenuation of gentamicin ototoxicity by glutathione in the guinea pig in vivo. *Hearing Research, 77*, 81-87.

[104] Lautermann, J., McLaren, J., Schacht, J. (1995). Glutathione protection against gentamicin ototoxicity depends on nutritional status. *Hearing Research, 86*, 15-24.

[105] Arnold, W., Nadol, J.B., Weidauer, H. (1981). Temporal bone histopathology in human ototoxicity due to loop diuretics. *Scandinavian Audiology Suppl. 14*, 201-213.

[106] Rybak, L.P. (1993). Ototoxicity of loop diuretics. *Otolaryngological Clinics of North America, 26*, 829-844.

[107] Forge, A. (1981). Ultrastructure in the stria vascularis of the guinea pig following intraperitoneal injection of ethacrynic acid. *Acta Otolaryngologica, 92*, 439-457.

[108] Pike, D.A., and Bosher, S.K. (1980). The time course of the strial changes produced by intravenous furosemide. *Hearing Research, 3*, 79-89.

[109] Wangemann, P., Liu, J., Marcus, D.C. (1995). Ion transport mechanisms responsible for K+ secretion and the transepithelial voltage across marginal cells of stria vascularis in vitro. *Hearing Research, 84*, 19-29.

[110] Liu, J., Marcus, D.C., Kobayashi, T. (1996). Inhibitory effect of erythromycin on ion transport by stria vascularis and vestibular dark cells. *Acta Otolaryngologica, 116*, 572-575.

[111] Brummett, R.E. (1981). Effects of antibiotic-diuretic interactions in the guinea pig model of ototoxicity. *Reviews of Infectious Diseases 3 Suppl.* S216-223.

[112] Taylor, R.R., Nevill, G., Forge, A. (2008). Rapid hair cell loss: a mouse model for cochlear lesions. *Journal of the Association for Research in Otolaryngology, 9*, 44-64.

[113] Garetz SL, and Schacht J (1996) Ototoxicity: of mice and men. In: T. Van de Water , R.R. Fay, A.N. Popper. (Eds.). Clinical Aspects of Hearing. New York: Springer. pp. 116-154.

[114] Tange, R.A., Dreschler, W.A., Claessen, F.A., Perenboom, R.M. (1997). Ototoxic reactions of quinine in healthy persons and patients with Plasmodium falciparum infection. *Auris Nasus Larynx, 24*, 131-136.

[115] Boettcher, F.A., Bancroft, B.R., Salvi, R.J. (1990). Concentration of salicylate in serum and perilymph of the chinchilla. *Archives of Otolaryngology Head and Neck Surgery, 116,* 681-684.

[116] Stypulkowski, P.H. (1990). Mechanisms of salicylate ototoxicity. *Hearing Research, 46,* 113-145.

[117] Santos-Sacchi, J., Song, L., Zheng, J., Nuttall, A.L. (2006) Control of mammalian cochlear amplification by chloride anions. *Journal of Neuroscience, 26,* 3992-3998.

[118] Tunstall, M.J., Gale, J.E., Ashmore, J.F. (1995). Action of salicylate on membrane capacitance of outer hair cells from the guinea-pig cochlea. *Journal of Physiology, 485,* 739-752.

[119] Puel, J.L., Bobbin, R.P., Fallon, M. (1990). Salicylate, mefenamate, meclofenamate, and quinine on cochlear potentials. *Otolaryngology Head and Neck Surgery, 102,* 66-73.

[120] Kujawa, S.G., and Liberman, M.C. (2006). Acceleration of age-related hearing loss by early noise exposure: evidence of a misspent youth. *Journal of Neuroscience, 26,* 2115-2123.

In: Prevention of Hearing Loss
Editors: V. Newton, P. Alberti and A. Smith

ISBN: 978-1-61942-745-7
© 2012 Nova Science Publishers, Inc.

Chapter IV

Consequences of Hearing Impairment to the Individual and Society

*M. Kathleen Pichora-Fuller** and *Janet R. Jamieson*

Abstract

Hearing impairment is diagnosed medically but experienced socially. Whether a person is born with hearing impairment or acquires it in old age, it shapes the person's identity and social relationships. Reduced access to sound undermines communication and social interaction as well as posing risks to safety and compromising independence. The mismatch between the person and his or her social and physical context makes it difficult to achieve a wide range of goals. Associated feelings of loss of control and social exclusion increase stress and decrease ability to cope with a variety of life issues. The widespread consequences for the individual and society are best understood from an ecological or systems perspective. Solutions that restore balance in the system to enable the person to fulfill life goals must combine changes in behaviour along with the use of appropriate technologies and environmental modifications. Behavioral changes involve not only the individual with the hearing loss, but also the person's family members and other significant communication partners (e.g., teachers, co-workers, health profess-sionals). Ultimately, interventions should be evaluated in terms of their effects on the individual's quality of life and ability to fulfill goals and aspirations in a range of situations. Hearing loss in children affects linguistic, cognitive, and social development with implications for educational and eventual vocational success. Progressive or acquired hearing loss in working-aged adults is associated with lower incomes, under-employment and reduced productivity, whether the workplace is a factory or a board room, and whether the cause of hearing loss is a disease or noise or aging. In adults, as well as consequences to mental health, stress associated with hearing loss may exacerbate physical health problems. In addition, difficulty communicating may significantly increase the risk of preventable adverse events in healthcare or limit access to health education programmes designed to promote healthy lifestyles and prevent or manage various health conditions. Indeed, considering the aging of the population, the increasing prevalence of hearing loss with age, and the increasing co-existence of disabilities and

---

* Corresponding author: k.pichora.fuller@utoronto.ca.

chronic health problems with age, hearing loss must be situated in a broader social and health context within which its interactions with other disabilities and age-related health problems, such as vision loss and cognitive decline,can be addressed. Hearing loss is not only about ears; it has implications for the general well-being and health of persons across the life-span in just about every aspect of their lives.

Introduction

Hearing impairment is diagnosed medically but experienced socially. Hearing provides access to sound, enabling us to interact with the auditory world, monitor our own behaviours, and communicate. Sound provides us with information about our surroundings; for example, a siren warns us of an approaching ambulance and we hear rain on the roof or a doorbell ringing. Sound gives us feedback about our own actions; for example, we hear our steps as we walk along the sidewalk and an apple crunch as we bite into it. Inter-personal communication entails an exchange between a sender and a receiver of a message as they co-construct meaning in a given situational context. Hearing is critical to spoken communication because it enables individuals to receive the speech signal sent by other communicators, monitor their own speech production, and assess the acoustical characteristics of social (e.g., the excited voices of children playing at recess) and physical environments (e.g., the reverberation of a cathedral) in which communication occurs.

In addition to interpersonal communication, increasingly humans also interact with machines by speech. Computers can produce and recognize speech; for example, automated telephone interfaces ask for caller account numbers and respond to speech. While this human-machine information exchange seems to qualify as a type of rudimentary communication and it can be successful for accomplishing well-defined tasks, we do not expect to hold a dynamic and rewarding conversation with a computer because it is not a person. Human communication is more than simply producing or recognizing speech, or even exchanging necessary information; it is primarily a system for establishing and maintaining social relationships.Notwithstanding the limitations of human-machine communication, however, the use of the Internet and other advanced multi-modal communication technologies to enable communication between people in various personal or professional relationships may present new opportunities and challenges for people who have hearing impairment.

Communication is vital to the formation and maintenance of our individual personal identities and our social identities as members of groups with varying status and power in society. Thus, for individuals who have impaired hearing, reduced access to the auditory world and lost or atypical opportunities to communicate will have psychological and social consequences. Such consequences will influence their development and education, their ability to fulfill adult roles in society at home, at work, and in the community, and also their ability to maintain independence and preserve active lifestyles and good health in old age. In relation to health, those with hearing loss are at greater risk for psychosocial health problems across the lifespan [1]. They may also be disadvantaged when receiving health information or health services geared towards health promotion or the prevention and treatment of many health conditions because there is often a heavy reliance on spoken communication. The consequences of hearing impairment across the lifespan can be felt in just about any sphere of life that involves spoken communication and social interaction.

The World Health Organization (WHO) International Classification of Functioning (ICF) [2] provides a framework for understanding how hearing *impairment*(at the level of the body functions and structures) relates to a person's basic auditory capacities for performing tasks during *activities* and the person's *participation* in life roles given the supports or barriers associated with environmental and personal factors. The WHO ICF framework is also useful insofar as it provides a perspective within which to understand how hearing health care practice has changed in the past and how it will likely continue to evolve in the future (see Table 4.1). Over the last century, there has been a general shift in health care delivery from a predominantly bio-medical physical approach focused on the diagnosis and medical and surgical treatments for acute diseases to a more holistic bio-psycho-social-environmental approach focused on the prevention and management of chronic disorders. Consistent with this general trend in health care, at least in developed countries, the work of hearing health care professionals in medical settings until the mid-20th century was dominated by a focus on *impairment* (e.g., site of lesion assessment and medical or surgical treatments for conditions such as middle ear diseases). Later developments focused on methods to test and improve the capacities of listeners as they performed tasks required to engage in *activities*, with an emphasis on the understanding of speech (e.g., rehabilitative interventions to provide amplification and training for individuals with chronic sensorineural hearing loss). By the 1980s there was increasing interest in the psycho-social experiences of people and questionnaires were created to explore these consequences of hearing loss and to measure how they were altered by rehabilitation. More recently, practice has begun to address the *participation* issues of people who have hearing loss.

Against the general backdrop of progress in the field of health psychology over the last three decades, innovations in rehabilitation for people who have hearing impairment have taken a more holistic approach and embraced the notion of "enablement" whereby the clinician and patient interact in a partnership to identify the person's goals and needs and to plan appropriate action taking [1]. Moving beyond the walls of the clinic and the context of the clinician-patient relationship, rehabilitation of the person began to be re-conceptualized in terms of "accessibility." Accessibility is achieved when the person benefits from a system of solutions, including the use of personal technologies and behaviour changes, but also initiatives to minimize barriers and increase the supportiveness of the social and physical contexts where people need to hear to be able to participate fully.

Optimizing social supports involves extending intervention from the individual by involving the person's significant communication partners such as family members, peers, educators, co-workers and a wide range of health and other professionals.

Table 4.1. Relationship WHO ICF concepts to shifts in the focus of hearing health care

WHO ICF Concept	Level of Problem	Focus of Hearing Health Care
Impairment	Body	Diagnostic/medical
Activity	Person	Rehabilitation
Participation	Society	Accessibility

Optimizing the physical environment involves the development and implementation of standards for acoustics in the built environment and the use of assistive technologies in public venues such as in the educational, justice, and health care systems. Accessibility initiatives necessarily involve the formulation of new public policies and changes in culture very broadly. In this chapter, we combine a broad accessibility view with a lifespan perspective. We highlight some of the consequences of hearing loss to the individual and society, with more emphasis on childhood and old age because of the special vulnerabilities of these age groups.

Childhood

Factors Affecting Access to Communication and communication Development

Most children experience hearing loss of some degree during the years from birth through to the end of adolescence. For a small proportion of these children, the hearing loss is a permanent condition that has a pervasive effect on many aspects of development. For another, much larger (and, in some cases, overlapping) group of these children, the hearing loss is a transient, though sometimes long-term, condition, known as otitis media, which may also impact development in idiosyncratic but significant ways. Although the focus of this section is primarily the former group of children, that is, those with permanent hearing loss, particular mention will also be made of the prevalence and frequently noted long-term impacts of otitis media.

Permanent Hearing Loss

Permanent childhood hearing loss has a significant impact on development because children who are deaf and hard of hearing live in a world where sound plays an important role and where the majority of peers and adults who surround them hear normally. Thus, their interactions with the physical world differ from those of individuals with normal hearing because of comparatively reduced auditory access. In addition, their social interactions are altered both directly, because auditory communication is more difficult, and indirectly, because there may be differences in the modalities they utilize to learn about and experience the world.

Permanent hearing loss with an onset at or before birth or during early childhood is a low prevalence condition, at least in western countries where the demographics of childhood hearing loss have been documented [3]. There is some variability in the range of reported prevalence figures from one country to another, which may be accounted for by the criteria used to define educationally significant childhood hearing loss. For example, lower incidence figures are found when hearing loss is specified as an average pure-tone threshold greater than 40 dB HL, but the rate increases when children are included who have lesser degrees of impairment or unilateral impairment.

Most children have thresholds that are less than 45 dB HL (the average level of conversation); that is, they have levels of hearing impairment that are generally categorized as mild or moderate. Broadly speaking, these children have sufficient access to sound in the early years to develop functional listening and speaking abilities for interpersonal communication, although they may derive great benefit from technologies (such as hearing aids); these children may be viewed as hard of hearing. It was long thought that minimal degrees of hearing impairment did not have a significant impact on development; however, there is a growing body of evidence that there can be significant delays in language and social-emotional development for children with even mild bilateral [4] or unilateral [5] losses. Children with greater degrees of impairment, that is, those whose average pure-tone thresholds fall into the severe-to-profound or profound range, comprise a small proportion of the overall group of children with hearing impairment[6]. However, as will be discussed later, inaccessible language early in life often has a drastic effect on language, cognitive, and social-emotional development as well as educational outcomes. Without amplification or effective benefit from amplification, these children are primarily visual processors of information and they may be viewed as deaf. Over time, personal and group identities can be shaped in various ways by these differences in access to meaningful sound in the surrounding world. In this section, the broad term "children with hearing impairment" will be used to refer to the combined group of deaf and hard of hearing children from birth through the end adolescence.

It should be noted that parental hearing status is strongly implicated in babies' early access to language. Over 95% of deaf and hard of hearing children are born to hearing parents [7], most of whom did not expect the diagnosis. From this perspective, then, these children are in a minority position in terms of hearing status within their own families, even from the earliest days of infancy. A particular challenge of early intervention is to support hearing parents in their efforts to develop a meaningful communication approach with their infants. By contrast, the small subset of deaf and hard of hearing children who have Deaf parents are typically born into families where visual communication, primarily through the use of a natural sign language, is the norm. (The use of the capitalized 'Deaf' is used to denote a person's membership in Deaf culture, the primary indicator of which is one's use of a natural sign language as the primary means of communication.) For these children, early, visually-based, accessible reciprocal communication has been noted between Deaf mothers and their deaf babies [8], and it has also been noted that many Deaf parents adjust to their child's hearing loss more rapidly than hearing parents do; in fact, some Deaf parents may actually welcome the diagnosis [9].

From the perspective that childhood hearing loss poses a significant threat to mutual reciprocal communication and restricted access to the surrounding social world for many children with hearing impairment, it is not surprising that emotional stability or mental health issues have been noted among this population. In particular, children with greater degrees of impairment have been found to demonstrate lower mastery in many areas of social competence in relation to their hearing peers [10]. However, it is difficult to determine precisely the frequency of psychological problems in those who are deaf, especially children, because most assessment measures have been designed for and normed on those who have normal hearing. What is clear among the diverse population of individuals with hearing impairment who also have mental health or psychosocial issues is that the accessibility of specialized social services tailored to meet their communication needs is poor.

It is not uncommon for hearing impairment to co-exist with other disabling conditions, which contributes to the tremendous heterogeneity of this population. According to the Gallaudet Research Institute (GRI) Annual Survey of Deaf and Hard of Hearing Children and Youth, almost 40% of deaf and hard of hearing students (with all degrees of hearing loss) between the ages of 5 and 19 years in the United States have educationally relevant conditions in addition to hearing impairment [6]. The vast majority of these additional conditions have a direct and significant impact on communication and social interaction with others. For example, almost 35% of the students in the GRI survey have additional conditions such as blindness, developmental delay, learning disabilities, or autism. Overall, the effects of additional disabling conditions are not additive; rather, as Moors [11] stated, they exponentially compound the developmental challenges confronting an individual. In fact, the presence of two or more educationally relevant disabling conditions may result in the need for alternative approaches to communication and highly specialized professional intervention in education and habilitation.

Increasingly, at least in most western industrialized nations, children with permanent hearing losses are integrated into regular educational settings where they receive most, if not all, of their education with hearing peers [6], typically with support from teachers of the deaf and hard of hearing, speech-language pathologists, audiologists, educational interpreters, and/or other professionals. Nevertheless, given the challenges with mutually accessible communication, it is not unusual for integrated deaf and hard of hearing students to experience social difficulties "fitting in" with their hearing peers in the integrated setting - even on the school playground [12].Overall, the social implications of restricted communication access and ease of communication in the early years - at home, in the classroom and playground, and in the broader community - appear to have strong repercussions across domains.

Otitis Media

Otitis media (OM) and otitis media with effusion (OME, or 'glue ear') together represent one of the most common infections in children. In fact, OME is the most common cause of hearing loss in children from 6 months of age onward [13]. The fluctuating conductive hearing loss associated with OM and OME is usually mild to moderate (10 – 40 dB), and is caused by the build-up of fluid behind the eardrum, interfering with the transmission of sound to the inner ear. In most cases, OME clears up spontaneously and reduces significantly after the age of 5 years, but a small group of children may have persistent and longstanding cases of OME into the school years.

It has been suggested that OM- and OME-related hearing loss can cause behaviour problems and delay language acquisition, but actual research findings are not conclusive. For example, a meta-analysis of different types of studies indicated a small but negative impact of OM on language development, most pronounced among children with additional special needs, such as Down Syndrome [14]. Whereas one study [15] found no evidence of a significant relationship between a history of OME and children's later academic skills, another study[16] uncovered behavior and developmental effects of OME into the teen years. Overall, then, it may be that OME produces long-term effects in an idiosyncratic manner, impacting some children's development more strongly than that of others.

What remains uncontested is that large numbers of children are affected by OM and OME and they experience some difficulty hearing while they have the infection. From this perspective, the acoustic environment is of major importance for communication accessibility to all children, whether they are hard of hearing or typically hearing but occasionally affected by OM or OME [17]. Because speaking and listening are the primary modes of communication in teaching and learning and conversational discourse - at least in general educational settings - speech intelligibility is the major concern when considering room acoustics in childcare and school settings [18]. Overall, generally favourable listening conditions and one-to-one communication are characteristic of home settings and parent-child communication. By contrast, the group settings in which children often participate frequently have hostile acoustical conditions, whether at daycare, preschool, or elementary or secondary school. In fact, according to parent reports, the noise in classrooms contributes heavily to the social exclusion of children with hearing impairments [19]. Indeed, it is clear that optimal room acoustics are important for communication access for all students, regardless of hearing status.

Modalities of Communication

Among children with permanent hearing impairment, preference for a particular modality for communication can be shaped by both external and internal factors. In terms of external factors, differences in the relative availability of visual and auditory information may affect a child's use of vision and/or audition. On the one hand, typically developing hearing children, who have normal access to sound, show an early ability to process language using a simultaneous visual-auditory approach, whereby they can look at an object and hear spoken input about the object at the same time. In general, children who are able to access auditory information for communication tend to use an oral-aural approach that involves both vision and audition. Likewise, children who are hard of hearing tend to use a simultaneous visual-auditory approach to communication, at least to the extent that they primarily and effectively listen and speak. On the other hand, deaf children who either have not received amplification or have not derived benefit from it, tend to display a sequential visual processing approach to communication, in which they first look at an object and then look at their communication partner for visually available linguistic input about the object. In the case of deaf children who use sign language as their main means of communication, then, it is not so much their loss of hearing as it is their use of vision that defines their approach to interacting with the surrounding world. Individuals who are primarily visual processors of information tend to use an approach that maximizes visual input, such as some form of a natural sign language, Cued Speech, and/or speech reading. Finally, parental hearing status is strongly implicated in the choice of communication approach. Deaf and hard of hearing infants born to Deaf parents who are members of the Deaf community and who use sign language as their primary means of communication will learn that language from their first teachers, namely their parents.

Children with permanent hearing loss are also influenced by internal factors, such as neural plasticity. Sharma and her colleagues [20] found that the most sensitive period for central auditory development - the time when the central auditory pathways exhibit the most plasticity - is during the first 3 ½ years of life, and likely ends by age 7. The implication is that children with congenital deafness who receive cochlear implants before the age of 4 years, while their brains have the most ability to form connections for auditory processing, develop significantly better speech and language compared to children implanted later. Progressive hearing losses, that is, losses that progress from mild to more severe levels or from unilateral to bilateral, with a marked decline in functional auditory capabilities as the loss progresses, represent another internal factor that may influence choice of communication modality. In this instance, it seems reasonable for the child to experience the reduction of hearing as an emotionally significant loss, and hence it is also a challenge in terms of both emotional coping and possibly adjusting to reliance on other modalities for communication.

There may also be a shift in modality preferences across time and settings. For example, some children whose early preference was for visually-based information may derive substantial benefit from hearing aids or cochlear implants, and they may shift toward greater processing of information by audition. In addition, the environment can modulate the communication abilities of deaf or hard of hearing children; the noisier the environment, the less is the child's access to sound and the greater is his/her preference for the modality that provides ease of access to information (i.e., vision).It seems, then, that although children may have primary preferences for a specific modality of communication, they may also have secondary or temporary preferences, depending on personal, social and environmental factors.

Stages and Settings for Communication

The compromised ability to communicate with ease in a world in which the majority of persons can hear has significant consequences across the course of childhood, from infancy to the transition into young adulthood. During infancy, the impact of hearing loss strongly impacts family functioning. There are qualitative differences in the ways families experience the birth of a deaf or hard of hearing child, and, similarly, infants experience the environment around them in different ways depending on individual, family, and environmental factors. Early intervention, thus, may focus more on contextual factors, such as helping the parents to develop effective communication strategies with their child, rather than focusing solely on the infant.

During the preschool years, children move from parallel play to interaction with others. Near the end of the preschool years, hearing children typically develop the ability to interact with each other with a common purpose. It is critical for children to develop skills for entering into play with their peers, and in the preschool years much of this can be learned by watching. Increasingly, however, as children move into the school years, entry into group activities involves verbal skills. Hearing children learn these skills incidentally in large part by overhearing, whereas children with hearing impairments do not have easy access to incidental learning through audition, and their social skill development may be disrupted as a result. For example, some deaf and hard of hearing children in integrated schools have been found to start to display signs of social isolation when in the company of hearing peers at play time, but not when placed with their peers with hearing losses [12]. It may be, then, that it is not so much the case that some deaf and hard of hearing children do not develop social skills as it is that they develop a different, more visually-based set of social skills in comparison to their hearing peers.

There is a growing body of literature that underscores the unique challenges confronting adolescents with hearing losses as they struggle with their emerging sense of identity. For example, Israelite, Ower, and Goldstein [21] suggested that the experience of growing up in a world where others can hear contributes heavily to deaf or hard of hearing adolescents' identity construction. Some adolescents, who are functionally deaf in noisy environments but functionally hard of hearing in quiet settings, may feel that they are deaf or hearing, depending on the circumstances. This sense of being both deaf and hearing has also been described by some European adolescents who use cochlear implants and who describe themselves as deaf in some settings and at some times and as hearing in other situations [22]. This lack of clarity concerning identity may lead to a sense of not belonging fully in either group; an alternate explanation is that this dual identity may, in fact, be a sign of resilience if the individual can function comfortably in both groups. Warick [23], in a qualitative study of the experiences of hard of hearing post-secondary students, described these students as "visitors in the classroom," conveying a sense of their frustration in attempting to adapt and integrate into a world where the majority is hearing. Overall, then, it appears that hearing loss impacts social development pervasively across the span of development, but in different ways at different stages and in different settings.

Shifting Boundaries

Several new initiatives in research and practice, including early identification of hearing loss and early intervention, improvements in assistive listening and educational technology, and a variety of alterations in the social context, are having dramatic impacts on the lives of deaf and hard of hearing children and their families. However, it should be noted that these initiatives are largely restricted to economically developed, resource-rich nations. In the case of countries with developing economies, the current outlook for children with hearing losses is, unfortunately, bleak. It is difficult to ascertain the exact prevalence of childhood hearing loss within these countries, but Spencer and Marschark [3] have suggested that about twice as many children have hearing losses as are found in developed countries. Although the World Health Assembly [24] advocated a decade ago for the early identification of hearing loss for all infants and/or toddlers, the implementation of universal newborn hearing screening appears to be one clear demarcation between developed and developing nations.

The identification of hearing loss through universal newborn hearing screening conducted shortly after birth, followed by specialized early intervention, has swept through most western nations and is now the expected standard of care [24]. Many early hearing detection and intervention programmes follow the "1-3-6" model, where infants are screened by one month of age, identified by three months of age, and placed in early intervention by six months of age. Researchers have generally found very significant and positive developmental advantages for children following early diagnosis and intervention, compared to the sequelae for late-identified children across domains, including language [25]and the development of play [26].

It should be stressed that the positive outcomes following newborn hearing screening are a result of the partnership of early identification and effective early intervention. Although research on programme efficacy is ongoing, several characteristics of effective early intervention programmes for deaf and hard of hearing children and their families have consistently emerged, including the use of a family-centered approach, in which the family is the driving force behind all decisions, choices, and practices. However, a note of caution should be sounded: although early identification, early intervention, and early access to amplification have collectively been found to result in improved performance for infants in many broad aspects of language development [27], they do not eliminate all complexities that even a mild hearing loss may pose to the development of speech skills. The outcomes for deaf and hard-of-hearing children have improved dramatically, but there is still a strong, pressing, and continued need for specialized intervention.

Within the past decade, technological advances, such as cochlear implants and digital hearing aids, have provided children better access to meaningful sound at earlier stages of development than previously witnessed. The possibility - and frequent practice in western countries - of early identification and early amplification for deaf infants, often followed by early cochlear implantation (usually at around one year of age) for eligible deaf children, have contributed to a blurring of the conventional distinction between "deaf" and "hard of hearing" among many slightly older children. Consistent with this, Geers [28] reported that children with cochlear implants who were placed in oral programmes showed a more rapid average rate of language development and speech skill development than did their peers who used hearing aids. Nevertheless, many researchers have found that the average language abilities of implanted children are still below those of hearing peers [29,30]. Importantly, better hearing prior to implantation has been shown to be one key factor associated with better language outcomes [31].

There have also been important changes to the environment - both physical and social - surrounding children with hearing impairment, at least in developed countries. For example, there is increasing recognition of the important role of favorable classroom acoustics for all children, not just for children with hearing losses, and a corresponding press for the implementation of acoustical standards in school building codes. In this connection, the American National Standard Institute has set forth standards for classroom acoustics to be implemented in new or retrofitted schools [32]. Yet another contextual change concerns the impact of information technology, including the Internet and handheld communication devices, in providing timely visual access to information for deaf and hard of hearing people. Socially, the shift in societal attitudes toward persons with disabilities affects children with hearing impairment in ways that are difficult to quantify. Overall, it appears that children with hearing impairment have greater access to reciprocal communication with those who surround them -deaf, hearing, and hard of hearing - than ever before, and their increased participation in everyday life may help shape societal attitudes in a positive manner that reflects their abilities and potential. The enduring challenge is to work toward the provision of resources, services, and expertise that will empower children and youth with hearing losses in developing countries as well.

Adulthood

Factors Affecting Access to Communication and the Preservation of Communicative Competence

Children who have been affected by hearing loss during development will continue to experience various consequences of hearing loss throughout their lives. For some individuals, these consequences may be of minimal importance, whereas for others the consequences may be devastating. Some children with permanent hearing loss who have received special education or habilitation may become successful adults. Nevertheless, even those with mild hearing impairment may not achieve the same level of education as peers with normal hearing, in turn limiting their options for further education and choices of occupation [33].Even children who experienced temporary hearing loss due to conditions such as otitis media early in life may experience problems in central auditory processing throughout their lives, making them more susceptible as adults to the adverse effects of noise in communication situations [34]. Moreover, hearing loss may be an infrequently recognized health condition in some of the most vulnerable members of society. Some children who have more compromised social and cognitive development may enter the mental health and/or justice systems as adults; conversely, the segment of the population in the mental health and/or justice systems may be at greater risk for acquiring hearing loss than those in the general population because they often have a history of noise exposure or substance abuse [35,36]. In general, however, adults who grew up with hearing impairment will have incorporated it into their identities over the course of development. In contrast, those who acquire hearing loss or experience a progression of hearing loss as adults will need to re-define themselves as they adjust to hearing loss as a chronic disability.

There is considerable heterogeneity in when and how hearing loss affects adults, but in contrast to the small minority of children who have permanent hearing impairment, the majority of adults have impaired hearing by the time they reach the age of 75 years. The strong association between hearing loss and aging that prevails in society is not surprising given that the prevalence and severity of hearing loss increases markedly with age, starting in the fourth decade. For example, a recent UK study found that the prevalence of functionally significant hearing loss for which intervention is typically beneficial (>35 dB HL average of pure-tone thresholds at .5, 1, 2, and 4 kHz) increased from about 1/5 in the group aged 65 to 74 years old to 3/5 in the group aged 75 to 84 years and then to 9/10 in the group aged 85 years or older [37]. Importantly, in the next decade the proportion of the population over the age of 65 will be higher than ever before as the baby boom generation born following World War II retires from the workforce.

Insofar as peers are more likely to experience similar problems, hearing loss may be considered to be 'normal' for older adults even it is not 'normal' for adults in younger age groups. Nevertheless, it is well known that there can be a lag of a decade or more in seeking professional help for problems in hearing. Despite engineering advances, hearing aids are still not a perfect solution for restoring lost auditory abilities, and many adults who are considered to be candidates for them based on audiometric criteria still do not wear hearing aids. A relatively stable finding over several decades has been that amongst the non-technological reasons that hearing aids have not been used sooner or to their full potential are psychosocial factors such as lack of social support, the failure of the individual to come to terms with hearing loss, and/or perceptions of stigma associated with hearing aids [38].

As discussed in other chapters, adult onset hearing loss may occur due to diseases, genetic or environmental factors. Many of the perceptual consequences of hearing loss which affect an individual's ability to perform tasks or engage in activities are common to many aetiologies, but some depend on the site and extent of damage to the auditory system. Age-related hearing loss may result in damage to multiple structures in the peripheral and central auditory systems. The hallmark of presbycusis, the elevation of high-frequency audiometric thresholds, can result from damage to the cochlear outer hair cells (OHC) from noise or ototoxic drugs. Current knowledge of OHC pathology, its effects on perception, and many related issues pertaining to intervention can be generalized across the adult age range. However, the peripheral and central auditory systems of older adults may also be damaged in ways that are not typical in younger adults. It is important to understand the age-specific aspects of auditory function if progress is to be made in helping older listeners prevent and overcome their unique difficulties [39]. For example, in older adults, less precipitous hhigh-frequency loss may result from a decrease in the endocochlear potentialas a result of damage to the striavascularis [40]. In addition, neural degeneration may occur independently or with cochlear damage, sometimes with much less change in the audiogram [41], and it is possible that permanent neural damage may be the consequence of temporary noise-induced loss [42]. There is growing interest in finding better clinical tests to differentiate sub-types of presbycusis because determining the specific pathology may clarify, at least to some extent, why there is such heterogeneity in the ability of older adults to perceive speech in noise and communicate in complex listening situations.

Clearly, there are the direct effects of audiometric loss on communication, but even older adults who have nearly normal audiograms can experience significant communication problems in many everyday situations. As early as the fourth decade of life, difficulties are first noticed in challenging listening environments such as those encountered at work, at home, and in public places where there is noise or groups engage in multiple simultaneous activities.Similarly, in laboratory experiments they exhibit poorer performance on a range of psychoacoustic measures of supra-threshold processing and problems understanding speech in noise [40]. A general finding is that older adults with audiometric thresholds within normal clinical limits below 4 kHz need about a 3 to 4 dB better signal-to-noise ratio (SNR) to match the performance of younger adults. One possible explanation is that neural degeneration manifests as problems in coding the temporal properties of sound, thereby compromising capacities such as the segregation of voices in a multi-talker situation.

Cognitive demands may also contribute to the listening problems of older adults when there are multiple talkers or when attention may need to be divided between simultaneous tasks such as conversing while driving a car [40]. Furthermore, the extra effort required to concentrate when following speech in noise or during multi-tasking consumes cognitive resources, with the result being that even if words are correctly recognized they may not be stored in memory or understood as well as if they had been heard in quiet. Thus, age-related hearing problems can undermine cognitive processing and exacerbate apparent cognitive decline in memory and comprehension. Listeners experience stress and fatigue when they must sustain mental effort to listen. Conversely, as illustrated in Figure 4.1, it is possible that individuals with better cognitive abilities will cope better because they are able to use stored knowledge and contextual information to greater advantage to compensate for reduced auditory abilities [43]. Auditory aging, whether or not there are clinically significant changes in the audiogram, interacts with cognitive aging as older adults meet the challenges of everyday life. These links between auditory and cognitive processing observed in healthy aging are of even greater importance when older adults must contend with hearing loss in combination with cognitive impairment (see below).

Ongoing frustrations and failures when listening may prompt older adults to opt out of social interactions that demand too much sustained mental effort. There are well-known effects of hearing loss on quality of life for a large segment of the aging adult population.

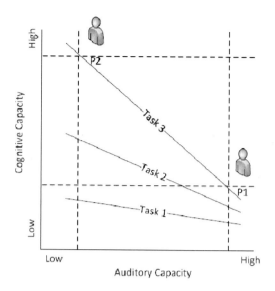

Figure 4.1. Tasks 1, 2 and 3 differ in difficulty and the need for auditory and cognitive capacities. Task 1 depends mostly on auditory capacity (e.g., detecting a sound), whereas task 2 depends more on cognitive capacity (e.g., comprehending a lecture), and task 3 depends even more on cognitive capacity (e.g., dividing attention during group conversation). Success corresponds to the area above the respective lines for each task. P1 is a person with normal hearing and slightly below average cognitive capacity who has sufficient combined capacities to be able to succeed on all three tasks. P2 is a person with hearing loss and high cognitive capacity who is able to succeed on all three tasks by using cognitive capacity (e.g., world and linguistic knowledge) to help compensate for deficits in auditory processing.

In terms of total disability-adjusted life-years (DALYs; a unit used by the WHO to measure the years of healthy life lost due to premature mortality and years lived with disability), adult-onset hearing loss ranked 15th in the world in terms of the global disease burden in 2002, and if only years lived with disability were assessed then hearing loss ranked second after depression [44]. Furthermore, communication has been identified as a key factor in population health and it has been related to longevity and years lived without disability [45].

There are indirect consequences of hearing loss on the older individual and society because age-related declines in hearing also interact with other age-related changes in health conditions. Population studies reveal dramatic increases with age in the prevalence of many disorders (hearing, vision, speech, language, cognition, emotion) that affect communication and social interaction. As well, there are increases in the prevalence of impairments in balance, mobility, touch, and dexterity that may increase barriers to communication. For example, reduced manual dexterity or tactile sensation may reduce ability to use some communication technologies such as small hearing aids. Multi-tasking may be too demanding; an example is a person is trying to listen while moving with the assistance of a walker or cane. Opportunities for social interaction may also be constrained by non-auditory health conditions; for example, those in wheelchairs may not be able to position themselves freely to optimize communication because seating locations are designated and some venues may not be accessible at all if the only entrance is by stairs. Thus, hearing problems may magnify the activity limitations and participation restrictions of older adults when combined with other health problems. Conversely, by preserving hearing abilities, some functional declines associated with other health problems may be offset. Ultimately, hearing may even be a critical factor in enabling older adults to maintain independent living, with associated cost savings for the health care system if the need for residential care is averted.

While the perceptual consequences of hearing loss may vary depending on how much and what type of hearing loss interferes with the ability to communicate, the emotional and social consequences depend more on personal and environmental factors than on the type and degree of hearing loss. Whether an adult discloses or attempts to conceal hearing loss, hearing-related communication problems may be compounded by negative stereotyping. As shown in Figure 4.2, there are bi-directional interactions between hearing loss and socio-emotional factors. Hearing problems can undermine social and emotional well-being with cascading negative effects on relationships and health in general. Conversely, those with higher levels of social support and emotional well-being may cope better as they adjust to living with a hearing loss and/or other health problems that combine to affect communication and participation.

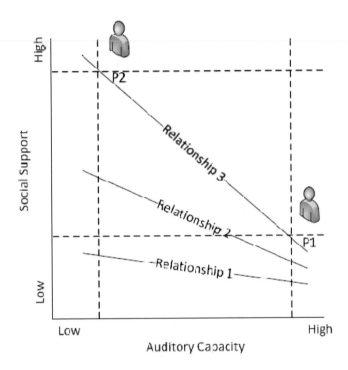

Figure 4.2. Relationships 1, 2 and 3 differ in their significance to the individual and the extent to which they rely on auditory communication and can be modulated by social support. Relationship 1 depends mostly on auditory capacity (e.g., a relationship between a receptionist and customers), whereas relationship 2 can be modulated to a greater extent by social support (e.g., a relationship between a person and friends belonging to the same bowling club), and relationship 3 can be modulated even more by social support (e.g., a family relationship between an adult son and his elderly mother with dementia). Success corresponds to the area above the respective lines for each relationship. P1 is a person with normal hearing and slightly below average social support who has sufficient combined capacities to be able to succeed in all three relationships. P2 is a person with hearing loss and high social support who is able to succeed in all three relationships because social support (e.g., help of a spouse) is available to help compensate for auditory deficits.

While it is obvious that parents play a central role in the life of a child who has a hearing loss, it may be less obvious how an adult's experiences of hearing loss affect and are affected by relationships with family members, including the spouse, children and grandchildren. Intergenerational communication may be especially challenging for people with hearing loss because use of contextual support may be less effective when a topic or terms are highly familiar to one generation but virtually unknown to another. In general, family solidarity turns the issues of the individual into family issues [46]. It is well-known that prompting by family members is a frequent predisposing factor that triggers action-taking for hearing loss. More importantly, the participation of family members in rehabilitation may be necessary to address the burden that hearing loss places on them. They may experience stress, anxiety, irritation, and frustration as they adjust their own lives in the process of understanding and accommodating the needs of the person who has hearing impairment [47]. The support of family members may be critical in helping the person who is hard of hearing to establish successful coping and adhere to treatments [1]. As reported by Kramer and colleagues, enablement in the workplace may also depend critically on the participation of others such as managers and co-workers in the rehabilitative process [1,43]. The support of significant others will be particularly important if the process of adjustment must be accelerated when hearing loss is sudden or if it must be prolonged because hearing loss is progressive.

In public situations, the adult with hearing loss will need to interact with strangers and these social interactions are likely to be mediated by stereotypes. Stigmatization may result from negative stereotypes. Perceptions of stigmatization fuel the denial of hearing problems and non-adherence to rehabilitative treatments [48]. Moreover, stigma due to hearing loss is entangled with ageism. Ageism in interactions, including interactions with health care providers, may reinforce feelings of incompetence and accelerate loss of communication competence [49]. In addition, stunning findings from social psychology have shown that a wide range of measures, including hearing thresholds [50]can be affected by age-related stereotypes. Thus, stereotypes can be applied negatively not only by non-members of a stereotype-group, but also by group members who may suffer from self-stereotyping. "Stereotype threat" refers to the risk of confirming a negative stereotype of a group with which one identifies [51].Another potentially important psychosocial factor is self-efficacy, or the confidence a person has in domain-specific abilities. Self-efficacy may influence performance in daily conversation, with the relevant domains being speech perception and language comprehension abilities. Self-efficacy has been shown to play an important role in the successful management of numerous health conditions; however, research directly focusing on self-efficacy related to listening abilities and hearing aid use has only recently begun to emerge [52,53].

As well as the social context, the acoustics and lighting characteristics of the physical environments in which adults communicate are tremendously important. Many adults with acquired hearing loss experience relatively little difficulty in ideal quiet listening conditions, whereas they find noisy situations to be challenging. Lighting is also important because visual cues are often useful to supplement auditory speech cues and to guide attention to objects in the environment. However, lighting and visual displays must also be designed taking into account the co-existence of age-related hearing and vision loss. Dual sensory losses may seriously limit the participation of those who also have mobility disabilities because cues enabling navigation are reduced and safety is compromised. Improvements in accessible design should be facilitated by the introduction of recent standards for accessibility related to impairments in both modalities [54].

Modalities of Communication

Once adulthood is reached, preferences for modalities of communication are usually well established, but as listening in noise becomes more challenging for older adults, they may rely increasingly on visual cues, including visual speech cues. Insofar as vision augments hearing in everyday bimodal communication, dual sensory loss will reduce the opportunities of an older adult to compensate by using the other modality. Indeed, Erber has suggested that both vision and hearing should be considered in determining hearing aid candidacy because improving hearing will be more important for those who have vision problems but they may have difficulty handling a small device if they cannot see it well [55].

As outlined previously in the section on childhood hearing loss, brain organization will depend on the extent to which the auditory and visual modalities are engaged by the person in performing regular tasks, including interpersonal communication and social interaction. It is now realized that the brain continues to be plastic into adulthood, and there is mounting evidence of brain re-organization associated with healthy aging, including reorganization related to sensory decline. The growing use of functional neuro-imaging has resulted in new knowledge concerning how networks in the brains of living humans serve complex high-level behaviours including perception, memory, attention, and language. Specifically, these methods have been used to investigate the auditory processing of distorted speech in adverse conditions by younger and older adults[56]. Event-related potential testing has also been used to investigate more time-sensitive aspects of brain activity in younger and older listeners [40].

Studies of age-related changes have repeatedly pointed to reduced symmetry in the activation of prefrontal cortex in older adults. When young and older adults perform tasks, including perceptual tasks, at the same level of proficiency, the general pattern is that older adults use more brain regions, including regions of both hemispheres. This functional reorganization, or plasticity, of the brain might result from dedifferentiation of brain function as a consequence of difficulty in activating specialized neural circuits, or it might result from compensatory adaptation to offset age-related neuro-cognitive declines; there is also evidence of a shift in the concentration of activity from posterior to anterior brain regions which is hypothesized to be associated with compensatory use of executive cognitive functions, memory and semantic processing to offset declines in sensory information processing [57]. Recent research on age-related changes in auditory processing of speech in noise is consistent with this general pattern of age-related brain reorganization [56].

The age-related shift in brain activity with reduced posterior activation and increased anterior activation may be a consequence of diminished sensory functioning in old age. Hearing declines with age, but there are also age-related declines in vision. Large-scale studies in the USA (Beaver Dam) and Australia (Blue Mountains) found that visual loss (defined as loss greater than 20/40 in the better eye) affected up to 1/20 in the age group 65 to 74 years old, increasing to up to 1/5 in the age group 75 to 84 years old, with about a quarter of the older group with vision loss having a moderate or severe degree of loss and losses that were more often due to pathologies such as macular degeneration that are not correctable with lenses [58, 59].Furthermore, compared to younger adults with vision loss, older adults have greater needs for assistance in activities of daily living and over 90% of seniors with vision loss require an aid or device; however, while the needs of about 10% of seniors remain unmet, the needs of over 20% of middle-aged people with dual sensory loss remain unmet [60]. By comparison, it has been estimated that over 2/3 of those with hearing loss who might benefit from a hearing aid have unmet needs [38].

The reduced abilities of older adults with dual sensory loss to use one modality to compensate for the other can also be complicated by disorders affecting the speech and language abilities of either those who have dual sensory loss or their communication partners. The effects of aphasia and dementia on communication are well known, but voice (and swallowing) problems are also common and affect quality of life because they reduce ability to talk and be understood as well as one's desire to communicate at all. For example, some disorders common in older people (e.g., Parkinson's) result in reduced motor speech abilities that reduce the production of auditory and visual cues for speech and emotion.

Cognitive and psychological disorders can also be exacerbated by or cause communication problems in older adults. In the UK, mood disorders such as depression were reported for 1/5 community living adults aged 65 to 74 years, increasing to over 1/4 for those aged 75 to 84 years, and to over 1/3 for those in the group aged 85+ years. A Canadian study found cognitive impairments in almost 1/6 of adults aged 75 to 84 years, almost 1/4 of those aged 85 to 89 years, over 1/3 of those aged 90 to 94 years, and over 1/2 of those aged 95+ years [61].Much more needs to be understood about how these psychological disorders interact with hearing loss (and also tinnitus) over the adult lifespan so that both better prevention and more appropriate intervention can be undertaken [1]. As summarized in a review by Pichora-Fuller in a collection of papers edited by Hickson, it is of great concern that the degree of dementia is significantly over-estimated in about 1/3 of cases if cognitive tests are conducted without versus with hearing aids, that hearing loss is found in up to 9/10 cases with dementia, and that hearing loss is more prevalent in those with dementia than in controls [43]. Even more striking findings are that hearing loss [62] and auditory speech processing problems [63] are predictive of future manifestation of dementia. Dual sensory loss is associated with even greater odds for cognitive decline and for functional decline on everyday activities over a four-year period [64]. Thus, multiple impairments can combine with hearing loss to challenge older communicators and their communication partners, including family, caregivers, and health professionals. Note that research is only just beginning to examine aging and related co-morbidities such as cognitive decline in persons whose primary language is sign language [65], and little is known about the effects of co-morbidities on older adults who use cochlear implants. Interestingly, research suggests that fluent bilinguals may be less susceptible to cognitive decline because using multiple languages enhances their cognitive executive functions [66] so it may turn out that there are similar benefits for those who are bilingual in spoken and signed languages. Clearly, a more integrated approach to assessment and management of older adults is required and hearing health professionals must play a more active role in geriatric health care teams.

Stages and Settings for Communication

The consequences of hearing loss to individuals vary across the lifespan because the contexts for communication vary with changing social goals and communication demands at different stages of adult development. Furthermore, rapid innovations in communication and information technologies are altering the ways in which adults of every age communicate in a wide range of contexts for a wide range of purposes (work, banking, shopping, entertainment, education, health care delivery, etc.). The mainstream adoption of these new technologies in society may exclude or present obstacles to older adults who must learn new ways of communicating, but they may also enhance or provide 'normal 'forms of visual or multi-modal communication (e.g., text messaging or email) or machine-mediated communication (e.g., speech-to-text converters) that could increase the inclusion of people with hearing loss who have difficulty with more conventional voice-based communication technologies (e.g., telephone) or face-to-face communication. These new technologies have expanded opportunities for social interaction through communication that can be asynchronous and independent of distance. Although younger generations grew up with the Internet, currently its use is increasing most rapidly amongst older adults. Intergenerational family communication online is becoming more and more common as grandparents learn to text to communicate with their adult children and grandchildren. Currently, over half of those aged 65 years old in the United States use the Internet [67].

Such 'virtual' settings for communication based on the Internet or mobile phones are also being developed for health promotion purposes and even to monitor those with chronic health conditions remotely in their homes without requiring attendance at clinics. In hearing health care, mobile devices can now be used to download applications for use by individuals to screen their own hearing, measure ambient noise levels, or obtain information about the availability of nearby hearing health care services. The relationship between people with hearing impairment and their hearing health care providers will continue to evolve with the introduction of follow- up and counselling appointments conducted by Internet, as well as the use of technology to enable a person to attach his/her hearing aid to a personal computer by connections such as USB so that it can be checked and adjusted remotely.

Working-aged adults may be affected by hearing loss in their occupational roles as well as in family roles such as being a spouse, parent or a caregiver for elderly parents. In the workplace, the hazards of noise exposure continue to affect industrial workers who must adopt behaviours such as using hearing protective equipment to prevent hearing loss. In addition, in the new knowledge economy of the information age in society, the increased importance of communication for workers has raised new challenges in the workplace for professionals and office workers who have hearing impairment. Especially in developing countries, the ubiquitous use of cell phones brings new opportunities for auditory and visual communication to those who did not previously have access to communication and information technologies. Furthermore, with the aging of the population, the age of the workforce now spans a wider range because mandatory retirement no longer exists in many jurisdictions. Thus, hearing in the workplace is an issue around the globe whether the workplace is a noisy factory or a quiet board room and whether the person has congenital deafness or presbycusis.

Workers with hearing loss are more likely than their counterparts with good hearing to have a low income or be underemployed [1].As reported by Kramer and colleagues, workers with hearing loss are more likely to take sick leave due to stress-related complaints such as fatigue, strain and burnout, although the days taken for sick leave due to other factors such as colds and flu were similar to the days taken by those with good hearing [43]. In general, the needs of workers with hearing loss are poorly understood by co-workers and management, and hearing loss in workers is associated with embarrassment, fear, distress, anxiety, feeling of loss of control, lack of energy, fatigue, and need for recovery after work [43].

Even outside of the workplace, hearing-related stress at work also has a negative effect on the self-image of workers and on their relationships with others, especially their spouses [1].Furthermore, the effects of hearing loss on working-aged adults with progressive losses may be devastating for a variety of reasons: adjustment at an earlier age may disrupt the realization of vocational ambitions and undermine the development of romantic and family roles, ongoing re-adjusting to increasing amounts of hearing loss may require continual learning of new ways of coping, and it may be difficult to adjust rapidly if the onset or progression of the loss is sudden. Progressive losses range from conductive losses such as otosclerosis that may be remediated by surgery or amplification, to sudden sensorineural hearing loss that may be remediated by cochlear implant, to even more complicated cases such as Usher Syndrome in which hearing, vision and vestibular losses co-occur and increase such that even those who use sign language may experience reduced communication over the course of adult development.

The ICF framework has been used to assess functioning in the workplace as an interaction between a worker's hearing impairment and contextual environmental and personal factors. Adopting an ecological approach that considers the needs of the person in context, the Vocational Enablement Protocol, a rehabilitation programme for workers with hearing loss employed in a wide range of job settings (most not requiring the use of ear protection) was developed and implemented [43]. As shown in Table 4.2, in keeping with an ecological approach, solutions could be sought through a combination of behaviour change, the use of technology, and/or environmental modification. These solutions could be implemented by one or more parties, including the person with hearing impairment, managers, co-workers, or various consulting professionals. Common recommendations for workers involved the use of hearing aids and/or assistive devices, work-related accommodations such as re-delegation of assignments, re-structuring of schedules and environmental modifications to reduce noise and distraction, counselling and communication training of the worker and significant others (including co-workers), and. for a few, vocational retraining or termination of employment [43].

Table 4.2. Example of how an ecological approach could provide a multi-component solution implemented by a worker with hearing loss and/or other parties

Component of Solution	Responsible Party	Example
Behaviour change	Manager	Revise schedule so meetings are booked in the morning when the worker with hearing loss is not fatigued
Technology	Worker with hearing loss	Use personal hearing aid during team meetings
Social environment modification	Co-workers	Circulate reports the day before the team meetings so material can be reviewed in advance
Physical environment modification	Consulting professionals	In the board room, improve acoustics by reducing ventilation noise and install and use a secure infra-red room system for use during meetings

This setting-specific delivery of rehabilitation effectively strives to make the workplace accessible to workers with hearing loss. Legislation to ensure accessibility for people with disabilities will put increasing pressure on hearing health care professionals to provide more such services outside of the four walls of the traditional clinical setting.

Given the importance of communication in the workplace today, hearing loss is likely becoming a greater factor influencing major decisions such as whether to retire early or extend work beyond the typical retirement age [1]. Ageism complicates decisions to seek help or take action by late-middle aged adults who have become aware of hearing problems because wearing a hearing aid may be seen as a marker for aging. The association between aging and hearing loss may be underscored when there is a connection between hearing loss and the decision to retire. Having made the decision to retire, hearing loss may influence the extent to which adults are able to adjust to life as a retired person, including establishing new social relationships and/or maintaining former relations when workers leave the workforce. More research concerning the relationship between hearing loss and adjustment to retirement is needed, especially because hearing loss is well-known to put older adults at risk for social isolation, which in turn may accelerate declines in other aspects of physical and mental health.

Hearing loss can compromise how well a person performs in basic activities of daily living (e.g., shopping) and discretionary social activities (e.g., socializing with friends). Furthermore, hearing loss may mask or exaggerate other health problems such as cognitive impairment because communication problems undermine accurate diagnosis and treatment. Loss of hearing could even jeopardize independence and ability to live alone and/or it could limit the options that might otherwise be available to seniors receiving health-related services provided in the home, day programmes or residential care facilities. Assessments of a person's competence to make decisions about personal care or finances may also be complicated by communication problems. Ultimately, even the delivery of palliative care can be undermined when the person who is dying cannot hear loved ones and/or when loved ones cannot hear the final words of the person who is dying.

The WHO ICF has inspired research to develop and evaluate many excellent programmes for older adults with hearing loss. A health promotion approach has been used to develop programmes to encourage community-living older adults to seek and take action for hearing-related problems (e.g., the "Keep on Talking" [68] and the "Active Communication Education" (ACE) programmes [69]). The "Hard of Hearing Club, "established as a hospital-based out-patient rehabilitation programme, focuses on social support to mitigate the consequences of social isolation in older adults [43]. Other programmes have used peer support to provide community-based services for older adults with hearing loss [70]. For adults living in residential care settings, an ecological approach guided the development of a programme to enhance accessibility by combining the use of technologies, environmental modifications, and behaviour change on the part of residents and staff [71]. The use of hearing aids [72] and environmental modifications such as reducing distracting sounds [73] have also been shown to reduce problem behaviours such as wandering in older adults with dementia. Despite the documented success of these programmes, they have not been widely adopted in regular practice, and other health care professionals who are not experts in hearing are usually unaware of the value of these interventions. Furthermore, although there are the clear connections between hearing loss and co-morbid health conditions, there is virtually no intervention research regarding the possible benefits of hearing rehabilitation in terms interactions with outcomes of treatments for other chronic disorders, the most obvious one being cognitive impairment.

Shifting Boundaries

Over the last two decades there have been parallel advances in our understanding of auditory aging as well as many other aspects of sensory and cognitive aging and how these issues are intertwined. In concert with the broader shift to health promotion and prevention, there has been a shift towards earlier identification of hearing loss in adults coupled with the design of programmes to promote earlier help-seeking and action-taking. The scope of interventions has also expanded by augmenting the provision of hearing aids with other solutions involving behaviour change on the part of the person with hearing loss, as well as significant others, and greater awareness of how to make communication environments more accessible. The shift has moved to more customization and bundling of solutions involving the three components: behaviour change, use of technology and environmental adaptation. These shifts go beyond the walls of hearing clinics, and the inclusion of other professionals and the public in the enterprise of accessibility is buoyed by more general attitudinal shifts in society and culture.

Traditionally, hearing health care professionals, who were sometimes focused more on the hearing loss than the person, designed generic intervention programmes for adults that often failed to appreciate how to tailor interventions to foster the psychosocial adjustment of the individual. Recent approaches to rehabilitation are more tailored to individuals and their social and physical context. An important shift has been to try to understand better how to facilitate behaviour change. For example, the need to incorporate stigma into audio logical assessment and intervention has been recognized. There is no doubt that auditory and psychosocial factors are related, but the nature of the relationship needs to be understood more fully to guide the design of new rehabilitative practices. Recent advances in the development of tools to measure and therapies to address psychological and social factors such as self-efficacy [74] may offer new ways to facilitate help-seeking and prevent relapse after treatment by keeping hearing aids on ears and out of drawers.

The shift to more customization is also reflected in trends in technology design. Conventional hearing technologies for adults were designed and fit using algorithms guided mostly by the audiogram but not other aspects of auditory or cognitive processing or by considerations of the auditory ecology of the person. Better differentiation of sub-types of presbycusis has implications for the realization of interventions ranging from the possibility of cell preservation or regeneration in the striavascularis to more sophisticated hearing aids incorporating signal processing and computational algorithms to compensate for reductions in central auditory and cognitive processing [39,40,75].

Although legislation concerning the rights and required accommodations for people with disabilities has been implemented over the last two or three decades in many countries, guidelines pertaining to hearing loss have been more difficult to specify than guidelines for other disabilities, likely because there are not easy generic solutions and architects are not adequately trained to build environments for people with sensory losses. To improve accessibility for people with sensory loss it is not so obvious how to achieve the equivalents to architectural requirements such as ramps or technological requirements such as elevators that provide obvious solutions for those who use wheelchairs. The issues of people who are hard of hearing have also been largely overlooked in emerging concerns about the need to create more accessible homes for older adults. Although there has been much work on preventing noise-induced hearing loss in the workplace, relatively little progress has been made regarding accommodation for workers who are hard of hearing in workplaces where noise is not a hazard. On a positive note, recent programmes illustrate how it is possible to implement interventions tailored to the individual needs of workers [1], and standards have been released recently [54]for acoustics and lighting to meet the communication needs of adults.

By striving for accessibility, such comprehensive approaches could greatly help in restoring the fit between the person with hearing loss and the social and physical context. The consequences of hearing loss to the individual and society should be reduced as this fit is improved. Furthermore, the increased mental effort faced by adults with hearing loss in everyday challenging listening conditions should be reduced, in turn reducing the risk that these individuals will opt to cope with hearing loss by withdrawing from social interaction. Rather, we hope that they will ultimately improve their ongoing participation in active, healthy lifestyles.

Conclusion

Across the entire lifespan, hearing impairment can have significant consequences for individuals, their family, peers, co-workers, and those with whom they interact on a wide range of professional and social relationships. Although there are widely recognized consequences of hearing loss to many aspects of child development, development continues throughout adulthood and hearing loss may pose challenges in different ways at different points in time and in different contexts. Hearing health care is evolving in harmony with more general trends in education, health care and in society more generally. Accordingly, there is an increasing awareness of how well-being must be understood in terms of the connection between biological and psychosocial factors as they are influenced by social and physical contexts. Technological change has opened new vistas for researchers, clinicians and people with hearing impairment. Recent technological innovations now allow us to understand better the multi-factorial interactions in brain networks during complex behaviors such as communication, how to assess hearing loss earlier and with more specific measures, and how to design better signal processing that is compatible with the explosion in use of information and communication technology in society. There is no doubt that future advances in hearing health care will only take us further in these directions so that the all too often negative consequences of hearing loss to the individual and society can be surmounted.

References

[1]   Stephens, D. and Kramer, S.E. (2010). *Living with hearing difficulties: The process of enablement.*Chichester, UK: Wiley-Blackwell.

[2]   World Health Organization (2001).International Classification of Functioning, Disability and Health (ICF). Geneva: World Health Organization.

[3]   Spencer, P.E. and Marschark, M. (2010). *Evidence-based practice in educating deaf and hard-of-hearing students*. New York: Oxford University Press.

[4]   Blair, J., Peterson, M. E., Viehweg, S. H. (1985).The effects of mild sensorineural hearing loss on academic performance of young school-age children.*Volta Review, 93,* 87-93.

[5]   Lieu, J. E. (2004). Speech-language and educational consequences of unilateral hearing loss in children.*Archives of Otolaryngology – Head and Neck Surgery, 130,* 524-530.

[6]   Gallaudet Research Institute. (2011). *Regional and National Summary Report of Data from the 2009-10 Annual Survey of Deaf and Hard of Hearing Children and Youth.*Washington, DC: GRI, Gallaudet University.

[7]   Mitchell, R. and Karchmer, M. (2004). Chasing the mythical ten per cent: Parental hearing status of deaf and hard of hearing students in the United States. *Sign Language Studies, 4,* 138-163.

[8]   Meadow-Orlans, K., Spencer, P., Koester, L. (2004.).*The world of deaf infants: A longitudinal study.* New York: Oxford University Press.

[9]   Schein, J. D. (1989). *At home among strangers.* Washington, DC: Gallaudet University Press.

[10]   Greenberg, M. and Kusché, C. (1989).Cognitive, personal and social development of deaf children and adolescents. In: M.C. Wang, M.C. Reynolds and H.J. Walberg (Eds.), *Handbook of Special Education: Research and practice* (Vol. 1, pp. 95-129). Oxford: Pergamon Press.

[11]   Moores, D. (2001). *Educating the deaf* (5th ed.). Boston, MA: Houghton-Mifflin Company.

[12]   Brunnberg, E. (2005). The school playground as a meeting place for hard of hearing children. *Scandinavian Journal of Disability Research, 7,* 73-90.

[13]   Higson, J.and Haggard, M. (2005). Parent versus professional views of the developmental impact of a multi-faceted condition at school age: Otitis media with effusion ("glue ear"). *British Journal of Educational Psychology, 75,* 623-643.

[14]   Roberts, J.E., Rosenfeld, R.M., Zeisel, S.A. (2004). Otitis media and speech and language: A meta-analysis of prospective studies. *Pediatrics, 113,* E238-E248.

[15]   Roberts, J.E., Burchinal, M.R., Zeisel, S.A. (2002). Otitis media in early childhood in relation to children's school-age language and academic skills.*Pediatrics, 110,* 696-706.

[16]   Bennett, K.E., Haggard, M.P., Silva, P.A., Stewart, I.A. (2001).Behaviour and developmental effects of otitis media with effusion into the teens.*Archives of Disease in Childhood, 85,* 91-95.

[17]   McKellin, W.H., Shahin, K., Hodgson, M., Jamieson, J., Pichora-Fuller, K. (2007).Pragmatics of conversation and communication in noisy settings.*Journal of Pragmatics, 39,* 2159-2184.

[18]   Picard, M. and Bradley, J.S. (2001). Revisiting speech interference in classrooms. *Audiology, 40,* 221-244.

[19]   Jamieson, J.R., Zaidman-Zait, A., Poon, B.T. (2011). Family support needs as perceived by parents of preadolescents and adolescents who are deaf or hard of hearing. *Deafness & Education International, 13,* 110-130.

[20]   Sharma, A., Dorman, M.F.,Spahr, A.J. (2002). A sensitive period for the development of the central auditory system in children with cochlear implants: Implications for age of implantation. *Ear and Hearing, 23,* 532-539.

[21] Israelite, N., Ower, J., Goldstein, G. (2002). Hard-of-hearing adolescents and identity construction: Influences of school experiences, peers, and teachers. *Journal of Deaf Studies and Deaf Education*, 7, 134-148.

[22] Wheeler, A., Archbold, S., Gregory, S., Skipp A. (2007). Cochlear implants: The young people's perspective. *Journal of Deaf Studies and Deaf Education*, 12, 303–316.

[23] Warick, R. (2004). Visitors in the classroom: The academic experiences of students who are hard of hearing (pp. 108-137). In: L. Andres and F. Finlay (Eds.). *Student affairs: Experiencing higher education*. Vancouver BC:University of British Columbia Press.

[24] World Health Organization. (2001). *Guidelines for hearing aids and services for developing countries*. Geneva: World Health Organization.

[25] Yoshinaga-Itano, C., Sedey, A.L., Coulter, B.A., Mehl, A.L. (1998).Language of early- and later-identified children with hearing loss.*Pediatrics*, 102, 1168-1171.

[26] Yoshinaga-Itano, C., Snyder, L., Day, D. (1998).The relationship of language and symbolic play in children with hearing loss.*The Volta Review*, 100, 135-164.

[27] Moeller, M.P. (2000).Early intervention and language development in children who are deaf and hard of hearing.*Pediatrics*, 106, 1-9.

[28] Geers, A. (2006). Spoken language in children with cochlear implants. In: P. Spencer and M. Marschark (Eds.), *Advances in the spoken language development of deaf and hard-of-hearing children* (pp. 244-270). New York: Oxford University Press.

[29] Connor, C., Hieber, S., Arts, H.A., Zwolan, T. (2000). Speech, vocabulary, and the education of children using cochlear implants: Oral or total communication? *Journal of Speech, Language, and Hearing Research*, 43, 1185-1204.

[30] Holt, R. and Svirsky, M. (2008). An exploratory look at pediatric cochlear implantation: Is earliest always best? *Ear and Hearing*, 29, 492-511.

[31] Svirsky, M., Robbins, A., Kirk, K., Pisoni, D., Miyamoto, R. (2000). Language development in profoundly deaf children with cochlear implants. *Psychological Science*, 11, 153-158.

[32] American National Standard. (2002). *Acoustical performance criteria, design requirements, and guidelines for schools* (ANSI Publication S12.60-2002). Melville, NY: Acoustical Society of America.

[33] Teasdale, W.W. and Sorensen, M.H. (2007). Hearing loss in relation to educational attainment and cognitive abilities: A population study. *International Journal of Audiology*, 46, 172-175.

[34] Maruthy, S. and Mannarukrishnaiah, J. (2008, April 2). Effect of early onset otitis media on brainstem and cortical auditory processing.*Behavioral and Brain Functions*, 4,17. Available from: URL: http://www.ncbi.nlm.nih.gov/pmc/articles/PMC 2323396 /(Accessed 17 July 2011).

[35] Dahl, M. (1994). Hard-of-hearing inmates in penitentiaries.*Journal of Speech Language Pathology and Audiology*, 18, 217-277.

[36] Fusick, L. (2008). Serving clients with hearing loss: Best practices in mental health counseling. *Journal of Counseling and Development*, 86, 102-110.

[37] Davis, A., Smith, P., Ferguson, M., Stephens, D., Gianopoulos, I. (2007). Acceptability, benefit and costs of early screening for hearing disability: A study of potential screening tests and models. *Health Technology Assessment*, 11(42). Available from: URL: www.hta.ac.uk/project/1025.asp. (Accessed 24 February 2011).

[38] Kochkin, S. (2007).MarkeTrak VII: Obstacles to adult non-user adoption of hearing aids. *The Hearing Journal, 60,* 24-51.

[39] Gates, G.A. and Mills, J.H. (2005).Presbycusis. *The Lancet, 366,* 1111-1120.

[40] Gordon-Salant, S., Frisina, R.D., Popper, A., Fay, D. (Eds), *The aging auditory system: Perceptual characterization and neural bases of presbycusis,* Berlin:Springer Handbook of Auditory Research.

[41] Walton, J.P. (2010). Timing is everything: Temporal processing deficits in the aged auditory brainstem. *Hearing Research, 264,* 63-69.

[42] Kujawa, S.G. and Liberman, M.C. (2009). Adding insult to injury: Cochlear nerve degeneration after "temporary" noise-induced hearing loss. *The Journal of Neuroscience, 29,* 14077-14085.

[43] Hickson, L. (Ed.). (2009). *Hearing care for adults.*Stäfa: Phonak.

[44] Cook, J., Frick, K.D., Baltussen, R., Resnikoff, S., Smith, A., Mecaskey, J., Kilima, P. (2006). Loss of vision and hearing.In: D.T Jamison, J.G. Breman, A.R. Measham, G. Alleyne, M. Claeson, D.B. Evans, P. Jha, A. Mills, P. Musgrove (Eds.),*Disease control priorities in developing countries* (2nd Edition, pp. 953-962). New York, NY: Oxford University Press and the World Bank.

[45] Arlinger, S. (2003). Negative consequences of untreated hearing loss: A review. *International Journal of Audiology, 42,* 2S17-21.

[46] Williams, A. and Nussbaum, J.F. (2001).*Intergenerational communication across the life span.*Mahwah, NJ: Lawrence Erlbaum Associates.

[47] Hétu, R., Jones, L., Getty, L. (1993). The impact of acquired hearing impairment on intimate relationships: Implications for rehabilitation. *Audiology, 32,* 363-381.

[48] Gagné, J.-P., Southall, K.,Jennings, M. B. (2009). The psychological effects of social stigma: Applications to people with acquired hearing loss. In: J. Montano and J. Spitzer (Eds.),*Adult AudiologicRehabilitation* (pp. 63-91). San Diego, CA: Plural Publishing.

[49] Ryan, E.B., Meredith, S.D., Maclean, M.J., Orange, J.B. (1995). Changing the way we talk with elders: Promoting health using the Communication Enhancement Model. *International Journal of Aging and Human Development, 41,* 89-107.

[50] Levy, B.R., Slade, M.D., Gill, T. (2006).Hearing decline predicted by elders' age stereotypes. *Journal of Gerontology BPsychological Sciences, 61,* 82-87.

[51] Schmader, T., Johns, M., Forbes, C. (2008).An integrated process model of stereotype threat effects on performance.*Psychological Review, 115,* 336-356.

[52] West, R.L. and Smith, S.L. (2007).Development of a hearing aid self-efficacy questionnaire.*International Journal of Audiology, 46,* 759-771.

[53] Smith, S.L., Pichora-Fuller, M.K., Watts, K.L., LaMore, C. (2011).Development of the Listening Self-Efficacy Questionnaire (LSEQ).*International Journal of Audiology, 50,* 417-425.

[54] International Organization for Standardization (ISO). No more squinting at small print or leaning forward to hear properly – thanks to new ISO standards. 2011. Available from: URL: www.iso.org/iso/pressrelease.htm?refid=Ref1397. (Accessed 3 February 2011).

[55] Erber, N.P. (2003). Use of hearing aids by older people: Influence of non-auditory factors (vision, manual dexterity). *International Journal of Audiology, 42*(Supplement 2),S21-S25.

[56] Peelle, J.E., Troiani, V., Wingfield, A., Grossman, M. (2010). Neural processing during older adults' comprehension of spoken sentences: Age differences in resource allocation and connectivity. *Cerebral Cortex,* 20, 773-782.

[57] Davis, S.W., Dennis, N.A., Daselaar, S.M., Fleck, M.S., Cabeza, R. (2007). Qué PASA? The posterior-anterior shift in aging. *Cerebral Cortex,* 18, 1201-1209.

[58] Attebo, K., Mitchell, P., Smith, W. (1996). Visual acuity and the causes of visual loss in Australia: The Blue Mountains Study. *Ophthalmology,* 103, 357-364.

[59] Caban, A.J., Lee, D.J., Gomez-Marin, O., Lam, B.L., Zheng, D.D. (2005).Prevalence of concurrent hearing and visual impairment in US adults: The National Health Interview Survey, 1997-2002. *American Journal of Public Health,* 95, 1940-1942.

[60] Gold, D. and Shaw, A. (2008). Characteristics and unmet needs of adults with vision loss in Canada: Interpretation of the participation and activity limitations survey, 2001. Report for Human Resources and Social Development Canada prepared by the CNIB, Toronto, Ontario, Canada.

[61] Ebly, E.M., Parhad, I.M., Hogan, D.B., Fung, T.S. (1994). Prevalence and types of dementia in the very old: Results from the Canadian Study of Health and Aging. *Neurology,* 44, 1593-1600.

[62] Lin, F.R., Metter, E.J., O'Brien, R.J., Resnick, S.M., Zonderman, A.B., Ferrucci, L. (2011). Hearing loss and incident dementia. *Archives Neurology,* 68, 214-220.

[63] Gates, G.A., Beiser, A., Rees, T.S., Agostino, R.B., Wolf, P.A. (2002). Central auditory dysfunction may precede the onset of clinical dementia in people with probable Alzheimer's disease. *Journal of the American Geriatric Society,* 50, 482-488.

[64] Lin, M.Y., Gutierrez, P.R., Stone, K.L., Yaffe, K., Ensrud, K.E., Fink, H.A., Sarkisian, C.A., Coleman, A.L., Mangione, C.M. (2004). Vision impairment and combined vision and hearing impairment predict cognitive and functional decline in older women. *Journal of the American Geriatrics Society,* 52, 1996-2002.

[65] University College London News.New study into dementia within the Deaf community. 2010. [cited 2010 February 24]. Available from: URL: http://www.ucl.ac.uk/news /news-articles/1002/10022401. (Accessed 24 February 2011).

[66] Craik, F.I.M. and Bialystok, E. (2005). Intelligence and executive control: Evidence from aging and bilingualism. *Cortex,* 41, 222-224.

[67] Jones, S. and Fox, S. (2009). PEW Internet Project Data Memo. Available from: URL: http://www.pewinternet.org/~/media//Files/Reports/2009/PIP_Generations_2009.pdf(A ccessed 5 July 2011).

[68] Worrall, L., Hickson, L., Barnett, H., Yiu, E. (1998). An evaluation of the *Keep on Talking*program for maintaining communication skills into old age.*Educational Gerontology,* 24, 129-140.

[69] Hickson, L., Worrall, L., Scarinci, N. (2007). A randomized controlled trial evaluating the *Active Communication Education* program for older people with hearing impairment. *Ear and Hearing,* 28, 212-230.

[70] Dahl, M. (1997). *To Hear Again*: A volunteer program in hearing health care for hard-of-hearing seniors. *Journal of Speech-Language Pathology and Audiology,* 21, 153-159.

[71]   Pichora-Fuller, M.K. and Robertson, L. (1997). Planning and evaluation of a hearing rehabilitation program in a home-for-the-aged: Use of hearing aids and assistive listening devices. *Journal of Speech Language Pathology and Audiology, 21,* 174-186.

[72]   Palmer, C.V., Adams, S.W., Bourgeois, M., Durrant, J., Ross, M. (1999).Reduction in caregiver-identified problem behaviors in patients with Alzheimer disease post-hearing-aid fitting.*Journal of Speech Language Hearing Research, 42,* 312-328.

[73]   Bellelli, G., Frisoni, G.B., Bianchetti, A., Boffelli, S., Guerrini, G.B., Scotuzzi, A., Ranieri, P., Ritondale, G., Guglielmi, L., Fusari, A., Raggi, G., Gasparalti, A., Gheza, A., Nobili, G., Trabucchi, M.(1998). Special care units for demented patients: a multicenter study. *Gerontologist, 38,* 456-62.

[74]   Smith, S.L. and West, R.L. (2006). The application of self-efficacy principles to audiologic rehabilitation: A tutorial. *American Journal of Audiology,* 15, 46-56.

[75]   Rudner, M., Foo, C., Rönnberg, J., Lunner, T. (2009). Cognition and aided speech recognition in noise. *Scandinavian Journal of Psychology, 50,* 395–403.

In: Prevention of Hearing Loss
Editors: V. Newton, P. Alberti and A. Smith

ISBN: 978-1-61942-745-7
© 2012 Nova Science Publishers, Inc.

Chapter V

Overall Strategies of Prevention

Andrew W. Smith[*]

Abstract

Prevention is an action to stop a disease or disability from occurring or progressing in an individual or in a population. Large public health initiatives only began in the 19th century, when it was realized that the health of individual members of society is profoundly influenced by society's collective characteristics. Primordial prevention targets prevention of the risk factors themselves, mainly via health education to promote lifestyle changes. Primary, secondary and tertiary prevention arrest the progression of hearing loss through impairment, disability and handicap. However newer understanding from the International Classification of Functioning, Disability and Health (ICF) and the UN Convention on the Rights of Persons with Disabilities (CRPD) links the medical and social models of disability with a more positive approach ("function and structure" rather than "impairment, "activity" rather than "disability", "participation" rather than "handicap") and the involvement of environmental and personal factors. The rights of persons with disabilities are not incompatible with prevention, provided their rights and dignities are recognized.

A strategy for effective prevention makes changes in the population as a whole and not just in the high-risk minority. This occurs through mass public health initiatives or changes in behaviour that target key risk factors. More data needs to be gathered on the burden caused by risk factors for hearing loss as well as on the size of the burden around the world. This is being addressed by the new Global Burden of Disease initiative.

Reducing hearing loss by relatively small amounts in the many people in a population with mild, moderate and moderately severe hearing loss will have a greater effect on the burden than targeting the few with severe or profound loss. The World Health Organisation (WHO) and other organizations are adopting this approach in order to set up large-scale interventions to make a difference in populations.

Excessive noise is an important risk factor for hearing loss; effective population interventions are needed against this and other high frequency causes of hearing loss and generic risk factors such as poverty, poor personal hygiene, and inaccessible health care.

[*] Corresponding author: andrew.smith@LSHTM.ac.uk.

The most effective vehicle for these interventions is Primary Ear and Hearing Care, using WHO manuals for training in developing countries.

The principles and methods of prevention for particular causes have been publicised by WHO and others. Priorities for action include adopting a comprehensive approach, instituting multisectoral action and enabling sustainable development. Surveillance and monitoring ensures that interventions are effective and that their cost-effectiveness must be compared. However available resources to address hearing loss are still inappropriately small compared to other NCDs, despite its huge cost to society, and its effects on equity.

Introduction

Prevention has different meanings for different people. Prevention is action before an event or situation to stop it occurring. It is derived from the Latin *praevenire* meaning precede, anticipate, hinder. In the health field, prevention usually means an action or intervention to stop a disease or disability from occurring or progressing in an individual or in a population that exhibits identifiable risk factors, often associated with different risk behaviours. It includes measures to reduce the consequences of the disease or disability.

This chapter reviews the general principles and practice of prevention and relates them to hearing loss. It first reviews the history of prevention from Hippocrates to the present. The next section defines the different levels of prevention used in the health and related fields, from the recently introduced primordial prevention, through primary, secondary and tertiary prevention, and rehabilitation. The section concludes with a discussion of recent understanding of the meaning of disability and prevention in the context of the WHO International Classification of Functioning, Disability and Health (ICF) and the UN Convention on the Rights of Persons with Disabilities (CRPD). This then links to a brief section on the ethics of prevention, especially as they relate to people with hearing loss and deafness.

The largest section of the chapter discusses in detail the strategies for prevention, especially in relation to the population strategy of prevention, and the importance of addressing risk factors. It also reviews the work and impacts of prevention of hearing loss by bodies such as WHO and WWHearing – World-Wide Hearing Care for Developing Countries.

The possibilities for and consequences of prevention of hearing loss are intimately related to health economics and social equity and these topics are discussed in the two final sections.

History of Prevention

From the historical viewpoint, Hippocrates of Kos (*ca.* 460 BC – *ca.* 370 BC) was the first person in the Western World recorded to have promoted the concept of prevention of disease through living a healthy life. Just treating, or covering up symptoms of illness was foreign to him. He insisted that prevention from disease was the primary focus of healthcare, achieved through a diet of nutritional food and exercise to prevent sickness and improve one's overall health [1]. He also advised anyone coming to a new city to enquire whether it was likely to be a healthy or unhealthy place to live, depending on geography or water supply, and on the behaviour of its inhabitants. The Romans understood that proper diversion of human waste was necessary for public health in urban areas. Variolation to prevent smallpox was carried out in India in the 8th century and soon after in China. Interventions to prevent disease were often carried out in ignorance of the mechanism: thus, when parts of cities were burned during the plague in 14th century cities, this killed the rats and their flea population (the true vectors of *Yersinia pestis*), whereas the belief that removing bodies of the dead would stop the epidemic, in practice had no effect.

The modern era of public health and prevention began in the West in the late 18th century when Edward Jenner demonstrated that vaccination with cowpox produced immunity to smallpox. Later, in the 19th century, John Snow was the first to use an epidemiological approach to investigate an outbreak of cholera in London. He made the apparently decisive public health intervention to stop it by removing the handle of the Broad Street pump which supplied the contaminated water to the local population.

Possibly the most revolutionary public health initiative in modern history – the *Public Health Act* of 1848 in England, facilitated the building of water supplies and sewerage systems. Despite its profound, positive effects, the main motivating force in its adoption was not social justice, but a desire to reduce dependence on public relief. However, long-term financing allowed local jurisdictions to plan public works systematically instead of building them gradually, ensuring a significant impact on population health.

This notion that healthiness is a characteristic of populations, which had disappeared for two millennia after Hippocrates, was also revived by Durkheim, the 19th century French sociologist. He wrote that the suicide rate varied between countries and was influenced by the collective characteristics of whole societies.

As Rose wrote in 1992 in his seminal work, *The Strategy of Preventive Medicine*, "...in order to grasp the principles of public health one must understand that society is not merely a collection of individuals but is a collectivity[1], and the behaviour and health of its individual members are profoundly influenced by its collective characteristics and social norms" [2].

Definitions of Prevention

There are several categories or levels of prevention, according to where in the causal chain they intervene (Figure 5.1). The concept and major part of this model was developed in the first classification of disability by WHO – the International Classification of Impairments, Disabilities and Handicaps, published in 1980; [3].

Although this model can be helpful to understand where in the natural history of health conditions the different levels of prevention act, it is now recognized that it focuses only on the medical model of disease, and tends to ignore the social context and environmental aspects of health conditions and disabilities.

These limitations have been addressed in the International Classification of Functioning, Disability and Health (ICF) [4], which can be seen as the successor or second edition of the 1980 classification, except that it has a different title in order to draw attention to its new approach to classification.

---

[1] A group or community of people bound together by common beliefs or interests.

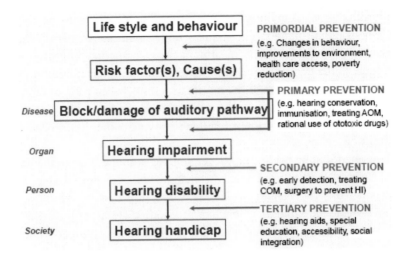

Figure 5.1. Interventions at different levels of prevention along the causal chain for hearing loss.

1) Primordial Prevention

Primordial prevention is defined as prevention of risk factors themselves; thus it consists of actions and measures that inhibit the emergence of the social, economic and cultural patterns of living that are known to contribute to an elevated risk of disease. It deals with the mitigation of risk factors and risky behaviours. This type of prevention rests mainly on public education, lifestyle messages, the influence of the media, legislation and government policy, and is very dependent on the commitment and determination of individual governments, and effective non-governmental organizations and lobby groups. There is a need to modify not only risk factors and risky behaviour but also such risky conditions as poverty, powerlessness and lack of social support. Thus, this is a different approach from the strategy for actual risk modification as part of the primary prevention strategy, which would be applicable at population and clinical level. [5,6,].

Primordial prevention usually begins in childhood when behaviour that is risky to health begins. Parents, teachers and peer groups have an important role here in imparting health education to children. Since this can prevent risk factors from appearing in the first place, it might be expected to be highly cost-effective. However this supposition has not been tested. Ursoniu, who has promoted the concept of and actions for primordial prevention, lists actions for smoking prevention as a good example of this [6]. These principles could be fairly readily transformed into actions for primordial prevention of noise-induced hearing loss, or for the risk factors of infectious causes of hearing loss, such as meningitis.

2) Primary Prevention

This consists of actions to avoid or remove the cause of a health problem in an individual or a population before the problem arises. It includes health promotion and specific protection (for example, HIV education) [7]. The purpose is to limit the incidence of disease by controlling causes and risk factors [6]. It involves two often complementary strategies –

targeting high risk in individuals resulting from specific exposure and targeting average risk in the whole population [2] (see section on Strategies later in this chapter). Primary prevention can intervene to prevent an impairment at 2 places in the causal chain (Figure 5.1), namely to prevent a risk factor causing a disease or prevent a disease or health condition causing a disability (e.g. immunisation against the meningococcus, *Neisseria meningitidis* to prevent meningitis, or early treatment of the meningitis to prevent the complication of sensori-neural hearing loss [8]).

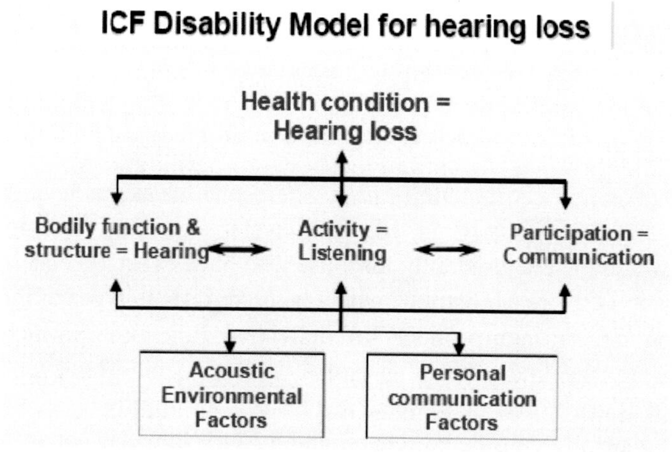

ICF Disability Model for hearing loss

Health condition =
Hearing loss

Bodily function &
structure = Hearing ⟷ Activity = Listening ⟷ Participation = Communication

Acoustic Environmental Factors   Personal communication Factors

Figure 5.2. Interpreting the new ICF disability model for hearing loss [adapted from 4]..

3) Secondary Prevention

This comprises actions to detect a health problem in an individual or a population at an early stage of its natural history, facilitating cure, or reducing or preventing spread, or reducing or preventing its long-term effects [7]. Neonatal hearing screening is an example of secondary prevention.. Secondary prevention targets the period between disease onset and time of "usual" diagnosis and aims to reduce prevalence. It can be applied only to a disease with a natural history that includes an early period when the disease is easily identified and treated so that progression to a more serious stage is stopped [6].

4) Tertiary Prevention

This includes actions to reduce the impact of an already established disease by restoring function and reducing disease related complications [7] (for example, provision of hearing aids or cochlear implants and special education to children with severe to profound hearing loss). Tertiary prevention is equivalent to rehabilitation.

The World Report on Disability [7] defines *rehabilitation* as "a set of measures that assist individuals who experience, or are likely to experience, disability to achieve and maintain optimal functioning in interaction with their environments".

MEDICAL MODEL	+	SOCIAL MODEL
• PERSONAL problem	+	SOCIAL problem
• medical care	+	social integration
• individual treatment	+	social action
• professional help	+	individual & collective responsibility
• personal adjustment	+	environmental manipulation
• behaviour	+	attitude
• care	+	human rights
• health care policy	+	politics
• individual adaptation	+	social change

Figure 5.3. The medical and social models of disability compared [adapted from 4].

The term "habilitation" is sometimes used where such measures help those who acquire disabilities congenitally or early in life to develop maximal functioning. The term "rehabilitation" would then be used only for those who have experienced a *loss* in function. If "habilitation" is not used, "rehabilitation" would be used for both types of intervention.

Rehabilitation targets improvements in individual functioning which should include making changes to the individual's personal environment. However barrier removal initiatives against hearing loss at societal level, such as improving acoustics in a public building, are not generally considered rehabilitation, since they are not specifically targeting individuals requiring rehabilitation. Often, rehabilitation occurs for a specific period of time, but can involve single or multiple interventions delivered by an individual or a team of rehabilitation workers, and may be needed from the acute phase through to post-acute and maintenance phases.

Rehabilitation involves identifying a person's problems and needs, relating these to relevant factors of the person and the environment, defining rehabilitation goals, planning and implementing the measures, and assessing the effects. Educating people with disabilities is essential for developing knowledge and skills for self-help, care, management, and decision-making. When families or close friends are partners in the rehabilitation process, the person with the disability experiences better health and functioning [9].

Disability and Prevention Defined in the ICF and the UN CRPD

Both the International Classification of Functioning, Disability and Health (ICF) [4] and the UN Convention on the Rights of Persons with Disabilities (CRPD) [10, 11] view disability as the outcome of complex interactions between health conditions and features of an individual's physical, social, and attitudinal environment that hinder their full and effective participation in society (Figure 5.2 shows these interactions specifically for hearing loss). Many people will experience disability temporarily or permanently at some point in their lives. Most who survive to old age will be increasingly disabled in their final years [12].

Traditionally, people with disabilities have been seen as conforming to a medical model (Figure 5.3). Disability has been equated only with an individual's personal health status, impairment, or capacity limitation. This one-sided, medicalised view fails to address the social factors, discrimination, prejudice, and inaccessibility that prevent full participation and contribute to the overall disability experience. Disability is also a social issue and by addressing these barriers, society can provide individuals with disabilities the opportunity to exercise their rights on an equal basis with all others. Both the medical and social models should be taken into account for people with disabilities [11]. Both these aspects are summarised in Figure 5.3.

In the International Classification of Functioning, Disability and Health (ICF) [4] the only responses to a search for "prevention", or "prevent", in the ICF online at http://apps.who.int/classifications/icfbrowser/ produced the following results. No reference was found when searching on "public health".

- *e5800 Health services.* Services and programmes at a local, community, regional, state or national level, aimed at delivering interventions to individuals for their physical, psychological and social well-being, such as health promotion and disease *prevention* services, primary care services, acute care, rehabilitation and long-term care services;
- *d5702 Maintaining one's health.* Caring for oneself by being aware of the need and doing what is required to look after one's health, both to respond to risks to health and to *prevent* ill-health,
- *e1 CHAPTER 1 PRODUCTS AND TECHNOLOGY.* The ISO 9999 classification of technical aids defines these as "any product, instrument, equipment or technical system used by a disabled person, especially produced or generally available, *preventing,* compensating, monitoring, relieving or neutralizing" disability..
- *e580 Health services, systems and policies.* Services, systems and policies for *preventing* and treating health problems, providing medical rehabilitation and promoting a healthy lifestyle. *Exclusion: general social support services, systems and policies (e575)*

Ethics of Prevention

Signatories to the UN Convention on the Rights of Persons with Disabilities (CRPD) [10], in Article 25, (see Box 5.1) recognize that "persons with disabilities have the right to the enjoyment of the highest attainable standard of health" and the right to have health care "as provided to other persons including ...population-based public health programmes", and "including early identification and intervention as appropriate and services designed to minimize and prevent further disabilities".

The World Report on Disability states (page 8) that primary prevention of health conditions does not come within the scope of the CRPD, but that the WHO and World Bank "...consider primary prevention as crucial to improved overall health of countries' populations".

"Viewing disability as a human rights issue is not incompatible with prevention of health conditions as long as prevention respects the rights and dignity of people with disabilities, for example, in the use of language and imagery [12].

Preventing disability should be regarded as a multidimensional strategy that includes prevention of disabling barriers as well as prevention and treatment of underlying health conditions" [13].

Box 5.1. Article 25, on Health, in UN Convention on the Rights of persons with Disabilities [10]. Articles relating specifically to prevention are in *italics*

States Parties recognize that persons with disabilities have the right to the enjoyment of the highest attainable standard of health without discrimination on the basis of disability. States Parties shall take all appropriate measures to ensure access for persons with disabilities to health services that are gender sensitive, including *health-related rehabilitation.*

In particular, States Parties shall:

(a) Provide persons with disabilities with the same range, quality and standard of free or affordable health care and programmes as provided to other persons, including in the area of sexual and reproductive health and *population-based public health programmes;*

(b) Provide those health services needed by persons with disabilities specifically because of their disabilities, including *early identification and intervention* as appropriate, and *services designed to minimize and prevent further disabilities,* including among children and older persons;

(c) Provide these health services as close as possible to people's own communities, including in rural areas;

(d) Require health professionals to provide care of the same quality to persons with disabilities as to others, including on the basis of free and informed consent by, inter alia, raising awareness of the human rights, dignity, autonomy and needs of persons with disabilities through training and the promulgation of ethical standards for public and private health care;

(e) Prohibit discrimination against persons with disabilities in the provision of health insurance, and life insurance where such insurance is permitted by national law, which shall be provided in a fair and reasonable manner;

(f) Prevent discriminatory denial of health care or health services or food and fluids on the basis of disability.

However, "people who identify themselves as Deaf (note the capital "D") belong to a proud and distinctive culture group known as the Deaf culture".

They "do not identify as having a disability or see themselves as experiencing a limitation. Instead, they identify as a member of a cultural and linguistic group" [14]. A resolution by the World Federation of the Deaf (WFD) in 1999 [15] stated that "Deaf people are a cultural and linguistic minority with a right to their native sign language as their mother tongue".

They may not accept the notion of prevention, especially primary prevention, whereas people who are hard of hearing are keen to promote research into prevention [16].

Strategies of Prevention

Medical care has been and largely still is targeted at the needs of sick individuals and how to treat them; this traditional approach has more recently been extended to identifying risk and preventing disease and disabilities in individuals. However, as Rose said in 1992 [2]: "The radical strategy is to identify and if possible to remedy the underlying causes of our major health problems. It then commonly emerges that those we wish to help...represent simply the extreme of a continuous distribution of risk or behaviour; when different populations are compared, the distribution is seen to shift up or down as a coherent whole. The essential determinants of health in a society are thus to be found in its mass characteristics: the deviant minority can only be understood when seen in its societal context, and effective prevention requires changes which involve the population as a whole. ....The health of society is integral and the supposedly 'normal' majority needs to accept responsibility for its deviant minority – however loth it may be to do so." Rose worked mainly on the epidemiology and prevention of cardiovascular disease, although his ideas have spread into many fields of health care. They have not been applied to hearing loss but it would be instructive to assess whether they could be and if there would be any benefit from doing so.

The Importance of Risk Factors

A risk factor has been defined as a behaviour, life-style, or environmental exposure, or an inborn or inherited characteristic which from epidemiological evidence is associated with a health-related condition which it is known to be important to prevent [17]. The total burden of disease in a community depends on the numbers of people exposed to a particular risk factor, i.e. the population distribution of the risk factor.

The new current Global Burden of Disease study is an independent, international initiative which brings together WHO, various academic institutions and relevant experts [21]. One of its guiding principles as it assessed [18, 19] and currently re-assesses the global burden [20, 21] is that estimates of the disease and injury burden caused by exposure to major risk factors are likely to be a much more useful guide to policies and priorities for prevention than a "league table" of the disease and injury burden. The 1990 GBD study represented a major advance in the quantification of the impact of diseases, injuries, and risk factors on population health globally and by region. Government and non-governmental agencies alike have used its results to argue for more strategic allocations of health resources to disease prevention and control programmes that are likely to yield the greatest gains in terms of population health. The results have also greatly increased understanding of the basic descriptive epidemiology of diseases and injuries worldwide [22]. If these principles were applied to hearing loss, there could be a substantial benefit because the results could provide justification for the allocation of much greater resources to this neglected field than has occurred up to now. A step in this direction is the inclusion for the first time of an expert group on hearing loss in the GBD 2010 initiative [23] (see Chapter 1).

Another step has been some attempts to set out the various risk factors for hearing loss such as found in recent publications e.g. (1) chapter 50 on "Loss of Vision and Hearing" of the 2006 WHO/World Bank publication "Disease Control Priorities in Developing Countries" [24] which adopted the risk factor approach for all the health conditions it addressed. These have been listed as items 1-9 in Box 5.2; (2) The position statement of the US Joint Committee on Infant Hearing in 2007 lists risk indicators in an appendix [25] and these are listed as items 10-19 in Box 5.2 (item 20 is from another source [26]).Risk factors have some causative effect even though the mechanism may or may not be known, and risk indicators are proxies for the actual risk factors .

Box 5.2. RISK FACTORS AND RISK INDICATORS for Hearing Loss
No.'s 1-9 are risk factors at all ages, taken from Cook at el 2006 [24]
(6-9 are risk factors for upper respiratory tract infections, otitis media, measles and meningitis.) No.'s 10-19 are risk factors or risk indicators for neonates & infants taken from the 2007 position statement of the US Joint Committee on Infant Hearing [25].

1. Noise
a. Noisy occupations (e.g. manufacturing, construction, farming industries; military; traffic police, musicians, especially in developing countries)
b. Certain lifestyles (e.g. personal stereos, clubbing, noisy toys, fire-crackers)
c. Some hobbies & sports (e.g. hunting, shooting clubs, motor racing).
2. Ototoxic chemicals and drugs; (risk may be potentiated by noise exposure)
3. Smoking may be a risk factor for high-frequency hearing loss,
adding to the effect of noise
4. Offspring of consanguineous marriages
5. Certain ethnic groups may be at higher risk of developing COM
6. Poverty,
7. Poor access to health care,
8. Poor hygiene, and
9. Overcrowding,
10. Care giver concern.
11. Positive Family history.
12. Neonatal intensive care admission with oxygenation, ventilation, ototoxic drug therapy, hyperbilirubinemia with exchange transfusion.
13. In utero infections, e.g. cytomegalovirus (CMV), herpes, rubella, syphilis, and toxoplasmosis.
14. Some craniofacial anomalies,
15. Syndromes associated with hearing loss or progressive or late-onset hearing loss
16. Various neurodegenerative disorders,
17. Culture-positive bacterial or viral meningitis.
18. Head trauma, requiring hospitalization.
19. Chemotherapy.
20. Low birth-weight, low Apgar scores (Vohr and others 2000 [26]).

However, in comparison to other health fields such as amongst other chronic non-communicable diseases, there has been very little information-gathering to measure the burden of hearing loss caused by exposure to these risk factors. What has been done is that the burden, in disability-adjusted life years, DALYs, of the total envelope of adult onset hearing loss has been estimated and published by WHO [27] together with the burden of hearing loss contributing to the total burden of certain causes (meningitis and otitis media) [28]. All these estimates, together with that for child-onset hearing loss, are being determined more accurately in the GBD-2010 study, using results of more recent reviews of surveys of prevalence of hearing impairment [29,30] This is also covered in Chapter 2. In future it will be necessary also to collect population-based cause-specific and risk-factor specific data for hearing loss for the major factors listed in Box 5.2 in different countries and regions, despite the difficulties of doing so in the field.

The High-Risk Strategy

To identify all individuals at high risk, it is necessary to undertake some kind of screening procedure. Each risk factor is measured as a continuous score, and the distribution is then dichotomised to identify a high-risk group, comprising individuals who will qualify for an intervention and the rest of the people tested are classed as "normal" and left in peace. This will relieve the high-risk status of the deviant minority without troubling the rest of the population. This makes sense to those targeted and to those left alone and can be easily "sold" to them by their physician. The majority of the population do not attend screening in order to find out everything that is wrong with them, but to seek reassurance that they are healthy, and can carry on as before without any need for interventions. The minority who receive an intervention need support and follow-up for them to carry on in the programme and not revert to the behaviour patterns of the majority. However, this high-risk strategy is not particularly effective in public-health terms, as will be shown in the next section.

The Population Strategy of Prevention

Now to return to Rose's idea about preventing the greatest burden of disease [2]. Caring for and treating sick individuals, preventing illness in high-risk individuals, donating to appeals for famine relief all target needy minorities. It is much more difficult to raise support for collective action against the underlying causes of the problem, because the public's, and most politician's perception of need is in personal rather than population terms.

Unfortunately, for a number of reasons, Rose has shown that the high-risk preventive strategy, although effective for the individuals concerned, can make no more than a marginal impact on the overall problem in the population [2]. Most of the cases will arise among the many at lower risk rather than the few at high risk, so that if many people each receive a little benefit, the total benefit will be large. Only if a problem is confined to an identifiable minority and if it can be successfully controlled in isolation, is the high-risk approach adequate, provided it is maintained as long as its causes persist. It would appear likely that hearing loss is generally not suitable, from a population point of view, to be controlled by the high-risk approach, and it would be preferable to adopt the population strategy of prevention.

However, there is probably not as yet sufficient population-based data to plot and compare the population distribution of hearing thresholds in many different populations, which would be needed to demonstrate the effectiveness of this approach. If this supposition is correct, the average hearing level in a particular population would predict the prevalence of disabling hearing impairment, just as average alcohol consumption in a society predicts the prevalence of heavy drinkers or average blood pressure predicts the prevalence of hypertension. There is likely to be more effect on the burden of hearing loss in a population or society by reducing hearing loss by relatively smaller amounts in many people with mild, moderate and moderately severe hearing loss than by targeting those with severe or profound loss.

This is the approach adopted by organizations such as WWHearing – World-Wide Hearing care for Developing Countries in collaboration with WHO. The mission of WWHearing is to provide affordable and effective hearing aids on a very large scale to children and adults with moderate and moderately severe hearing loss but not to focus on those with more severe hearing loss. WWHearing has successfully completed pilot projects in India [31] and China [32] to provide hearing aids to adults and children respectively. The results demonstrate that appropriately trained and supervised community health workers or teachers of deaf children can find people in the community who would benefit from a hearing aid, and fit and follow them up correctly. Concurrent studies carried out economic analysis on the provision of hearing aids and showed this was least costly at the primary level of health care than at higher levels [33, 34] . Another pilot study developed a more streamlined hearing aid delivery model than available currently at government clinics in Brazil, and another fitted four hundred hearing aids, and carried out hearing-impairment training for community healthcare workers in the Philippines [35].

There are various free hearing aid programmes in western countries, such as in Denmark and the United Kingdom, and these could also provide useful information on the effectiveness of such approaches. A model project called Hearing Express is now being developed and is designed to administer quality hearing health services to large volumes of individuals through financially sustainable outlets in developing countries. These services include affordable and rapid screening, diagnostics and hearing aid services. [36] This approach is also embodied in the WHO Guidelines on Hearing Aids and Services for Developing Countries [37]. In addition to its work specifically on hearing aids and services, WWHearing, in its collaboration with WHO, has recently developed a comprehensive programme – called Audio 2020 – which includes in its action plan a component to promote and implement activities for prevention of hearing loss. [38]

The objective of the population approach is to control the underlying determinants of ill health and in this way to reduce population incidence rates. An example of a specific area in prevention of hearing loss could be in prevention of noise-induced hearing loss (NIHL). Changes in incidence of a health condition such as NIHL may reflect population-wide distributional shifts in associated risk factors, and a small shift in distribution may have a large effect on the individuals falling into the highly vulnerable tail of the distribution of the population with hearing loss. Thus mass health education and hearing conservation programmes will be needed to combat the increasing levels of social and industrial noise in developing countries and the consequent noise induced hearing loss (see Chapters 12 and 13 dealing with Industrial Hearing Conservation and Social and Community Noise respectively). Other risk factors for hearing loss such as poverty, poor personal hygiene, lack of access to health care are readily amenable to the population strategy of prevention, and are likely to have an effect even though the exact causal chain may not be known. The actual interventions against these risk factors are more likely to be in the socio-economic and political sphere than in the medical one. Some of these types of strategy may be very long-term in producing significant effects, and other short-term strategies may be needed as well, in the interim.

WHO Strategies for Prevention

The population strategy for prevention, described above, has not yet been implemented against hearing impairment by WHO or by other organizations, as far as is known. Some tentative steps have been made in that direction.

In order to further develop the public health approach to prevention, WHO has grouped different causes of hearing loss according to their frequency (see Figure 5.4 and [24]). In a programme for prevention, those causes with high and moderate frequency and effective means of prevention and control need to be targeted. From a public health perspective, those with lower frequency should be ignored even if there is an effective method of prevention or control and even though for the individuals concerned these may mean significant disability. Of course this argument only applies to the public health programme and alongside this there should be adequate provision put in place locally to diagnose and manage the lower frequency causes producing significant hearing loss. These issues are highly relevant in the spread of universal neonatal hearing screening programmes that make early diagnosis of infant hearing loss especially where severe or profound. Development of such programmes needs to be looked at from a public health perspective as well as an individual one.

WHO is developing a series of effective strategies for prevention against ototoxic drugs, chronic otitis media, noise induced hearing loss, infant hearing screening, and has already developed guidelines for hearing aids for developing countries [37]. For these other interventions, expert reports have been produced and guidelines are being considered.

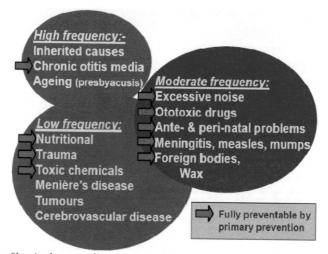

Figure 5.4. Main causes of hearing loss according to their usual frequency and preventability by primary prevention.

The most cost-effective vehicles for providing these interventions include primary ear and hearing care, as part of a national or district programme for prevention. Most interventions against ear and hearing disorders can be implemented at the primary level by trained primary ear and hearing care (PEHC) workers or primary health care (PHC) workers or their equivalent. If these interventions are used on a large scale they will have a major impact on the burden of ear disease and hearing loss. The WHO Training Resource For Primary Ear And Hearing Care [39], launched in 2006, was developed in order to train the large numbers of PEHC and PHC workers that would be needed. It consists of 4 practical, interactive manuals at three levels of training. It has been translated from the original English into Spanish, French, and Chinese and translated and adapted into various local languages.

It has been launched and utilised for training in countries such as Nigeria, Kenya, Colombia, and China and in others, such as India, the manuals have been adapted and translated for local training, which forms part of the new National Programme for Prevention and Control of Deafness (NPPCD) (see Chapter 17). However, no proper evaluation of its effectiveness as a training tool has yet been undertaken, and this is urgently needed.

The components of a national or district programme for prevention are listed in Box 5 3. They will also link to habilitation and rehabilitation programmes, community based rehabilitation, and provision of hearing aids services and educational services. Prevention and control measures with clear evidence of effectiveness and high cost-effectiveness should be adopted and implemented. Population-wide interventions must be complemented by individual health-care interventions.

Box 5.3. Components of a Programme for Prevention of Hearing Loss

- Primary Ear and Hearing Care
- Health Education
- Surveillance & treatment of infectious diseases
- Immunisation
- Maternal health, ante-, peri-natal care
- Screening & early detection for hearing impairment
- Genetic counselling
- Hearing Conservation
- Hearing Aids provision & services
- Educational services
- Appropriate secondary & tertiary services
- Training & refresher courses for all levels
-

Preventing Chronic Diseases – The Stepwise Framework

In 2005, WHO published the report "Preventing Chronic Diseases – a vital investment.[41]. Part 4 of this report included the *Stepwise framework*, a flexible and practical approach to assist ministries of health in balancing diverse needs and priorities while implementing evidence-based interventions against Chronic Diseases such as those recommended by the WHO. The framework is guided by a set of principles based on a public health approach to chronic disease prevention and control. Even though deafness and hearing impairment are not usually thought of as chronic diseases, the WHO Programme of Prevention of Deafness and Hearing Impairment is included in the Department of Chronic Diseases and Health Promotion, and this report and many others from this Department are relevant for prevention of hearing loss.

Causes	Primary	Secondary	Tertiary
Prenatal causes			
Rubella	Immunisation	Early detection by screening all or high-risk groups and treatment, if available	Hearing aids
Syphilis	Health education, Treatment of the mother		
Toxoplasmosis	Health education, treatment of the mother		Special education
Iodine deficiency	Nutrition, Supplementation		
Ototoxicity	Avoidance, rational use		Rehabilitation
Genetic causes	Health education, Counselling, identification of carriers		
Congenital malformations		Surgery, when appropriate	
Perinatal causes			
Low birth weight	Nutrition, ante-natal care	Early detection by screening all or high-risk groups and treatment, if available	Hearing aids
Birth trauma, hypoxia	Improved birth practice		Special education
Cytomegalovirus	Personal hygiene, health education		
Jaundice	Detection, management of at-risk groups		Rehabilitation
Ototoxicity	Avoidance, rational use		
Noise	Reduction, avoidance, Conservation		
Childhood causes			
Otitis externa Foreign bodies	Personal hygiene, Health education	Treatment, removal	Surgery
Chronic otitis media	Personal hygiene Better living conditions, Proper management of URTIs, better nutrition, breast feeding		Hearing aids Special education
Measles, mumps	Immunization	Health education for early recognition, prompt treatment Case follow-up	Rehabilitation as appropriate
Meningitis	Prophylaxis, Immunization	Early treatment	
Ototoxicity	Avoidance, Rational use		
Adult causes			
Excessive Noise	Health education/promotion, Conservation Legislation, reduction	Change of environment' Early detection, surgery	Hearing aids (Special education)
Ototoxicity	Health education/ promotion, avoidance legislation, rational use		
Otosclerosis	Counselling		Rehabilitation
Trauma	Health education/ promotion, legislation, helmets, seat belts		
Presbyacusis	Avoid ototoxics, excessive noise		

Figure 5.5. Interventions for primary, secondary and tertiary prevention against the main causes of hearing loss.

The national government of a country usually provides the unifying framework for chronic disease prevention and control, and it should ensure that actions at all levels and by all stakeholders are mutually supportive. Policies and plans should focus on common risk factors and cut across specific diseases. Population-wide and individual interventions should be combined and milestones are set for each step and level of intervention, with emphasis on reducing health inequities. Most countries will not have the resources to do everything implied by the overall policy at once; the activities selected first should be those that are immediately feasible and likely to have the greatest impact for the investment (i.e. the most cost-effective) . WWHearing has adapted the stepwise framework to focus on prevention of hearing impairment and provision of hearing aids [42].

WHO Global Status Report on Non-Communicable Diseases (NCDs) 2010

This important report [43] sets out options for both population-wide interventions, largely aimed at prevention, and individual interventions, aimed at early detection and treatment to reduce progression to severe and costly complications. It identifies primary health care as the best framework for implementing its recommended interventions on an adequate scale. Urgent priorities for better health include strong health-care systems, with reliable surveillance and monitoring, and full engagement of non health sectors, industry, civil society, and other partners, since causes often lie beyond the control of public health authorities.

Its recommendations are intended to cover major NCDs (cardiovascular diseases, cancers, diabetes and chronic lung diseases), and none mention deafness or hearing. However, many are relevant for prevention of hearing loss. To demonstrate this, some of the "Priorities for action" (report page 7) have been adapted in the following passage and could be utilised so as to relate to hearing loss. The report itself states that many of the approaches and opportunities for tackling these NCDs are relevant to others not addressed in the report.

Priorities for action In common with other NCDs, the numbers and burden of hearing loss have been rising in recent years, and likewise there is more knowledge and understanding of its prevention and management. More than half of the burden of hearing loss is preventable. Appropriate actions are also needed against hearing loss in the areas of *surveillance, prevention,* and *health care* which should also be part of a national programme. Those actions include:

- *A comprehensive approach:* Risk factors for hearing loss often begin early in life and continue throughout adulthood. To reverse the increasing burden of hearing loss requires a comprehensive approach that targets the whole population and includes both prevention and management interventions.
- *Multisectoral action:* Government, civil society and the private sector must work together and provide support for the prevention and management of hearing loss. Multiple sectors including non-health sectors must be brought together for successful action based on international experience and previous lessons learnt. Guidelines on promoting intersectoral action are included in Chapter 7 of this report [43].

- *Sustainable development:* The increasing burden of hearing loss has a negative impact on human and social development. Its prevention should be a priority in national development initiatives and an integral part of poverty reduction programmes.
- *Surveillance and monitoring:* Measuring the burden of hearing loss is crucial to reversing it. Specific measurable indicators must be adopted and used worldwide and surveillance for hearing loss should be integrated into national health information systems. Essential components of surveillance comprise: a) monitoring exposures (risk factors); b) monitoring outcomes (cause-specific disability rates); c) monitoring health system responses, including national capacity to prevent hearing loss (i.e. policies, plans, infrastructure, human resources, access to health care including medicines and devices).

Currently, resources allocated to all aspects of hearing loss (research, prevention, management) are inappropriately small in comparison to the size of the burden, even in comparison to those for other NCDs which are themselves under-funded.

Economics of Prevention

Hearing loss substantially affects social and economic development in communities and countries. Ruben, taking into account rehabilitation, special education, and loss of employment, estimated the cost to the U.S. economy in 1999 of communication disorders (hearing, voice, speech, and language disorders) at between US$176 billion and US$212 billion (2004 dollars; 2.5–3 percent of the gross national product of the United States in that year). Hearing loss accounted for about one-third of the prevalence of these communication disorders [44]. In a more recent study, the real financial costs of hearing loss in Australia were estimated to total U.S.$8,600 million (or 1.4% of the gross domestic product), with 57% of these costs associated with loss in productivity [45].

These costs are huge so one would expect that funding preventive interventions would be a good investment. However, as Harrop-Griffiths pointed out: "Prevention...makes moral sense but may not always make economic sense. The saving to society as a result of prevention should outweigh the cost of that prevention". Prevention interventions "must be aimed at disorders of hearing and balance which are relatively common, of a severity to cause significant disability....and potentially avoidable by simple straightforward measures involving minimal financial cost" [46].

A Bethesda Conference task force of the American College of Cardiology considered economic costs in relation to heart disease but in so doing re-iterated some basic principles. Extracts from their report have been paraphrased in the next three paragraphs so as to be relevant for hearing loss, [47].

Any society with finite resources has to determine which interventions and programmes have the most value. This can be done by determining which interventions yield the best extra or incremental benefits, such as the most quality-adjusted life-years [QALYs], relative to the extra resources (costs) required to produce those benefits.

Cost-effectiveness analysis is widely used for economic analysis of medical strategies and interventions. It compares incremental costs and benefits, usually by a cost-effectiveness ratio (cost per unit of health outcomes achieved). This enables the ranking of the relative value of different options. When common definitions of health outcomes are employed, the opportunity costs of various choices can be compared. ("Opportunity costs" are the value forgone by devoting resources to a given activity rather than to their best alternative use.). A societal perspective should be adopted in which all costs and benefits are taken into account, regardless of whom they affect in order to minimise the effect that a party in the treatment decision has to lose in order that someone else might gain. In the evaluation of preventive services, it is important to value appropriately the transition from being well to being ill or developing a disability, and not underestimating the preference for wellness.

Measuring indirect costs. These are resources expended that are not directly related to medical care and include days lost from work, time diverted from other (non-work) productive activity, dollars devoted to care-giving activities, the value of caregiver time when provided outside the labour force (e.g., by family caregivers), or lost enjoyment associated with the intervention. (e.g., losing the pleasure associated with smoking as a result of adherence to a smoking cessation regime). These costs can be considerable and must be fully accounted for since they may offset much of the investment in the preventive intervention.

The methods of Economic Analysis are further pursued in Chapter 15: Economic Aspects.

Case Study: Hearing Conservation Programme Costs

In 2006 there were more than 445,000 veterans receiving compensation for hearing loss associated with military service in the US, and 395,000 receiving compensation for service-related tinnitus. The cost of compensation to the US Department of Veterans Affairs in that year was more than $1.2 billion, plus a further $290 million for hearing aids and audiological services [48].

A recent article in the Army Times newspaper stated that noise exposure in the military was of such concern to Congress that in 2002 it directed the Veterans Administration to contract with the Institute of Medicine National Academies to review noise exposure in the military from World War II to the present. Hearing protection has been standard issue for combat forces since 2002, but Army Audiologists informed the newspaper that one in four soldiers returning home report hearing loss, dizziness or ringing in the ears [49].

The total cost of safety and health programmes in Industry is difficult to compute. Hearing conservation is a system of healthcare and the total costs include not only monitoring, sound reduction, provision of personal hearing protection, undertaking of hearing tests, record keeping and the staff required to perform these tasks, but also resources for the programme and loss of revenue from lost working hours while testing and education take place. Against this must be set the savings from a hopefully more productive workforce, with fewer injuries.

The cost of compensation usually includes the provision of hearing aids, their maintenance and replacement. According to a study by Eurogip [50], the cost of hearing loss due to noise represents about 10 % of the total cost of compensation of occupational diseases (period 1999–2001).

That is, from 2.5 % of the total cost of compensation in Denmark, to over 13.9 % in Germany to 29.9 % in Italy. Total costs include increased absenteeism from stress [51] and lower level employment or higher unemployment amongst hard of hearing people.

Social Equity

An issue that should not be ignored is social equity, and is perhaps best considered here. The recent WHO Global Status Report on NCDs [43], in a section called "Impact on Development" (Executive Summary page 2) stated that "People of lower social and economic positions fare far worse than people of higher social positions; the factors determining social positions are education, occupation, income, gender and ethnicity. There is strong evidence for the correlation between a host of social determinants, especially education, and prevalent levels of NCDs and risk factors." This certainly includes hearing loss [52, 53, 54]

WHO recently addressed the issue of social equity in detail through appointing the WHO Commission on Social Determinants of Health, chaired by Sir Michael Marmot [55]. It covers all aspects of health and ill-health and its findings fully apply to prevention of hearing loss.

Thus, the report of the commission stated that "social inequity manifests across various intersecting social categories such as class, education, gender, age, ethnicity, disability, and geography. It signals not simply difference but hierarchy, and reflects deep inequities in the wealth, power, and prestige of different people and communities. People who are already disenfranchised are further disadvantaged with respect to their health" (Page 18)

In addition "Social stratification likewise determines differential access to and utilization of health care, with consequences for the inequitable promotion of health and well-being, disease prevention, and illness recovery and survival." (Page 49)

The Commission concluded that the following actions must be done in order to build health-care systems based on principles of equity, disease prevention, and health promotion:

- Build quality health-care services with universal coverage, focusing on Primary Health Care.
- Strengthen public sector leadership in equitable healthcare systems financing, ensuring universal access to care regardless of ability to pay.

In order to build and strengthen the health workforce, and expand capabilities to act on the social determinants of health, the following actions are needed:

- Invest in national health workforces, balancing rural and urban health-worker density.
- Act to redress the health brain drain, focusing on investment in increased health human resources and training and bilateral agreements to regulate gains and losses".

Conclusion

Prevention is an action to stop a disease or disability from occurring or progressing in an individual or in a population. Primordial prevention targets the prevention of the risk factors and primary, secondary and tertiary prevention arrest the progression of hearing loss through impairment, disability and handicap. WHO now links the medical and social models of disability with a more positive approach that includes addressing environmental factors and personal factors. The rights of persons with disabilities are not incompatible with prevention.

The best strategy for effective prevention makes changes to key risk factors in the population as a whole and not just the high-risk minority. More data needs to be gathered on the burden caused by risk factors for hearing loss as well as on the size of the burden in different populations around the world. Reducing hearing loss by relatively smaller amounts in the many people in a population with mild, moderate and moderately severe hearing loss has a larger effect on the burden than targeting the few with severe or profound loss. The most effective vehicle for most population interventions would be through Primary Ear and Hearing Care, using the WHO manuals on this topic for training. Actions against noise-induced hearing loss should be included amongst these interventions.

Priorities for action include adopting a comprehensive approach, instituting multisectoral action and enabling sustainable development. Surveillance and monitoring is essential to ensure that interventions are effective. It is also important to compare their cost-effectiveness.

Available resources to prevent hearing loss remain inappropriately small, despite its huge cost to society, and its effects on equity.

References

[1]   Armstrong, R. (2011). A Brief History of Healthcare, how did we get it so wrong, where do we go from here? Available from: http://www.nofinishlineblog.com/a-brief-history-of-healthcare-how-did-we-get-it-so-wrong-where-to-we-go-from-here.html (Accessed 12 August 2011).

[2]   Rose, G., Khaw, K-T., Marmot, M. (2011). Rose's Strategy of Preventive Medicine. Oxford: Oxford University Press, 2008. Also on-line at Oxford Scholarship Online. Oxford University Press. Available from: http://www.oxfordscholarship.com/ oso/public/content/publichealthepidemiology/9780192630971/toc.html (Accessed 24 July 2011).

[3]   International Classification of Impairments, Disabilities and Handicaps . (1980). Geneva: World Health Organization.

[4]   International Classification of Functioning, Disability and Health (2002).Geneva: World Health Organization. Available from: http://www3.who.int/icf/icftemplate.cfm (Accessed 30 July 2011).

[5]   Heart and Stroke Foundation of Canada. (2003). The growing burden of heart disease and stroke in Canada. Available from: http://www.cvdinfobase.ca/cvdbook/ CVD_En03.pdf (Accessed 12 August 2011).

[6]   Ursoniu, S. (2009). Primordial prevention, developing countries and the epidemi-ological transition: thirty years later. *Wien Klin Wochenschr,121,* 168-172.

[7]   World Health Organisation, World Bank. (2011). World Report on Disability. WHO, Geneva 2011. Available from: http://www.who.int/disabilities/world_report/2011/en/index.html.

[8]   Smith, A., Bradley, A. K., Wall, R. A., McPherson, B., Secka, A., Dunn, D. T., Green wood, B.M. (1988). Sequelae of epidemic meningococcal meningitis in Africa. *Trans actions of the Royal Society of Tropical Medicine and Hygiene, 82,* 312–320.

[9]   Storbeck, C., Pittman, P. (2008). Early intervention in South Africa: moving beyond hearing screening. *International Journal of Audiology, 47,* Suppl 1 S36-S43. doi:10.1080/14992020802294040 PMID:18781512.

[10]   UN Convention on the Rights of Persons with Disabilities (CRPD). adopted on 13 December 2006 during the sixty-first session of the General Assembly by resolution A/RES/61/106. Available from: http://www2.ohchr.org/english/law/disabilities-convention.htm (Accessed 30 July 2011).

[11]   Officer, A., Groce, N. (2009). Key concepts in disability. *The Lancet, 374,* 1795-1796.

[12]   Lollar, D.J., Crews, J.E. (2003). Redefining the role of public health in disability. *Annual Review of Public Health, 24,*195-208. doi:10.1146/annurev. publhealth. 24.100901.140844 PMID:12668756.

[13]   Coleridge, P., Simonnot, C., Steverlynck, D. (2010). *Study of disability in EC Development Cooperation.* Brussels: European Commission.

[14]   World Federation of the Deaf (WFD). What is Deaf culture? (2011). Available from: http://www.wfdeaf.org/our-work/focus-areas/deaf-culture-2 Accessed on 25 October 2011.

[15]   Resolution of the XIII World Congress of the World Federation of the Deaf (Brisbane, Australia, 25-31 July 1999). Available from: http://www.policy.hu/flora/congress.htm (Accessed 30 July 2011).

[16]   International Federation of Hard of Hearing Young People (IFHOHYP). (2002). Declaration on Genetic Research. Page 10 of booklet "What is IFHOHYP", IFHOHYP, St Petersburg.

[17]   Last, J. (2001). A Dictionary of Epidemiology, (4th Ed.) New York, USA: International Epidemiology Association.

[18]   Murray, C.J.L., Lopez, A.D., (Eds.). (1996).The Global Burden of Disease: a comprehensive assessment of mortality and disability from diseases , injuries and risk factors in 1990 and projected to 2020, (1st ed.). Cambridge, MA: Harvard University Press.

[19]   The global burden of disease: 2004 update. (2008). Geneva: World Health Organi-zation.

[20]   Global Burden of Disease Study. (2010). On-going project: Links to information (1) WHO: Available from: http://www.who.int/healthinfo/global_burden_disease/GBD_2005_study/en/index.html (Accessed 1 August 2011).

[21]   Global Burden of Disease Study. (2010). Available from: http://www.globalburden. org/index.html (Accessed 1 August 2011).

[22]   Lopez A, .Mathers C, Ezzati M, Jamison D, Murray C (Eds.). (2006). *Global burden of disease and risk factors.* Oxford: Oxford University Press and World Bank.

[23]   Mackenzie, I., Smith, A. (2009). Deafness – The neglected and hidden disability. *Annals of Tropical Medicine and Parasitology, 103,* 565–571.

[24] Cook, J., Frick, K.D., Baltussen, R., Resnikoff, S., Smith, A., Mecaskey, J. and Kilima, P. (2006). Loss of vision and hearing. *In*: Jamison, D. T., Breman, J. G., Measham, A. R., Alleyne, G., Claeson, M., Evans, D. B., Jha, P., Mills, A., Musgrove, P.(Eds.), Disease Control Priorities in Developing Countries, (2nd Ed, pp. 953–962). New York, NY: Oxford University Press.

[25] Year 2007 Position Statement: Principles and Guidelines for Early Hearing Detection and Intervention Programs. (2007). Joint Committee on Infant Hearing. *Pediatrics,120*;898. DOI: 10.1542/peds.2007-2333. Available from: http://pediatrics. aappublications.org/content/120/4/898.full.html (Accessed 1 August 2011).

[26] Vohr, B.R., Widen, J.E., Cone-Wesson, B., Sininger,Y.S., Gorga, M.P., Folsom,R.C., Norton, S.J. (2000). Identification of Neonatal Hearing Impairment: Characteristics of Infants in the Neonatal Intensive Care Unit and Well-Baby Nursery. *Ear and Hearing, 21*, 373–382.

[27] Changing History: The World Health Report 2004, Statistical Annex Table 3. (2004).Geneva:World Health Organisation. Available from: http://www.who.int/ whr/2004/annex/topic/en/annex_3_en.pdf. (Accessed 1 August 2011).

[28] Smith A, and Mathers C. (2006). Epidemiology of Infection as a Cause of Hearing Loss. In: Infection and Hearing Impairment. V. Newton, P. Vallely, London: Whurr/Wiley.

[29] Pascolini, D. and Smith, A. (2009). Hearing impairment in 2008: a compilation of available epidemiological studies. *International Journal of Audiology, 48*, 1–13.

[30] Stevens, G.A., Flaxman, S., Brunskill, E., Mascarenhas M,, Mathers, C.D., Finucane, M.M. (2011). Global and regional hearing impairment prevalence: an analysis of 42 studies in 29 countries. *European Journal of Public Health.* doi: 10.1093/eurpub/ckr176

[31] Development, Implementation and Evaluation of a Community Based Hearing Aid Service. (2009). Report by Departments of Otorhinolaryngology and Community Health Christian Medical College, Vellore and Scheffelin Institute Of Health - Leprosy And Research Centre Karigiri. WWHearing Executive Committee. Unpublished Document available from the Secretary, at asmith@wwhearing.org

[32] Technological Report: Measuring the Outcomes and Cost-Effectiveness of Hearing Aid Programs for Marginalized Hearing Impaired Children in Guangxi province and Beijing, China. (2008). Report by Pilot Team from China Rehabilitation Research Centre for Deaf Children (CRRCDC) to WWHearing Executive Committee. Unpublished Document available from the Secretary, at asmith@wwhearing.org.

[33] Baltussen, R., Li, J., Wu, L., Hui Ge, X., Teng, B., Sun, X., Han, R., Wang, X., McPherson, B. (2009).Costs of screening children for hearing disorders and delivery of hearing aids in China . *BMC (BioMed Central) Health Services Research*, 9, 64 doi:10.1186/1472-6963-9-64. Available from: http://www.biomedcentral.com/1472-6963/9/64

[34] Baltussen, R., Vinod, A., Monica, P., Balraj, A., Job, A., Norman, G., Joseph, A. (2009). Costs and health effects of screening and delivery of hearing aids in Tamil Nadu, India: an observational study BMC (BioMed Central) *Public Health, 9*, 135 doi:10.1186/1471-2458-9-135. Available from: http://www.biomedcentral.com/1471-2458/9/135

[35] WWHearing Affiliated Projects. Available from: http://www.wwhearing.org/affiliated-projects/ (Accessed 24 September 2011).

[36] Hearing Express Model Project. WWHearing website (page called Make Hearing Matter). http://www.wwhearing.org/hearing-express/ (Accessed 10 August 2011).

[37] World Health Organisation Guidelines on Hearing Aids and Services for Developing Countries.(2004).(2nd Ed.), Geneva: World Health Organisation. Available from: http://whqlibdoc.who.int/publications/2004/9241592435_eng.pdf (Accessed 10 August 2011).

[38] AUDIO-2020 - the global initiative of WWHearing in collaboration with the World Health Organization (WHO). Available from: http://www.wwhearing.org/audio-20-20/. (Accessed 25 September 2011).

[39] World Health Organization. (2006). Primary Ear and Hearing Care Training Resource. Basic Level, Intermediate Level Students Workbook, Intermediate Level Trainers Manual, Advanced Level. Geneva: World Health Organisation. Download manuals from: http://www.who.int/pbd/deafness/activities/hearing_care/en/index.html (Accessed 2 August 2011)

[40] World Health Organisation. (1991). Report of the Informal Working Group on Prevention of Deafness and Hearing Impairment Programme Planning. Document WHO/PDH/91.1. Geneva: World Health Organisation.

[41] World Health Organisation. (2005). Preventing Chronic Diseases – a vital investment. Geneva: WHO. Available from: http://www.who.int/chp/chronic_disease_report/part1/en/index17.html (Accessed 2 August 2011).

[42] WWHearing. (2007). Affordable Hearing Aids a stepwise framework. 2007 Geneva: WWHearing. Unpublished Document available from the Secretary, at asmith@wwhearing.org.

[43] World Health Organisation. (2011). Global status report on Non-Communicable Diseases 2010, Geneva: World Health Organization. Available from: http://whqlibdoc.who.int/publications/2011/9789240686458_eng.pdf (Accessed 24 September 2011).

[44] Ruben, R. (2000). Redefining the survival of the fittest: communication disorders in the 21st century. *The Laryngoscope, 10*, 241-245.

[45] Anon. (2006). Listen, Hear: the Economic Impact and Cost of Hearing Loss in Australia. Canberra: Access Economics.

[46] Harrop-Griffiths, K. (Year) The prevention of hearing and balance disorders. In: A.G. Kerr, (Ed.) Scott, Brown's Otolaryngology, (6th Ed., pp. 2/8/1-26)). .

[47] Krumholz H, Weintraub, W. Bradford D, Heidenreich P, Mark D, and Paltiel A. (2002). Task Force #2—The Cost of Prevention. Can We Afford It? Can We Afford Not To Do It? *JACC.40*, 603-615.

[48] Saunders, G.H., Griest, S.E. (2009).Hearing loss in veterans and the need for hearing loss prevention programs. *Noise and Health, 11*, 14-21.

[49] Kennedy, K., Anderson, J.R., War is hell — on your hearing. Available from: www.armytimes.com/news/2010/04/offduty_hearing_042310w (Accessed 12 August 2011).

[50] EUROGIP.- Europe Groupement d'intérêt public - (2004). Costs and funding of occupational diseases in Europe - The European Forum of Insurances against Accidents at Work and Occupational Diseases: Eurogip-08/E August 2004. Available from: http://www.eurogip.fr/en/docs/Eurogip_cout_financement_2004_08E.pdf (Accessed 11 August 2011).

[51] Kramer, S., Kapteyn, T., Houtgast, T., (2006). Occupational performance: Comparing normally-hearing and hearing-impaired employees using the Amsterdam Checklist for Hearing and Work. *International Journal of Audiology, 45*, 503-512.

[52] Couzos, S. (2004). Practical measures that improve human rights– towards health equity for Aboriginal children. *Health Promotion Journal of Australia, 15*, 186-192. Available from: http://www.naccho.org.au/Files/Documents/HPJA%202004-3%2002-Couzos.pdf (Accessed 25 September 2011).

[53] Shield, B. (2005). Evaluation of the social and economic costs of hearing impairment. London South Bank University. Researched and written for www.hear-it.org, 2005.

[54] Kochkin, S., Marke, T. VIII. (2010). The efficacy of hearing aids in achieving compensation equity in the workplace. *Hearing Journal, 63*, 19-24,26,28. doi: 10.1097 /01.HJ.0000389923.80044.e6. Available from: http://journals.lww.com/thehearing - journal/ Fulltext/2010/10000/MarkeTrak_ VIII__The_efficacy_ of_hearing_aids_ in. 4. aspx#P92. (Accessed 25 September 2011).

[55] World Health Organisation. (2008). Closing the gap in a generation. Health equity through action on the social determinants of health. Final Report: Commission on Social Determinants of Health, Geneva: WHO Available from: http://whqlibdoc. who.int/publications/2008/9789241563703_eng.pdf (Accessed 12 August 2011).

In: Prevention of Hearing Loss
Editors: V. Newton, P. Alberti and A. Smith

ISBN: 978-1-61942-745-7
© 2012 Nova Science Publishers, Inc.

Chapter VI

The Role of Immunisation in the Prevention of Hearing Loss

*Peter S. Morris** and Amanda J. Leach*

Abstract

The Expanded Programme of Immunisation represents one of the great public health achievements of the last 50 years. In 1974, the programme established a core set of 6 vaccines (BCG, diphtheria, tetanus, pertussis, polio, and measles) and a coverage target of 90% by 1990. The contribution of immunisation to early childhood mortality and disability has been substantial. With 20 vaccine preventable diseases now being addressed, immunisation will continue to reduce poor outcomes associated with infection (including hearing loss) throughout the world.

To date, the largest gains in the prevention of severe to profound sensorineural hearing loss have come from the measles and rubella vaccines, and the protein-conjugated bacterial meningitis vaccines (targeting Hib, pneumococcal and mening-ococcal disease). Most of the mild and moderate conductive hearing loss in the world is associated with otitis media. To some extent, OM is a vaccine preventable disease. In the future, the development of otitis media vaccines (or combinations of vaccines) that reduce colonisation and protect against common respiratory bacterial and viral pathogens has the potential to dramatically reduce the frequency of mild and moderate hearing loss in young children.

The World Health Organization (WHO) estimates that around 4% of the world's population has a hearing disability and 6% have a hearing impairment [1, 2]. The majority of these individuals live in developing countries. In this setting, preventable or treatable infection remains the most important cause of disease.

In developed countries with comprehensive health systems, rates of acquired hearing impairment in children should be decreasing [3]. Bacterial meningitis is on the decline [4] and chronic middle ear infections associated with permanent hearing loss is uncommon (affecting <1% of the population) [5]. The contribution of immunisation to these improvements has been substantial.

* Corresponding author: peter.morris@menzies.edu.au.

Overall, the WHO estimates that around 50% of the burden of hearing impairment is preventable [1]. In this chapter, we consider how much hearing impairment is prevented by immunisation and how this may change in the future. The overall benefits of immunisation have been widely applauded: ... "With the exception of safe water, no other modality, not even antibiotics, has had such an effect on mortality reduction..." [6, 7]. However, the impact on specific disabilities (such as hearing impairment) is less clear.

How Immunisation Prevents Hearing Loss

Immunisation has the potential to prevent any hearing loss that occurs following infection. Generally, infection causes persistent hearing loss though one of the following diseases processes: i) congenital infection; ii) bacterial meningitis; iii) labyrinthitis; and iv) otitis media [8,9]. Infection may also be associated with hearing loss indirectly through the use of ototoxic antibiotics. Finally, although the exact mechanism is often unclear, hearing loss may also be one of the sequelae of a severe infection complicated by hypoxic, ischaemic or haemorrhagic brain injury, severe hypotension, encephalitis, or encephalopathy.

Congenital Infection

Congenital infection (or perinatal infection) is defined as infection that is transmitted from the mother to foetus or baby during pregnancy or child birth. Some of these infections (e.g. rubella, cytomegalovirus, toxoplasma and syphilis) may be associated with sensorineural hearing loss. The frequency and severity of the hearing loss will vary with the timing of infection and the causative infectious agent [10, 11]. Severe or profound hearing loss is most likely when infection occurs in the first trimester and if the infection is caused by rubella or cytomegalovirus (CMV) [10, 11].

Bacterial Meningitis

Bacterial meningitis is defined as inflammation of the protective membranes around the brain and spinal cord (the meninges) that occurs with a bacterial infection [11, 12]. The associated hearing loss is sensorineural and due to the development of suppurative labyrinthitis [13]. Spread of infection into the labyrinth occurs either: i) via the CSF though the cochlear aqueduct or internal auditory canal; ii) from pathogen also located in the middle ear that pass the oval or round windows; or iii) via the bloodstream in associated bacteraemia. The frequency and severity of hearing loss will vary with the type of infection, the severity of the infection, the age of the affected individual, and the causative infectious agent [12]. Severe or profound hearing loss is most likely in meningitis in a young child due to *Streptococcus pneumoniae* [14]. While many viral infections have been implicated in the development of sudden hearing loss through viral labyrinthitis (see below), hearing loss is not usually a complication of viral meningitis (although it can occur).

Bacterial meningitis is the most common cause of acquired sensorineural hearing loss in childhood and affects 3-18% of survivors [14]. Another 10% have transient hearing loss caused by direct damage to the cochlea, labyrinth, or 8th nerves either as bacterial invasion or associated with the inflammatory response [15]. The hearing loss in bacterial meningitis occurs relatively early (within 48 hours) and may recover or progress over the next 2-6 weeks [15].

Labyrinthitis

Infectious labyrinthitis can be suppurative or non-suppurative [11, 12]. Suppurative infections are usually bacterial and associated with meningitis (see above) or severe otitis media or mastoiditis (see below). Non-suppurative infections are usually viral. These non-suppurative infections are responsible for some of the 5-30 individuals per 100,000 who develop sudden onset sensorineural hearing loss each year [16]. For the majority of individuals affected by this condition, the aetiology is never elucidated [17]. The most commonly implicated viruses are mumps, herpes, CMV, measles, influenza, and Epstein-Barr virus (EBV) [17]. The associated hearing loss is sensorineural and its frequency and severity will vary with the type of infection, the severity of the infection, the age of the affected individual, and the causative infectious agent. Severe or profound hearing loss is most likely in severe viral labyrinthitis in an adult due to herpes virus. The hearing loss associated with labyrinthitis may be temporary or may persist (or progress) over time [16].

Otitis Media

Otitis media (OM) is defined as infection or inflammation of the middle ear space. OM is usually associated with the presence of a middle effusion which is responsible for the initial conductive hearing loss [18, 19]. The hearing loss is usually mild (~25dB) and only clinically significant if it is persistent and affects both ears. Otitis media is best regarded as a spectrum of disease. There are 4 common presentations of active infection: i) otitis media with effusion (OME); ii) acute otitis media without perforation (AOMwoP); iii) acute otitis media with perforation (AOMwiP); and iv) chronic suppurative otitis media (CSOM) [20]. OME and AOM are associated with both viral and bacterial infections. Bacterial infection can occur following an initial viral infection. More than one virus or bacterium can be involved in a single infection. The most important bacterial aetiological agents are *Streptococcus pneumoniae* (pneumococcus), *Haemophilus influenzae* and *Moraxella catarrhalis* [18, 19]. Viruses implicated in the development of OM include: respiratory syncytial virus (RSV), influenza, rhinovirus, adenovirus, parainfluenza virus, and human metapneumovirus. If the initial AOM is associated with perforation of the tympanic membrane and this infection persists over many weeks, the TM perforation increases in size and a diagnosis of chronic suppurative OM is appropriate [18, 19, 20]. CSOM is associated with more significant hearing loss (around 35 dB). Unfortunately, this condition is associated with more complex mixed infection (with opportunistic pathogens *Pseudomonas*, *Proteus* and *Staphylococcus* species frequently isolated) and can be difficult to treat [5, 18]. The WHO recommends that if CSOM affects more than 4% of population, it should be regarded as a public health emergency [22].

Such high rates of CSOM are seen in some developing countries and disadvantaged populations (especially Indigenous populations) [20]. CSOM contributes the largest burden of preventable persistent hearing loss and hearing disability throughout the world [22].

Ototoxic Antibiotics

The association between antibiotic use and hearing loss has been recognised since the beginning of the antibiotic era. While streptomycin was shown to be a highly effective treatment for tuberculosis from 1944 onwards, many treated patients developed sensorineural hearing loss or vestibular impairment [8]. Hearing loss occurs as a result of damage to the more sensitive outer cochlear hair cells. It is usually bilateral and irreversible. It is now recognised that there is an associated genetic susceptibility and some families have more than one member affected [23]. In some countries, where aminoglycosides (like streptomycin and gentamycin) are freely available or prescribed without careful monitoring, antibiotic use is regarded as an important cause of preventable severe hearing impairment. While neonates and children are less often affected than adults, currently available data from developed countries cannot exclude a hearing impairment after treatment in as many as 1-2% of neonates and young children [24]. Macrolide antibiotics (like erythromycin and azithromycin) have also been associated with hearing loss [11]. This hearing loss occurs much less often than with aminoglycosides and is usually temporary. Vancomycin is a glycopeptide antibiotic that is used to treat oxacillin resistant staphylococcal infections. Reports of associated hearing loss have occurred in adults with either high serum levels or concurrent use of aminoglycosides.

A Brief History of Immunisation

Immunisation is defined as "Rendering a person or animal immune to certain infections by the process of injecting either antigen or a serum containing specific antibodies." 'Active immunisation' involves exposure to an antigen to stimulate a protective antibody response while 'passive immunisation' involves injection of preformed antibodies. The term 'vaccination' was used originally to describe use of the smallpox vaccine prepared from vaccinia virus infection (cowpox). Today, its meaning is synonymous with immunisation.

The World Health Organization (WHO) estimates that around 14% of the global under 5 mortality is vaccine preventable. The strength of immunisation is the ability to prevent serious diseases at relatively low cost. This is particularly attractive in countries where access to modern medical care is either limited or hard to access. Every country in the world now has some form of immunisation programme [25]. National (or universal) immunisation schedules describe those vaccines that are delivered to the whole population. Each country also has a list of other vaccines that are indicated for selected high-risk individuals (or populations) or are available for purchase.

The Smallpox Story [26]

As far as we know, immunisation was first used as a large scale intervention to prevent smallpox. Smallpox vaccination is now the model of successful infection control. In the middle ages, smallpox affected 10-20% of European populations. Of those affected by the more severe form of the disease, around 30% died. At that time, a practice of 'variolation' (deliberate skin infection with the pustules of someone infected with smallpox) was occurring in China and some parts of Europe. Variolation was associated with development of pustules in the area inoculated but a much milder associated illness and considerably lower risk of death (although death did occur in 1-2%). An English country doctor, Edward Jenner, pursued and publicised the observation that milkmaids who had been infected with cowpox (due to vaccinia virus) were resistant to varioloation and smallpox. He agreed with others before him that exposure to cowpox was protective and proposed that deliberate exposure might prevent disease. In 1796, he began his experiments when he vaccinated an 8 year old child and then repeatedly exposed him to smallpox. His case series of 23 vaccinated patients was published in 1800. It prompted great interest in vaccination in Europe and North America. However, protection did not come without risks. Cross-infection and contamination were not understood, and deliberate infection with pus from cowpox pustules could be complicated by infection with other pathogens (including smallpox).

In recognition of Jenner's work, Louis Pasteur labelled the general process of inoculation to prevent disease as 'vaccination'. The impact of Jenner's efforts on public health was dramatic. Life expectancy in regions with effective vaccination programmes began to increase. By the middle of the 19th century, the UK had a national smallpox vaccination programme. In 1960, the smallpox vaccine programme was expanded globally by the WHO. In 1979, the WHO declared that smallpox had been eradicated.

The Global Initiative

In 1948, vaccines in widespread use in developed countries included smallpox, diphtheria, tetanus and pertussis [27, 28]. In that year, the first combination vaccine covering diphtheria, tetanus and pertussis was made available (known as DTP or triple antigen). In 1955, polio vaccine was licensed in the USA. Global immunisation became a focus of the WHO when it approved a strategy to eradicate smallpox in 1959. Its initial plan of mass vaccination was broadened to include case finding and appropriate management through the Intensified Smallpox Eradication Programme in 1967 [26]. The WHO continued to support greater use of BCG, diphtheria, tetanus, pertussis vaccines. In 1974, the launch of the Expanded Programme of Immunization (EPI) established a core set of 6 vaccines (BCG, diphtheria, tetanus, pertussis, polio, and measles) and a coverage target of 90% by 1990 [29]. At that time, less than 5% of the world's population had been vaccinated against these diseases. More recently, the WHO and partners also facilitate greater use of 8 new and underused vaccines (hepatitis B, *Haemophilus influenzae* type b, mumps, pneumococcus, rotavirus, rubella, yellow fever, and Japanese encephalitis). In the future, this list will expand and may include some of the 6 other currently available vaccines (human papillomavirus, meningococcus, influenza, rabies, hepatitis A, typhoid and varicella vaccines). Overall, there are now 20 vaccine preventable diseases being addressed with available vaccines around the world.

Recent improvement in the global vaccine initiative have been a consequence of economic growth, reduced cost and increased availability of vaccines, and substantial increases in funding for programme in developing countries [7]. Since 2000, the GAVI Alliance (Global Alliance for Vaccination and Immunisation) has dramatically increased funding for vaccine delivery [30]. This has been associated with a steady increase in vaccine coverage in poorer countries.

The complexity of the immunisation schedule has also increased over the last 20 years. In Australia, the number of diseases prevented by approved vaccines in the national schedule has increased from 7 in 1991 to 15 in 2011 [28]. Similar increases are described in all developed countries. Although the emphasis is still on early childhood, there are now vaccines for adult health problems as well. Hepatitis B and human papillomavirus (HPV) vaccines have been proven to prevent cancer [7]. In the future, we may also accept that some chronic diseases are preventable by vaccination.

Childhood Immunisation Schedule

Examples of typical universal immunisation programmes are shown in Table 1 [31]. In some places, a total of 8 vaccines are delivered in the first 6 months of age (infant vaccines) and another 5 are delivered between 6 months and 5 years of age (early childhood vaccines). Currently, only HPV immunisation begins in late childhood. Polysaccharide pneumococcal vaccine and influenza vaccine are often given as part of the universal immunisation schedule for older members (e.g. >65 years) of the population.

In developing countries, it is now possible to expand the number of vaccines included in the universal national schedule. This is largely due to a series of recent innovative funding initiatives. These initiatives use a business model to support the introduction of more expensive early childhood vaccines (into relatively poor countries) through market shaping, co-funding, and collaboration with pharmaceutical companies through advance market commitments (that allow vaccines to be purchased at dramatically lower cost) [7, 30, 32].

Important Adverse Events Associated with Immunisation

A major challenge to immunisation programmes is ensuring that health intervention do more good than harm. This is particularly important for preventive interventions where healthy individuals are exposed to an intervention to prevent an illness that they may never get (or get in such a mild form that it is of no consequence). Since immunisation requires deliberate exposure to an antigen that is sufficient to cause an immune response, adverse events are common [28]. These should be anticipated and discussed with the family. For several vaccines, 10-20% of vaccinated children experience side effects within 24 hours (pain or swelling at the site of injection, fever, and rash occur most frequently) [28]. The measles-mumps-rubella vaccine (MMR) is associated with a rash and fever 5-12 days after immunisation in 5-15% of children 28]. More serious reactions like anaphylaxis may affect up to 1 in 300,000 children and usually have an onset within 15 minutes of immunisation [28].

One of the paradoxes associated with immunisation is that once a population is almost completely (and effectively) immunised against an infection, the risk of acquiring disease becomes very low [33]. In these circumstances, the most important benefit of immunisation is protection of any unimmunised members of the community (especially young infants) and anyone who is immuno-compromised. For the immunised individual, the direct benefit is reduced (because the risk of disease is reduced) while the potential side effects have not changed. This paradox has been seen with polio immunisation using the live oral vaccine. In the USA from 1985 to 2000 (prior to the introduction of inactivated polio vaccine- IPV), nearly all cases (around 8 per year) were vaccine associated paralytic polio (VAPP) [33].

Eligibility for Immunization

Vaccines are designed to be suitable for use in all individuals at risk of infection. However, there are some important exceptions. In some circumstances, immunisation has reduced effectiveness [28] - inappropriate age (e.g. some vaccines not protective in neonates and/or infants), previous immunisation within 4 weeks, and previous treatment with blood products or immunoglobulin. In addition, there are some circumstances where there is an increased potential for side effects- allergy, previous severe reaction, pregnancy, or use of live vaccines in immuno-compromised individuals. Anaphylaxis is the only absolute contraindication to immunisation [28].

Current Global Immunisation Coverage

Data on vaccination coverage is collected for all countries and is available for download at http://www.who.int/immunization_monitoring/data/en/ [31]. Overall coverage for the most important performance indicators (DPT3- 3rd dose by 1st birthday and measles containing vaccine- 1 dose by 2nd birthday) was 82% in 2009 [25]. Of the 193 member countries in the WHO, 122 have achieved 90% coverage of DTP3, and 157 have achieved 80%. The data are similar (but not quite as good) for measles (see Figure 1). There are fewer data on seroconversion, so actual protection associated with vaccination programmes is less well described [25]. Overall, the reported coverage for measles and DPT3 varies from 69-71% in the African region to 94-96% in the European region. In recent years, global coverage has increased steadily from 16-20% in 1980 to 82% in 2009 [25]. However, within some countries and for some vaccines, periods of reduced coverage occur. Unfortunately, this often leads to a sharp increase in disease.

Challenges Facing Vaccination Programmes

Globally, there are 2 important barriers to complete coverage: i) lack of resources to allow production, storage, transportation, and delivery of immunisation according to the recommended schedule; and ii) refusal of parents to participate in the immunisation programme [25, 34, 35]. The lack of resources is most important in developing countries while a conscious decision to refuse vaccination is most problematic in developed countries. Managing the impact of 'conscientious objectors' will become increasingly important over time as more countries can afford a comprehensive immunisation programme that is free to families [35, 36].

While delivery of an effective immunisation programme may appear simple, there are many issues to be considered: i) the cost of each vaccine; ii) local production or importation of vaccines; iii) appropriate storage and transport of vaccines; iv) effective delivery of vaccines; v) monitoring of vaccination status; vi) monitoring of side effects [7]. Dealing with all of these is challenging in resource poor settings. Most vaccines require an infant immunisation programme to achieve maximum protection. This is associated with multiple health care visits in the first few months of life. Since this is when children are most at risk of serious illness, the immunisation schedule is often incorporated into an early childhood surveillance programme [37].

The large variability in vaccine delivery between countries has been appreciated for some time. A strategy to address disparities in immunisation coverage within the same country was introduced in 2002. The RED Initiative (Reaching Every District) aims to ensure that every district with a population of around 1 million achieves immunisation coverage of at least 80% for the 6 core vaccines [7, 38, 39]. The RED approach recommends using data on infant immunisation to prioritise districts (and regions within districts) with low immunisation uptake. Where improvement is needed, the initiative concentrates on the following 5 components of successful programmes: i) regular outreach services; ii) on-site support and training; iii) community links with service delivery; iv) using monitoring data for action; and v) better management of human and financial resources [7, 38]. Vaccines are often provided as part of local health days and can also be given with vitamin A, zinc, insecticide-treated bed nets, and anticipatory guidance. Clearly, with a more holistic approach health benefits may extend beyond those attributable to the immunisation service.

Appropriate Storage and Transport of Vaccines (the 'Cold Chain')

Most vaccines need to be stored at 2-8 degrees (promoted as "Strive for Five" in Australia) [28]. This is done to ensure that the antigen (usually a protein) that elicits the immune response is not structurally affected by freezing or overheating. The requirement for refrigeration has important implications for both storage and transport. As countries need to deliver vaccines to remote regions that often lack basic infrastructure, lack of suitable carriers and storage capacity can be a major barrier. The development of vaccine vial monitors (VVMs) has helped programme identify problems with their cold chain [37]. The monitors also increase flexibility for use of vaccines outside the cold chain, and reduce vaccine wastage. In the future, we are likely to see more use of relatively thermostable vaccines (like hepatitis B) outside of the cold chain, and the mass production of vaccines that do not require refrigeration [7, 40]. Additionally, new vaccines that can be taken orally, by nasal spray, and by transdermal patch are likely to be less reliant on temperature stability [7].

Evidence of Effectiveness for Established Vaccines

In this era of evidence-based practice, it has become increasingly important to assess the data used for decision-making. For this chapter, we have searched the Medline database to indentify publications that have assessed the impact of immunisation on hearing loss. We looked for evidence of reduction of risk of hearing loss, congenital infection, bacterial meningitis, labyrinthitis, and otitis media. We prioritised systematic reviews (especially Cochrane reviews) and randomised controlled trials published since 2000 for evidence of effect. Since none of the currently available vaccines were developed or tested with prevention of hearing loss as their primary focus, we accepted that the amount of data available (or accessible via our search strategy) was likely to be limited (and any estimates would be imprecise). We also recognise that many of the vaccines assessed were introduced more than 50 years ago and consequently important studies may not be accessible through the Medline database. This should be taken into account when considering the evidence. We did not specifically look for studies on antibiotic-associated ototoxity or hearing loss associated with severe infection not associated with onset in utero, meningitis, or ear diseases (including labyrinthitis and otitis media).

Vaccine efficacy is usually described as 1-RR (relative risk) i.e., if the relative risk of infection after immunisation, RR=0.1 then the vaccine efficacy is 90%. If herd immunity occurs, vaccine efficacy will underestimate the number of cases of disease that are prevented. The public health impact of an immunisation programme (the number of cases prevented) will be determined by the underlying risk of disease combined with vaccine efficacy (plus any additional herd immunity effects). While vaccine efficacy is usually assumed to be fairly consistent across different populations, underlying risk of disease varies substantially in different settings for most infections.

Search Strategy

The Medline database was accessed using PubMed and the following Medical Subject Heading (mesh) search terms:

i   (immunisation[mesh] OR vaccines[mesh]) AND (hearing loss[mesh] OR "congenital infection" OR "perinatal infection" OR "intrauterine infection" OR "transplacental infection" OR meningitis[mesh] OR ear diseases[mesh])

ii   (immunisation[mesh]) combined with the specific infectious disease mesh was used to identify the evidence of effectiveness and the current published literature on vaccine under development.

iii Evidence of effectiveness was identified through the combination of i) and ii) above with the following search terms "AND (clinical trial[pt] OR systematic[sb] OR clin evid[journal])". We also searched the Cochrane Library (Wiley Publishing) and Clinical Evidence (BMJ Publishing). The last search was conducted on July 9th 2011.

BCG Vaccine

The Bacille Calmette-Guerin (BCG) vaccine is a live strain of mycobacterium bovi that protects against *Mycobacterium tuberculosis* (TB) [11]. It has been used since 1921.

Tuberculosis infects around 8 million individuals each year worldwide and is the most common vaccine preventable cause of death (see Table 1). BCG immunisation is usually given as a single dose in the neonatal period in countries (or regions or populations) with high rates of tuberculosis.

Manifestations of TB infection include pulmonary and extra-pulmonary disease. The association with hearing loss is a common complication of tuberculous meningitis. In some settings [11, 41, 42], it will also be due to the use of streptomycin [43]. This antibiotic is no longer part of recommended standard treatment regime for uncomplicated tuberculosis. However, streptomycin and other aminoglycosides are still used as additional second-line therapies in multi-drug-resistant TB infection (MDR-TB) [44].

Sensorineural hearing loss is estimated to occur in 10-30% of tuberculous meningitis survivors [45]. The extent that this is due to infection or a complication of antibiotic treatment (or both) is not clear. Tuberculous otitis media has also been described [46]. This is believed to be uncommon.

We identified no Cochrane review but several other systematic reviews [47 – 50]. Evidence of the effectiveness of BCG vaccination is clear but the estimates of protection are inconsistent. Overall, trials of the vaccine have found inconsistent and modest levels of protection (around to 50%) [47 – 51]. Prevention of more severe infection (miliary TB and meningitis) appears to be greater than protection against any TB infection [50]. There are no data directly related to prevention of hearing loss.

Measles-Mumps-Rubella Vaccine (MMR)

Measles is one of the universal 6 core vaccines and was first introduced in 1969 [27, 28]. The measles-mumps-rubella vaccine (MMR) is a combination attenuated live vaccine that was introduced in developed countries in 1971. In some countries, varicella is also included in the combination (MMRV). Prior to the introduction of combination vaccines, measles and rubella had existed as single vaccines that were widely used. While many countries now use MMR or MMRV, many developing countries have elected to delay the introduction of rubella vaccination until they are confident they will achieve high rates of coverage. The WHO currently recommends that a country should achieve >80% coverage of measles containing vaccine before introducing a rubella containing vaccine [37]. The reason for this is that failure to achieve high coverage may paradoxically result in more women reaching child bearing age susceptible to rubella infection (by reducing opportunities for natural protection through infection in early childhood). In these circumstances, introduction of rubella vaccination in childhood could lead to an increase in congenital rubella syndrome.

Prior to the introduction of these immunisations, measles, mumps and rubella were all common childhood illnesses [11, 12]. Everyone would expect to be exposed to these viruses at some point in their life (usually in early childhood). Both measles and rubella were included in the 6 classical infectious disease exanthems of childhood (first and third disease).

The clinical manifestations of measles infections include fever, rash, conjunctivitis, and bronchitis [11, 12]. Around 1% of infected children have illnesses complicated by encephalitis and around 1 in 1,000 develop subacute sclerosing panencephalitis (SSPE) as a long-term complication [11, 12]. In developing countries, the mortality associated with measles in young children is substantial [37]. The hearing loss associated with measles is likely to occur through labyrinthitis. Before 1950, measles was thought to be responsible for 4-20% of childhood sensorineural hearing loss in developed countries [11]. Overall, around 0.1% (or 1 in 1,000) children with measles will develop sensorineural hearing loss. Studies conducted in developing countries before vaccination improved also found very high rates [52]. The hearing loss is mild/moderate in 55% and 45% have a profound loss. Presumably the rapid reduction in measles mortality over the last decade has been accompanied by reductions in hearing loss as well [7, 53].

Measles has also been associated with otitis media (occurring in around 9%) and otosclerosis [11]. While a causal relationship between measles infection and otosclerosis has not been proven, supporting evidence includes reduction in otosclerosis following widespread measles vaccination and identification of measles DNA and RNA in otosclerotic stapes footplates [54].

The clinical manifestations of rubella include fever and rash [11, 12]. Rubella has milder but similar features to measles. This led to its other name, German measles (from 'germane to measles'). While rubella is usually a mild illness is children and adults, it can be devastating for the unborn foetus. Congenital rubella infection can result in stillbirth, microcephaly, intellectual disability, epilepsy, blindness, and sensorineural hearing loss. Congenital infection is most likely to have severe consequences when it occurs in the first trimester. In countries that introduced the vaccine, rates of congenital rubella syndrome have decreased by 99% [37]. Overall, 5-25% of women of child bearing age are susceptible to infection [11, 12]. In those infected, sensorineural hearing loss occurs in 68-93%. It is usually bilateral, profound, and sometimes progresses.

The clinical manifestations of mumps infection include fever, rash, parotitis and orchitis [11, 12]. Occasionally mumps is complicated by aseptic meningitis. Hearing loss associated with mumps is likely to occur through labyrinthitis and it is often unilateral (80%) [11, 12]. Overall, hearing loss affects around 0.05% (i.e. 1 in 2000).

The MMR vaccine is currently usually given as a single dose at around 12 months of age with a booster in late childhood [28]. Some developing countries still give the measles vaccine alone and may still give this early at 6-9 months of age. In these settings, the aim is to protect the infant from overwhelming measles infection in the months leading up to their first birthday.

We identified one Cochrane review and several non-Cochrane systematic reviews [58, 59]. The Cochrane review did not find evidence of effectiveness of the vaccine from the small number of published randomised controlled trials but concluded that changes in incidence data associated with vaccination are consistent with the vaccine being highly effective [37, 55]. Countries effectively vaccinating children before 1 year of age can anticipate a vaccine efficacy of around 85% [57, 58]. The systematic reviews did not specifically look at the impact on hearing loss.

Haemophilus Influenzae Type B Vaccine

Haemophilus influenza type b (Hib) was the first infection to be prevented by the widespread use of a protein-conjugated vaccine [11, 12]. By attaching the polysaccharide capsule to an immunogenic protein, young children are able to generate a B cell response and produce anti-capsular antibodies on re-exposure. Hib infection is an important cause of disease in young children. Prior to the introduction of immunisation, Hib was the most frequent cause of meningitis and bacteraemia in infants [11, 12]. The clinical manifestations of infection include sepsis, bacteraemia, meningitis, epiglottitis, pneumonia, cellulitis (especially peri-orbital cellulitis), arthritis, and osteomyelitis [11, 12]. The association with hearing loss is most likely to occur through meningitis and associated inflammation of the cochlea. Hib meningitis is complicated by sensorineural hearing loss in around 3-8% of affected children [14]. Nearly all invasive Hib disease occurs in young children.

The infant Hib conjugate vaccine is available as single vaccine or as part of a combination vaccine that includes the triple antigen (diphtheria, tetanus and pertussis). The schedule usually consists of 3 doses given in the first 6 months of life with a booster after 12 months [28]. Herd immunity contributes additional protection through the impact of immunisation on nasopharyngeal colonisation [11, 12]. In countries with successful immunisation programme rates of early childhood meningitis and epiglottitis have been dramatically reduced [11, 12].

We identified one Cochrane review (withdrawn 2009) and several non-Cochrane systematic reviews [60 – 62]. While the reviews were consistent in finding that immunisation was associated with large reduction in Hib disease, there was little information on the impact on hearing. The overall vaccine efficacy estimated from the trials was around 80%. A recently published review of the global burden of Hib disease highlighted the very large number of deaths, meningitis and pneumonia cases. This review did not include hearing loss as an outcome [63].

Pneumococcal Vaccine

There are currently 2 forms of pneumococcal vaccine in widespread usage. There is a polysaccharide vaccine that includes 23 (of around 90) pneumococcal serotypes. This is used most commonly to prevent invasive pneumococcal disease and pneumonia in adults (11,12). In addition, there are conjugate pneumococcal vaccines where 7-13 serotypes are conjugated to a protein [11,12]. Protein conjugation makes the vaccine immunogenic in infants. If affordable, 3 doses of the conjugate vaccine should be given early in the first year of life [28].

Pneumococcal disease affects a large proportion of all populations. Clinical manifestations of infection include sepsis, bacteraemia, meningitis, pneumonia, bronchitis, sinusitis, otitis media, arthritis, and osteomyelitis [11, 12]. The association with hearing loss is most likely to occur through meningitis and otitis media. Pneumoccoccal meningitis has a relatively high risk of sensorineural hearing loss (from 9-19%) [14].This disease can affect all ages but rates are highest in the very young and elderly. The polyvalent polysaccharide vaccine is recommended in many developed countries to be given as a single dose in adults at risk (including those aged 65 years or older [28]. In the past, repeat vaccination after 5 years has been used. Concerns about increasing rates of local reactions meant this practice is no longer recommended. The infant pneumococcal conjugate vaccine schedule usually consists of 3 doses given in the first 6 months of life with a booster after 12 months [28]. We identified three Cochrane reviews and several non-Cochrane systematic reviews [64 – 68]. The impact of the vaccine on meningitis and bacteraemia was substantial (vaccine efficacy 80-90%). Unfortunately the impact on AOM was less impressive (vaccine efficacy 6%) due to serotype replacement by non-vaccine serotypes [65]. Larger benefits for AOM were seen in the trial that used the 11 valent conjugate vaccine conjugated to the protein D of *Haemophilus influenzae* due to protection against *Haemophilus* infection and reduced pneumococcal serotype replacement [69]. Further studies assessing the impact of this vaccine (now 10-valent, following removal of serotype 3 due to potential negative vaccine efficacy for this serotype) on otitis media are in progress. Conjugate pneumococcal vaccination was also associated with a reduction in insertion of tympanostomy tubes (vaccine efficacy 20%) [70]. Importantly, the vaccine was also associated with a reduction in invasive pneumococcal disease (and some degree of non-vaccine serotype replacement) in adults through its herd immunity effect [67]. A recent review of the global burden of pneumococcal disease found that invasive pneumococcal infection was responsible for around 11% of all childhood mortality in children less than 5 years old [71]. This review did not assess the impact of the vaccine on hearing loss.

Meningococcal Vaccines

There are several different meningococcal vaccines currently in use. There are 13 serogroups of *Niesseria meningiditis* [11, 12]. The common six A, B, C, Y, W135 and 29E are responsible for >99% of disease [11, 12]. Overall the risk of meningococcal meningitis is around 1 per 100,000 in developed countries [11, 12]. However, different serotypes cause disease with different frequencies in different settings. The most common manifestations of meningococcal infection are sepsis and meningitis [11, 12]. Young children and adolescents are at most risk. Very high rates of disease occur episodically as epidemics (serotype A) in the African meningitis belt across the top of Africa. Hearing loss associated with meningococcal disease is most often associated with meningitis (although this complication is less common than other forms of bacterial meningitis). Permanent sensorineural hearing loss affects up to 3-7% of infected children [14]. There are several different meningococcal vaccines in use around the world. In the USA (and many other developed countries), conjugate meningococcal serotype C vaccine is given at 12 months [28]. In New Zealand, an epidemic of serotype B was managed with a strategy that included use of a specifically developed vaccine [72]. In Africa, use of a vaccine that includes serotype A is recommended. In 2010, a low-cost vaccine developed specifically for the African meningitis belt was released (MenAfriVac) [73]. We identified two Cochrane reviews and several non-Cochrane systematic reviews [74 – 77]. The polysaccharide serotype A vaccine has been shown to be highly protective (vaccine efficacy 95%) in children and adults >5 years of age (and possibly younger). The conjugate serotype C vaccine is immunogenic when given in infancy but clinical outcome data have not been collected in randomised controlled trials. In countries when meningococcal serotype C conjugate vaccine is being used, there have been reductions in rates of disease of around 90%. None of the reviews addressed the impact on meningococcal vaccines on hearing.

Varicella Vaccine

Varicella infection can be associated with sudden onset facial nerve palsy (Bell's palsy). Hearing is usually not affected. However, when facial palsy is due to recurrence of varicella infection (Ramsay Hunt syndrome), hearing loss can occur. Varicella is also known to affect 1-5 per 100,000 pregnancies. Around 5% of women with no history of previous infection are susceptible. If infection occurs at 8-20 weeks, around 1-2% of babies will be affected. Although CNS abnormalities are a recognised component of syndrome, sensorineural hearing loss has not been described often [78].

We identified no Cochrane reviews specifically addressing the effectiveness of routine early childhood vaccination. There was a Cochrane review on post exposure vaccination and other reviews which estimated vaccine efficacy (>95% with 2 dose schedule) [79, 81]. None of the reviews considered the impact on hearing loss.

Influenza Vaccines

Influenza virus vaccine exists in both killed and live attenuated forms. Influenza infection has been associated with sudden onset sensorineural hearing loss (11,16). Currently, it is unclear whether the infection is truly causal or just coincidental. More importantly (in terms of the global burden of hearing loss), influenza infection is also known to be associated with otitis media [82].

In the USA, influenza vaccine is now part of the universal schedule. In most other developed countries, use is limited to specific high risk groups. In 2009, with concerns about an influenza pandemic due to a new H1N1 strain, new vaccines were developed over a short period of time and more widespread vaccination occurred [83].

We identified one Cochrane review and several non-Cochrane systematic reviews [82 – 84]. The impact on hearing loss was not specifically assessed. The impact on otitis media has been reported but the results are inconsistent. It would appear that influenza vaccine protects against AOM associated with influenza infection if it is given before the influenza season and the vaccine includes the circulating strain. Overall, the impact is likely to be modest because most illnesses (including influenza-like illnesses) with associated AOM are not due to influenza virus [85].

Other Vaccines on the Universal Immunisation Schedule

Associations between diphtheria, tetanus, pertussis, polio, yellow fever, Japanese encephalitis infection and hearing loss have also been described. Although these infections are not regarded as important causes of hearing loss (and reports are uncommon), the dramatic impact of immunisation on these life-threatening and disabling infections may also have reduced rates of sensorineural hearing loss by a small amount.

Vaccines in Development

Prevention of all important infections by immunisation is likely to be possible within the next 100 years. Already, research studies of relevance to immunisation have been conducted for all clinically important infections. These studies include basic epidemiology, immunogenicity, development of animal models, and clinical trials. Infections that are common, associated with important complications, and generate a protective immune response after a single exposure, are the most suitable vaccine candidates. None of the vaccines in development meet all of these criteria.

Prior to approval for general use, researchers must establish that the proposed vaccine is immunogenic, safe and effective. Currently, evidence of safety and efficacy usually requires a large scale randomised controlled trial in the first instance, with safety confirmed through ongoing monitoring. Once a vaccine has been shown to be safe and effective, further modification may be assessed though immunogenicity studies if there are accepted serological determinants of protection. Vaccines that are already being evaluated in clinical trials are the ones most likely to be more widely available in the near future.

Otitis Media Vaccines (Spn, Hi, Mc, RSV)

Otitis media is one of the most common infections of childhood (see above). Both the pneumococcal and influenza vaccines have been shown to reduce otitis media but their effects have been modest [65;82;84]. The most significant development in recent years has been the Czechoslovakian trial that reported a 30% reduction of both pneumococcal and non-typable *Hemophilus* otitis media infections confirmed by tympanocentesis [69]. Overall there was a reduction of AOM (as diagnosed by the research team) by 30%. This is considerably more than the other conjugate pneumococcal vaccine studies that assessed OM. However, because the rates of infection were relatively low in this study, the absolute benefits of the vaccine were similar to the other studies.

Immunisation animal models for all 3 common bacterial otitis pathogens (pneumococcus, *Hemophilus* and *Moraxella*) have been developed [86]. However, to date, none of these candidate vaccines have progressed to human clinical trials. An oral non-typable *Haemophilus* vaccine has been developed and tested in several RCTs summarised in a Cochrane review [87]. Reductions in rates of acute bronchitis have been described in different populations. The impact on OM in children has not been assessed.

Immunisation that protects against viral infection that often leads to otitis media is another direction of research activity [85]. While influenza immunisation can prevent acute otitis media, this is not a common otitis pathogen [82, 84]. Respiratory syncytial virus (RSV) is the viral pathogen most likely to directly lead to middle ear inflammation and rhinovirus is the most frequent upper respiratory tract pathogen. RSV vaccines have been evaluated in clinical trials but unfortunately, rather than being protective, immunisation was associated with a more severe subsequent RSV infection [88]. The specific impact on OM was not described. We did not identify any recent rhinovirus trials.

CMV Vaccine

The cytomegalovirus (CMV) is a member of the herpes virus family. CMV infections are common and often asymptomatic. Infection occurs throughout the world. Clinical manifestations consist of a generalised febrile illness similar to Epstein-Barr (EBV) infection [11, 12]. The most important association between CMV infection and hearing loss is through congenital infection. Currently, CMV is the most common recognised congenital infection and occurs in around 1% of pregnancies [10]. Congenital CMV infection is most likely when the unborn foetus is exposed at around 10 weeks gestation. In the USA, around 40,000 babies are infected each year [11]. Of these 90% are asymptomatic and 10% are symptomatic. Hearing loss affects 7% and 60% of these groups respectively. Hearing loss is progressive in 50% and onset is delayed (up to 18 months).

The development of a CMV vaccine has been considered a priority for some time. Studies of passive immunisation during pregnancy have demonstrated that presence of antibodies improves outcomes [89]. In 2009, a phase II RCT of 300 pregnant women demonstrating 50% protection from infection was published [90]. This study represented a major advance. It confirms that vaccination in pregnancy is likely to be effective and that it appears safe. Unfortunately, the protection against infection was only modest. Greater benefits in terms of subsequent disease are still possible. In addition, modification of the formation of the vaccine may also increase immunogenicity and protection from infection.

Toxoplasmosis Vaccine

Toxoplasma gondii is a protozoan parasite. It can infect warm-blooded animals and the cat is its primary host. Toxoplasma infections are common and often asymptomatic [11, 12]. Infection occurs throughout the world and is most common in individuals exposed to domestic cats or undercooked meat. Toxoplasma infection can also cause a generalised febrile illness similar to Epstein-Barr (EBV) infection. The most important association between toxoplasma infection and hearing loss is through congenital infection [91]. Congenital toxoplasma infection is most likely when the unborn foetus is exposed at around 10 weeks gestation [10, 11]. Around 1 in 1,000 to 3,000 pregnant women are affected. In these affected pregnancies, around 10-15% of children will develop sensorineual hearing loss. The hearing loss may not be present at birth and can be progressive. Importantly, any subsequent hearing loss can be prevented with treatment with pryimethamine and sulphonamide immediately after birth [91].

Toxoplasma vaccines have been developed and used in livestock (eg. Sheep and pigs). They appear to be safe and effective. Although there is research into the development of vaccines able to protect against toxoplasma infection, we did not identify any clinical trials. This suggests that availability of an effective vaccine within the next 20 years is unlikely.

Syphilis Vaccine

Syphilis is caused by a bacterial spirochete, *Treponema pallidum*. The infection is sexually transmitted and has a wide range of clinical manifestations [11, 12]. Hearing loss associated with syphilis is most likely following congenital infection. It can also occur following acquisition in adulthood (and subsequent labyrinthitis) if not treated.

Globally, the WHO estimates that around 1.5% of all pregnancies are complicated by infection with syphilis [92, 93]. Around 40-80% of syphilis exposed foetuses are adversely affected. In many developing countries, it is estimated that syphilis is associated with up to 25% of stillbirths and 11% of neonatal deaths. Relatively high rates of congenital syphilis occur in sub-Saharan Africa (with 4-15% of pregnant infected in some antenatal clinics) and well as in selected populations in Central and South America and South East Asia [94]. In contrast, congenital syphilis infection affects around 1 in 10,000 pregnant women in developed countries [11]. One third to two thirds of infected infants are asymptomatic at birth.

Sensorineural hearing loss due to syphilis is reported to occur in 30-40% and is a late manifestation [11]. It usually appears after 2 years of age and can be prevented if the child is treated before 3 months of age. Infants who are infected in utero can be asymptomatic at birth but develop features of syphilis over time ("the sins of the father"). Sensorineual hearing loss, notched incisor teeth and interstitial keratitis were characteristic of congenital syphilis in Hutchison's original description. However, treatment with penicillin greatly reduces the risk of congenital infection and progressive disease. In the only systematic review of prospective inception cohort studies, Chau only found one eligible study [95]. Interestingly, all 75 babies confirmed to have congenital syphilis (and who received appropriate treatment) had normal hearing. It would appear that, in a setting where diagnosis is made early and treatment given appropriately, the risk of sensorineural hearing loss is much less than previously described.

Although there is research into the development of vaccine able to protect against syphilis infection, we did not identify any clinical trials. This suggests that availability of an effective vaccine within the next 20 years is unlikely.

Herpes Simplex Vaccine

Herpes simplex virus (HSV) type 1 is a DNA virus that is most often associated with cold sores. Occasionally it can cause herpes stomatitis in children, encephalitis, or labyrinthitis [11, 12]. Both herpes encephalitis and labyrinthitis can lead to sensorineural hearing loss. Congenital herpes infection can also be associated with hearing loss but it is not a common complication [96].

Although there is research into the development of vaccine able to protect against HSV1 infection, we did not identify any recent clinical trials. This suggests that availability of an effective vaccine within the next 20 years is unlikely. However, there have been trials of HSV2 vaccine [97 – 99]. To date, these have assessed the risk of reactivation and genital infection rather than protection of the unborn foetus from congenital infection.

HIV Vaccine

Human immunodeficiency virus (HIV) is a retrovirus that (over time) leads to life-threatening immunodeficiency [11]. HIV infection can be associated with hearing loss either directly (via labyrinthitis, through its effect on the immune response and increased susceptibility to otitis media, labyrhinthitis and meningitis, or as a side effect of the long-term drug therapy currently necessary to ensure survival [11]. HIV infection is also known to cause facial palsy (although this is rare). Overall, hearing problems appear common (affecting more than 20%). Currently, the underlying cause is uncertain and more research is needed [100].

A large number of phase 1 and phase 2 clinical trials of HIV vaccines have been published [101 102]. To date, evidence of protection has been limited but promising. Most of the trials have focussed on development of antibodies and protection against future infection. The few that have examined clinical outcomes have not specifically described the impact on hearing loss.

Malaria and Non-Specific Febrile Illness

Hearing loss may occur following any life threatening condition.[103] Severe infections may lead to hypoxic, ischaemic or haemorrhagic brain injury, severe hypotension, encephalitis, or encephalopathy. All of these complications can affect hearing. In developing countries, the underlying aetiology of hearing loss after illness is not always clear. Empirical treatment is based on the clinical features rather than a clear diagnosis. A sick febrile infant may have sepsis, malaria, pneumonia, or meningitis. In some settings, haemorrhagic fever illnesses will also be considered in the differential diagnosis. Distinguishing between these conditions without access to further investigations can be challenging. Severe malaria (including cerebral malaria) may be an important cause of acquired hearing loss either as a complication of the illness or as a consequence of the use of quinine or chloroquine [104]. Fortunately, the newer more effective artemether combination medications have a more favourable side effect profile. Similarly, sepsis or severe pneumonia may cause hearing loss either as a complication of the illness, as a result of unrecognised meningitis, or through the use of aminoglycoside medications. In some cases, empirical treatment may require the use of more than one ototoxic medication.

Summary

The Expanded Programme of Immunisation represents one of the great public health achievements of the last 50 years. Its contribution to early childhood mortality and disability has been substantial. In developed countries, historically important diseases like diphtheria, tetanus, polio, measles, congenital rubella, and Hib meningitis are hardly seen and other forms of bacterial meningitis are also greatly reduced. As immunisation coverage (and financial support for immunisation programmes) expands in developing countries, a similar change in the epidemiology of early childhood infection will occur. Immunisation will continue to reduce poor outcomes associated with infection throughout the world.

The prospects for prevention of sensorineural and conductive hearing loss are best considered separately. Since 70-90% of severe and profound sensorineural hearing loss is not infectious in origin, immunisation will only form part of the sensorineural hearing loss prevention strategy. To date, the largest gains in the prevention of severe to profound sensorineural hearing loss have come from the measles and rubella vaccines, and the protein-conjugated bacterial meningitis vaccines (targeting Hib, pneumococcal and meningococcal disease). In the future, the largest gains are likely to come from i) more widespread use of currently available vaccines; ii) more effective meningitis vaccines (protecting a greater range of pneumococcal and meningococcal serotypes); iii) a more effective tuberculosis vaccine; iv) development and implementation of CMV and HIV vaccines.

Most of the mild and moderate conductive hearing loss in the world is associated with otitis media.

To some extent, OM is a vaccine preventable disease. Currently, immunisation with pneumococcal conjugate vaccine (especially when conjugated to *Haemophilus* protein D) and influenza vaccine can only prevent a small proportion of acute otitis media episodes. However, this may prove important in reducing high rates of chronic suppurative otitis media seen in certain populations (Indigenous children in developed countries, and disadvantaged populations in developing countries).

In the future, the development of otitis media vaccines (or combinations of vaccines) that reduces colonisation and protect against common respiratory bacterial and viral pathogens has the potential to dramatically reduce the frequency of mild and moderate hearing loss in young children.

Conclusion

Immunisaiton prevents hearing loss through the reduction of congenital infection, bacterial meningitis, labyrinthitis, and otitis media. Over the last 40 years, we have seen immunisation coverage for the 6 core vaccine preventable diseases increase from around 5% to 80%.

As all countries expand their universal immunisation schedule, the benefits of vaccination will increase. More effective meningitis, tuberculosis, and otitis media vaccines, and the development of CMV and HIV vaccines will reduce the global burden of hearing loss even further.

Table 6. 1. Worldwide burden of vaccine preventable disease and comparison of universal immunisation schedule in USA, India and Botswana[31]

Infectious agent	Estimated incidence (100,000's-2004)	Estimated mortality (1000's- 2004)	USA	India	Botswana
Tuberculosis	78	1,464		✓	✓
Diphtheria	0.34	5	✓	✓	✓
Pertussis	184	254	✓	✓	✓
Tetanus	2.5	105	✓	✓	✓
Polio	0.02	?	IPV	OPV	OPV
Measles	270	424	✓	✓	✓
Mumps	5.4	?	✓		
Rubella	?	196	✓		
Hepatitis B	57	105	✓	✓	✓
Hib[*]	25	386	✓		
Pneumococcus	145	826	✓		
Meningococcus	?	340	✓		
Varicella	?	?	✓		
Hepatitis A	14	?	✓		
Influenza	40	375	✓		
Rotavirus	?	527	✓		
HPV[**]	4.9	247	✓		

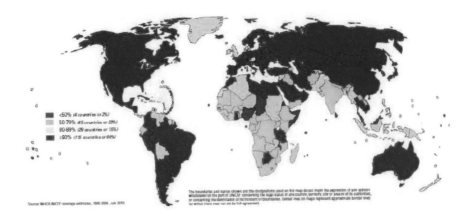

Figure 6.1. Immunisation coverage with measles-containing vaccines in infants, 2009. (Map produced as part of the UNICEF/WHO Immunisation Summary, 2011 edition.) [25].

References

[1]   Jamison, D. T., Breman, J. G., Measham, A. R. Alleyne, G, Claeson, M.,Evans, D. B., Jha, P., Mills A., Musgrove P. A co-publication of Oxford Uet al.(2006). Disease Control Priorities in Developing Countries. (2nd ed.) Washington (DC): The International Bank for Reconstruction and Development/The World Bank Group.

[2]   Mathers, C., Smith, A., Concha, M. (2007).Global burden of hearing loss in the year 2000. Geneva: World Health Organisation.

[3]   Smith, R. J., Bale, J. F., Jr., White, K. R. (2005). Sensorineural hearing loss in children. *Lancet;* 365, 879-890.

[4]   Thigpen, M. C., Whitney, C. G., Messonnier, N. E., Zell, E. R., Lynfield, R., Hadler, J. L. Harrison, L. H., Farley, M. M., Reingold, A., Bennett, N. M., Craig, A. S., Schaffner, W., Thomas, A., Lewis, M. M., Scallan, E., Schuchat, A; Emerging Infections Programs Network. (2011). Bacterial meningitis in the United States, 1998-2007. *New England Journal of Medicine,* 364, 2016-2025.

[5]   Verhoeff, M., Van der Veen, E. L., Rovers, M. M., Sanders, E. A., Schilder, A. G. (2006). Chronic suppurative otitis media: a review. *International Journal of Pediatric Otorhinolaryngology,* 70, 1- 12.

[6]   Plotkin, S., Orenstein, W., Offit, P. (2008).Vaccines. (5th ed.) Philadelphia: Saunders.

[7]   WHO, UNICEF, World Bank. State of the world's vaccines and immunization. 3rd ed. Geneva: World Health Organization; 2009.

[8]   Vallely, P. J., Klapper, P. E., Cleator, G. M. (2002). Infectious causes of paediatric hearing impairment. In: V. E. Newton (Ed.) Pediatric Audiological Medicine. London: Whurr Publishers;

[9]   Northern, J. L. and Downs, M. P. (2011). Hearing in Children. 5th ed. Baltimore: Lippincott Williams and Wilkins.

[10]   Remington, J. S., Klein, J. O., Wilson, C. B., Nizet, V., Maldonado, Y. (2011). *Infectious Diseases of the Fetus and Newborn.* 7th ed. Philadelphia: W.B Saunders.

[11] UpToDate. Waltham, M. A. UpToDate Inc.; 2011. Available from; www.uptodate.com (Accessed 22 October 2011).

[12] Feigin, R. D., Cherry, J. D., Demmler-Harrison, G. J., Kaplan, S. L (2009). Feigin and Cherry's Textbook of Pediatric Infectious Diseases. (6th ed.) Philadelphia: Saunders/ Elsevier.

[13] Kopelovich, J. C., Germiller, J. A., Laury, A. M., Shah, S. S., Pollock, A. N. (2011). Early prediction of postmeningitic hearing loss in children using magnetic resonance imaging. *Archives of Otolaryngology Head and Neck Surgery,* 137, 441-447.

[14] Edmond, K., Clark, A., Korczak, V. S., Sanderson, C., Griffiths, U. K., Rudan, I. (2010) Global and regional risk of disabling sequelae from bacterial meningitis: a systematic review and meta-analysis. *Lancet Infectious Diseases,* 10, 317-328.

[15] Richardson, M. P., Reid, A., Tarlow, M. J., Rudd, P. T. (1997). Hearing loss during bacterial meningitis. *Archives of Diseases in Childhood,* 76, 134-138.

[16] Schreiber, B. E., Agrup, C., Haskard, D. O., Luxon, L. M. (2010). Sudden sensorineural hearing loss. *Lancet,* 375, 1203-1211.

[17] Chau, J. K., Lin, J. R., Atashband, S., Irvine, R. A., Westerberg, B. D. (2010). Systematic review of the evidence for the etiology of adult sudden sensorineural hearing loss. *Laryngoscope,* 120, 1011-1021.

[18] Bluestone, C. D. and Klein, J. O. (2007). *Otitis Media in Infants and Children.* 4th ed. Philadelphia: W.B. Saunders.

[19] Rovers, M. M., Schilder, A. G., Zielhuis, G. A., Rosenfeld, R. M. (2004). Otitis media. *Lancet,* 363, 465-473.

[20] Morris, P. S. and Leach, A. J. (2009). Acute and chronic otitis media. *Pediatric Clinics of North America,* 56, 1383-1399.

[21] Rosenfeld, R. M. and Bluestone, C. D. (2003). Evidence-Based Otitis Media. (2nd ed.) Hamilton: B.C. Decker Inc.

[22] Report of a WHO/CIBA Foundation Workshop.(1996). Prevention of Hearing Impairment from Chronic Otitis Media. Geneva: World Health Organisation.

[23] Bitner-Glindzicz, M. and Rahman, S. (2007). Ototoxicity caused by aminoglycosides. *British Medical Journal,* 335,784-785.

[24] Matz, G. J. Aminoglycoside cochlear ototoxicity. (1993). *Otolaryngology Clinics North America,* 26, 705-712.

[25] World Health Organization. (2011). WHO vaccine preventable diseases: monitoring system. 2010 global summary. Geneva: World Health Organization.

[26] Fenner, F., Henderson, D. A., Arita, I., JeZek, Z., Ladnyi, I. D.(1988). Smallpox and its Eradication. Geneva: World Health Organization.

[27] The College of Physicians of Philadelphia. (2011).The History of Vaccines. A project of the College of Physicians of Philadelphia. Available from: http://www.history ofvaccines.org/. (Accessed 23 October, 2011).

[28] The Australian Immunisation Handbook.(2009). (9th ed). Canberra: The Australian Government Department of Health and Aging.

[29] Bland, J. and Clements, J. (1998). Protecting the world's children: the story of WHO's immunization programme. *World Health Forum,* 19, 162-173.

[30] GAVI Alliance. (2011).GAVI Alliance Progress Report 2010. Geneva: GAVI Alliance.

[31] WHO World Health Organization: Immunization VAB. (2011).WHO vaccine-preventable diseases: monitoring system 2010 global summary - National vaccines schedules. Available from: http://www.who.int/immunization_monitoring/en/global summary/ScheduleSelect.cfm. Geneva: World Health Organization. (Accessed 23 October, 2011).

[32] Clemens, J., Holmgren, J., Kaufmann, S. H., Mantovani, A. (2010), Ten years of the Global Alliance for Vaccines and Immunization: challenges and progress. *Nature Immunology,* 11, 1069-1072.

[33] Poliomyelitis prevention in the United States: introduction of a sequential vaccination schedule of inactivated poliovirus vaccine followed by oral poliovirus vaccine.(1997). Recommendations of the Advisory Committee on Immunization Practices (ACIP). *MMWR Recomm. Rep.* 1997; 46(RR-3):1-25.

[34] Wolfson, L. J., Gasse, F., Lee-Martin, S. P, Lydon, P., Magan, A., Tibouti, A., Johns, B., Hutubessy, R., Salama, P., Okwo-Bele, J. M. (2008). Estimating the costs of achieving the WHO-UNICEF Global Immunization Vision and Strategy, 2006-2015. *Bulletin of the World Health Organisation,* 86, 27-39.

[35] Lawrence, G. L., Hull, B. P., MacIntyre, C. R., McIntyre, P. B. (2004). Reasons for incomplete immunisation among Australian children. A national survey of parents. *Australian Family Physician,* 33, 568-571.

[36] Larson, H. J., Cooper, L. Z., Eskola, J., Katz, S. L., Ratzan, S. (2011). Addressing the vaccine confidence gap. *Lancet,* 378,526-535.

[37] World Health Organization, UNICEF (2009). The World Bank. State of the world's vaccines and immunization. (3rd ed.) Geneva: World Health Organization.

[38] Vandelaer, J., Bilous, J., Nshimirimana, D. (2008), Reaching Every District (RED) approach: a way to improve immunization performance. *Bulletin of the World Health Organisation,* 86, A-B.

[39] World Health Organization.(2007). Global Framework for Immunization Monitoring and Surveillance. Geneva: World Health Organization.

[40] Hipgrave, D. B., Maynard, J. E., Biggs, B. A. (2006), Improving birth dose coverage of hepatitis B vaccine. *Bulletin World Health Organisation,* 84, 65-71.

[41] Sonmez, G., Turhan, V., Senol, M. G., Ozturk, E., Sildiroglu, H. O., Mutlu, H. (2008). Relationship between tuberculous otomastoiditis and tuberculous meningitis. *Journal of Laryngology and Otology,* 122, 893-897.

[42] Kuan, C. C., Kaga, K., Tsuzuku, T.(2007). Tuberculous meningitis-induced unilateral sensorineural hearing loss: a temporal bone study. *Acta Otolaryngologica,* 127, 553-557.

[43] Lima, M. L., Lessa, F., Guiar-Santos, A. M., Medeiros, Z. (2006). Hearing impairment in patients with tuberculosis from Northeast Brazil. *Revista do Instituto de Medicina Tropical de Sao Paolo,* 48, 99-102.

[44] Duggal, P. and Sarkar, M. (2007). Audiologic monitoring of multi-drug resistant tuberculosis patients on aminoglycoside treatment with long term follow-up. *BMC Ear Nose Throat Disorders*, 7, 5.

[45] Van Well, G. T., Paes, B. F., Terwee, C. B., Springer, P., Roord, J. J., Donald, P. R., Van Furthi, A. M., Schoeman, J. F. (2009). Twenty years of pediatric tuberculous meningitis: a retrospective cohort study in the western cape of South Africa. *Pediatrics,* 123, e1-e8.

[46] Yaniv, E., Traub, P., Conradie, R. (1986). Middle ear tuberculosis--a series of 24 patients. *International Journal of Pediatric Otorhinolaryngology, 12*, 59-63.

[47] Barreto, M. L., Pereira, S. M., Ferreira, A. A. (2006). BCG vaccine: efficacy and indications for vaccination and revaccination. *Journal of Pediatrics* (Rio Journal), 82(3 Suppl.),S45-S54.

[48] Brewer, T. F. (2000). Preventing tuberculosis with bacillus Calmette-Guerin vaccine: a meta-analysis of the literature. *Clinical Infectious Diseases, 31* Suppl. 3, S64-S67.

[49] Colditz, G. A., Berkey, C. S., Mosteller, F., Brewer, T. F., Wilson, M. E., Burdick, E., Fineberg, H. V. (1995). The efficacy of bacillus Calmette-Guerin vaccination of newborns and infants in the prevention of tuberculosis: meta-analyses of the published literature. *Pediatrics, 96*, 29-35.

[50] Colditz, G. A., Brewer, T. F., Berkey, C. S., Wilson, M. E., Burdick, E., Fineberg, H. V., Mosteuer, F. (1994). Efficacy of BCG vaccine in the prevention of tuberculosis. Meta-analysis of the published literature. *Journal of the American Medical Association, 271*, 698-702.

[51] Aronson, N. E., Santosham, M., Comstock, G. W., Howard, R. S., Moulton, L. H., Rhoades, E. R. Harrison, L. H. (2004). Long-term efficacy of BCG vaccine in American Indians and Alaska Natives: A 60-year follow-up study. *Journal of the American Medical Association, 291*, 2086-2091.

[52] Wright, D. O. and Leigh, B. (1995).The impact of the Expanded Programme on Immunisation on measles-induced sensorineural hearing loss in the western area of Sierra Leone. *West African Journal of Medicine, 14*, 205-209.

[53] Wolfson, L. J., Strebel, P. M., Gacic-Dobo, M., Hoekstra, E. J., McFarland, J. W., Hersh, B. S. (2007). Has the 2005 measles mortality reduction goal been achieved? A natural history modelling study. *Lancet, 369*, 191-200.

[54] Karosi, T., Konya, J., Petko, M., Szabo, L. Z., Pytel, J., Jori, J., Sziklai, I. (2006). Antimeasles immunoglobulin g for serologic diagnosis of otosclerotic hearing loss. *Laryngoscope*,116, 488-493.

[55] Demicheli, V., Jefferson, T., Rivetti, A., Price. D. (2005). Vaccines for measles, mumps and rubella in children. *Cochrane Database Systematic Reviews*,(4), CD004407.

[56] Scott, P., Moss, W. J., Gilani, Z., Low, N. (2011). Measles vaccination in HIV-infected children: systematic review and meta-analysis of safety and immunogenicity. *Journal of Infectious Diseases, 204* Suppl. 1, S164-S178.

[57] Uzicanin, A. and Zimmerman, L. (2011). Field effectiveness of live attenuated measles-containing vaccines: a review of published literature. *Journal of Infectious Diseases, 204* Suppl. 1, S133-S148.

[58] Sudfeld, C. R., Navar, A. M., Halsey, N. A. (2010). Effectiveness of measles vaccination and vitamin A treatment. *International Journal of Epidemiology, 39*, Suppl. 1:i48-i55.

[59] Anders, J. F., Jacobson, R. M., Poland, G. A., Jacobsen, S. J., Wollan, P. C. (1996). Secondary failure rates of measles vaccines: a metaanalysis of published studies. *Pediatric Infectious Disease Journal, 15*, 62-66.

[60] Swingler, G., Fransman, D., Hussey, G. (2007). Conjugate vaccines for preventing Haemophilus influenzae type B infections. *Cochrane Database Systematic Reviews*, (2), CD001729.

[61] Griffiths, U. K. and Miners, A. (2009). Economic evaluations of Haemophilus influenzae type b vaccine: systematic review of the literature. *Expert Review of Pharmacoeconomic Outcomes Research,* 9, 333-346.

[62] Theodoratou, E., Johnson, S., Jhass, A., Madhi, S. A., Clark, A., Boschi-Pinto, C., Bhopal, S., Rudan, I., Campbell, H. (2010). The effect of Haemophilus influenzae type b and pneumococcal conjugate vaccines on childhood pneumonia incidence, severe morbidity and mortality. *International Journal of Epidemiology,* 39 Suppl. 1, i172-i185.

[63] Watt, J. P., Wolfson, L. J., O'Brien, K. L., Henkle, E., oria-Knoll, M., McCall, N., Lee, E., Mulholland, K., Levine, O. S., Cherian, T., Hib and Pneumococcal Global Burden of Disease Study Team. (2009). Burden of disease caused by Haemophilus influenzae type b in children younger than 5 years: global estimates. *Lancet,* 374, 903-911.

[64] Lucero, M. G., Dulalia, V. E., Nillos, L. T., Williams, G., Parreno, R. A., Nohynek, H., Riley, D., Maketa, H. (2009). Pneumococcal conjugate vaccines for preventing vaccine-type invasive pneumococcal disease and X-ray defined pneumonia in children less than two years of age. *Cochrane Database Systematic Reviews*, (4), CD004977.

[65] Jansen, A. G., Hak, E., Veenhoven, R. H., Damoiseaux, R. A., Schilder, A. G., Sanders, E. A. (2009). Pneumococcal conjugate vaccines for preventing otitis media. *Cochrane Database Systematic Reviews,* (2), CD001480.

[66] Moberley, S. A., Holden, J., Tatham, D. P., Andrews, R. M. (2008). Vaccines for preventing pneumococcal infection in adults. *Cochrane Database Systematic Reviews,* (1), CD000422.

[67] Hsu, H. E., Shutt, K. A., Moore, M. R., Beall, B. W., Bennett, N. M., Craig, A. S., Farley, M. M., Jorgensen, J. H., Lexau, C. A., Petit, S., Reingold, A., Schaffner, W., Thomas, A., Whitney, C. G., Harrison, L. H. (2009). Effect of pneumococcal conjugate vaccine on pneumococcal meningitis. *New England Journal of Medicine,* 360, 244-256.

[68] Pedersen, R. H., Lohse, N., Ostergaard, L., Sogaard, O. S. (2011). The effectiveness of pneumococcal polysaccharide vaccination in HIV-infected adults: a systematic review. *HIV Medicine,* 12, 323-333.

[69] Prymula, R., Peeters, P., Chrobok, V., Kriz, P., Novakova, E., Kaliskova, E., Kohl, I., Lommel, P., Poolman, J., Prieels, J. P., Schuerman, L. (2006). Pneumococcal capsular polysaccharides conjugated to protein D for prevention of acute otitis media caused by both Streptococcus pneumoniae and non-typable Haemophilus influenzae: a randomised double-blind efficacy study. *Lancet,* 367, 740-748.

[70] Lack, S., Shinefield, H., Fireman, B., Lewis, E., Ray, P., Hansen, J. R. Elvin, L., Ensor, K. M., Hackell, J., Siber, G., Malinoski, F., Madore, D., Chang, I., Kohberger, R., Watson, W., Austrian, R., Edwards, K. (2000). Efficacy, safety and immunogenicity of heptavalent pneumococcal conjugate vaccine in children. Northern California Kaiser Permanente Vaccine Study Center Group. *Pediatric Infectious Disease Journal*, 19, 187-195.

[71] O'Brien, K. L., Wolfson, L. J., Watt, J. P., Henkle, E., Oria-Knoll, M., McCall, N., Lee, E., Mulholland, K., Levine, O. S., Cherian, T.; Hib and Pneumococcal Global Burden of Disease Study Team. (2009). Burden of disease caused by Streptococcus pneumoniae in children younger than 5 years: global estimates. *Lancet,* 374, 893-902.

[72] Lennon, D., Jackson, C., Wong, S., Horsfall, M., Stewart, J., Reid, S. (2009), Fast tracking the vaccine licensure process to control an epidemic of serogroup B meningococcal disease in New Zealand. *Clinical Infectious Diseases,* 49, 597-605.

[73] Bishai, D. M., Champion, C., Steele, M. E., Thompson, L. (2011), Product development partnerships hit their stride: lessons from developing a meningitis vaccine for Africa. *Health Affairs (Millwood), 30,* 1058-1064.

[74] Patel, M., Lee, C. K. (2005). Polysaccharide vaccines for preventing serogroup A meningococcal meningitis. *Cochrane Database Systematic Reviews,* (1), CD001093.

[75] Conterno, L. O., Silva Filho, C. R., Ruggeberg, J. U., Heath, P. T. (2006). Conjugate vaccines for preventing meningococcal C meningitis and septicaemia. *Cochrane Database Systematic Reviews,* 3, CD001834.

[76] Prasad, K. and Karlupia, N. (2007). Prevention of bacterial meningitis: an overview of Cochrane systematic reviews. *Respiratory Medicine,* 101, 2037-2043.

[77] Pollabauer, E. M., Petermann, R., Ehrlich, H. J. (2005). Group C meningococcal polysaccharide-tetanus toxoid conjugate vaccine: a meta-analysis of immunogenicity, safety and posology. *Human Vaccination,* 1, 131-139.

[78] Mutton, P. E. (1995). Intra-uterine varicella or herpes zoster and childhood deafness. *Journal of Paediatric Child Health,* 31, 483.

[79] Macartney, K. and McIntyre, P. (2008). Vaccines for post-exposure prophylaxis against varicella (chickenpox) in children and adults. *Cochrane Database Systematic Reviews,* CD001833.

[80] Bayer, O., Heininger, U., Heiligensetzer, C., Von Kries, R. (2007). Metaanalysis of vaccine effectiveness in varicella outbreaks. *Vaccine,* 25, 6655-6660.

[81] American Academy of Pediatrics Committee on Infectious Diseases.(2007). Prevention of varicella: recommendations for use of varicella vaccines in children, including a recommendation for a routine 2-dose varicella immunization schedule. *Pediatrics,* 120, 221-231.

[82] Manzoli, L., Schioppa, F., Boccia, A., Villari, P. (2007). The efficacy of influenza vaccine for healthy children: a meta-analysis evaluating potential sources of variation in efficacy estimates including study quality. *Pediatric Infectious Disease Journal,* 26, 97-106.

[83] Abelin, A., Colegate, T., Gardner, S., Hehme, N., Palache, A. (2011). Lessons from pandemic influenza A(H1N1): the research-based vaccine industry's perspective. *Vaccine,* 29, 1135-1138.

[84] Jefferson, T., Rivetti, A., Harnden, A., Di Pietrantonj, C., Demicheli, V. (2008). Vaccines for preventing influenza in healthy children. *Cochrane Database Systematic Reviews* (2):CD004879.

[85] Nokso-Koivisto, J., Raty, R., Blomqvist, S., Kleemola, M., Syrjanen, R., Pitkaranta, A., Kilpi, T., Hovi, T. (2004). Presence of specific viruses in the middle ear fluids and respiratory secretions of young children with acute otitis media. *Journal of Medical Virology,* 72, 241-248.

[86] Cripps, A. W., Otczyk, D. C., Kyd, J. M. (2005). Bacterial otitis media: a vaccine preventable disease? *Vaccine,* 23, 2304-2310.

[87] Foxwell, A. R., Cripps, A. W., Dear, K. B. (2006). Haemophilus influenzae oral whole cell vaccination for preventing acute exacerbations of chronic bronchitis. *Cochrane Database Systematic Reviews* (4), CD001958.

[88] Kim, H. W., Canchola, J. G., Brandt, C. D., Pyles, G., Chanock, R. M., Jensen, K., Parrot, R. H. (1969). Respiratory syncytial virus disease in infants despite prior administration of antigenic inactivated vaccine. *American Journal of Epidemiology*, 89, 422-434.

[89] Nigro, G., Adler, S. P., La, T. R., Best, A. M. (2005). Passive immunization during pregnancy for congenital cytomegalovirus infection. *New England Journal of Medicine*, 353, 1350-1362.

[90] Pass, R. F., Zhang, C., Evans, A., Simpson, T., Andrews, W., Huang, M. L., Corey, L., Hill, J., Davis, E., Flanigan, C., Cloud, G. (2009). Vaccine prevention of maternal cytomegalovirus infection. *New England Journal of Medicine*, 360, 1191-1199.

[91] Brown, E. D., Chau, J. K., Atashband, S., Westerberg, B. D., Kozak, F. K. (2009). A systematic review of neonatal toxoplasmosis exposure and sensorineural hearing loss. *International Journal of Pediatric Otorhinolaryngoogy*, 73, 707-711.

[92] Schmid, G. P., Stoner, B. P., Hawkes, S., Broutet, N. (2007). The need and plan for global elimination of congenital syphilis. *Sexually Transmitted Diseases*, 34(7 Suppl.), S5-10.

[93] Blencowe, H., Cousens, S., Kamb, M., Berman, S., Lawn, J. E. (2011). Lives Saved Tool supplement detection and treatment of syphilis in pregnancy to reduce syphilis related stillbirths and neonatal mortality. *BMC Public Health*, 11 Suppl. 3:S9.

[94] Kamb, M. L., Newman, L. M., Riley, P. L., Mark, J., Hawkes, S. J., Malik, T., Broutet, N. (2010). A road map for the global elimination of congenital syphilis. *Obstetrics and Gynaecology International*, 2010.

[95] Chau, J., Atashband, S., Chang, E., Westerberg, B. D., Kozak, F. K. (2009). A systematic review of pediatric sensorineural hearing loss in congenital syphilis. *International Journal of Pediatric Otorhinolaryngology*, 73, 787-792.

[96] Westerberg, B. D., Atashband, S., Kozak, F. K. (2008). A systematic review of the incidence of sensorineural hearing loss in neonates exposed to Herpes simplex virus (HSV). *International Journal of Pediatric Otorhinolaryngology*, 72, 931-937.

[97] Corey, L., Langenberg, A. G., Ashley, R., Sekulovich, R. E., Izu, A. E., Douglas, J. M., Jr. Handsfield, H. H., Warren, T., Marr, L., Tyring, S., DiCarlo, R., Adimora, A. A., Leone, P., Dekker, C. L., Burke, R. L., Leong, W. P., Straus, S. E. (1999). Recombinant glycoprotein vaccine for the prevention of genital HSV-2 infection: two randomized controlled trials. Chiron HSV Vaccine Study Group. *Journal of the American Medical Association*, 282, 331-340.

[98] Stanberry, L. R., Spruance, S. L., Cunningham, A. L., Bernstein, D. I., Mindel, A., Sacks, S., Tyring, S., Aoki, F. Y., Slaoui, M., Denis, M., Vandepapeliere, P., Dubin, G.; GlaxoSmithKline Herpes Vaccine Efficacy Study Group. (2002), Glycoprotein-D-adjuvant vaccine to prevent genital herpes. *New England Journal of Medicine*, 347, 1652-1661.

[99] Bernstein, D. I., Aoki, F. Y., Tyring, S. K., Stanberry, L. R., St-Pierre, C., Shafran, S. D., Leroux-Roels, G., Van Herck, K., Bollaerts, A., Dubin, G.; GlaxoSmithKline Herpes Vaccine Study Group. (2005). Safety and immunogenicity of glycoprotein D-adjuvant genital herpes vaccine. *Clinical Infectious Diseases*, 40, 1271-1281.

[100] Chandrasekhar, S. S., Connelly, P. E., Brahmbhatt, S. S., Shah, C. S., Kloser, P. C., Baredes, S. (2000). Otologic and audiologic evaluation of human immunodeficiency virus-infected patients. *American Journal of Otolaryngology*, 21, 1-9.

[101] Kim, D., Elizaga, M., Duerr, A. (2007). HIV vaccine efficacy trials: towards the future of HIV prevention. *Infectious Disease Clinics of North America, 21,* 201-17.

[102] Barouch, D. H. and Korber, B. (2010). HIV-1 vaccine development after STEP. *Annual Review of Medicine,* 61,153-167.

[103] Halpern, N. A., Pastores, S. M., Price, J. B., Alicea, M. (1999). Hearing loss in critical care: an unappreciated phenomenon. *Critical Care Medicine,* 27, 211-219.

[104] Zhao, S. Z. and Mackenzie, I. J. (2011). Deafness: malaria as a forgotten cause. *Annals of Tropical Paediatrics,* 31, 1-10.

In: Prevention of Hearing Loss
Editors: V. Newton, P. Alberti and A. Smith

ISBN: 978-1-61942-745-7
© 2012 Nova Science Publishers, Inc.

Chapter VII

Nutrients and Hearing

Valerie E. Newton[*]

Abstract

Animal research and investigations with human subjects have indicated the possibility that certain nutrients added to the diet may prevent some types of hearing impairment or modify the degree of hearing loss developing. In this chapter the findings of several of these studies are outlined together with the use of fortification and supplementation strategies as preventative measures.

Introduction

Hearing impairment is a major contributor to the prevalence of disability in all countries and has many causes, not all of which are yet known. Whereas it has long been realised that nutritional deficiencies have an aetiological role, the extent to which nutrients are involved in hearing, and the apparent beneficial role of supplementation in the prevention or reduction of some types of hearing loss, has only been identified more recently. Animal experiments and human studies have helped to indicate some of the mechanisms involved. In particular, with oxidative stress being increasingly implicated in the causation of hearing loss, the fact that some nutrients are powerful antioxidants is increasing interest in their potential for hearing loss prevention [1].

Having a hearing loss has consequences for communication, education and social interaction, so clearly the use of appropriate nutrients in adequate dosage to prevent or reduce hearing loss could have a major effect upon the individuals concerned, and have economic benefits for countries introducing fortification or supplementation programmes. At the present time most of the research is based upon animal experimentation and not all findings have

---

[*] Corresponding author: val_newton@lineone.net.

subsequently been tested on human subjects, or the human studies have not had a large enough sample size for sufficient confidence in the efficacy of the treatment approach.

In this Chapter some of the research concerning nutrients which have a specific effect upon hearing will be outlined, and the role of supplementation and food fortification will be considered as preventative strategies.

Nutrients

Nutrients are substances required by the body for life and growth and can be classed as essential or non-essential. The term "essential" nutrients is used for those nutrients which are either not synthesised by the human body or are synthesised in inadequate amounts and have to be obtained from the diet. Proteins, carbohydrates, fats, minerals, vitamins and water are essential nutrients. "Non-essential" nutrients can be synthesised in the body but the synthesis, in some instances, depends upon adequate amounts of an essential nutrient. Proteins, carbohydrates and fats, known as macronutrients, are consumed in large quantities and are required by the body for energy; vitamins and minerals classed as micronutrients, are required in small quantities and are needed for metabolic processes.

The intake of nutrients required by healthy people has been determined by the Food and Nutrition Board, Institute of Medicine, USA which has set reference values - Dietary Reference Indicators[2].These include the Recommended Dietary Allowance (RDA), which is the average daily level of intake sufficient to meet the nutrient requirements of nearly all (97-98%) healthy people, Adequate Intake levels, where information is insufficient to calculate RDA, and the Tolerable Upper Intake Level of nutrients above which there is a danger of toxicity. It is, however, the bioavailability of ingested nutrients which is important rather than just the amount ingested. Bioavailability refers to the rate and degree to which a substance is absorbed and used by the body. This is influenced by a number of factors including genetic inheritance and other substances ingested such as drugs used for treatment purposes.

Nutrient Deficiencies

Nutrient deficiencies are seen most frequently in developing countries where there is widespread poverty. Some micronutrient deficiencies are also found in developed countries, particularly iodine deficiency. Most micronutrients are essential nutrients and iodine, vitamin A and iron are the most important micronutrients from a public health viewpoint. In 1991, as a request from the World Health Organisation (WHO) the Vitamin and Mineral Nutrition Information Database (VMNID) was set up and collected data on anaemia, vitamin A and iodine. Currently this database is being expanded to include data on zinc, iron and folate. In 2007, WHO estimated that two billion people were deficient in micronutrients with pregnant women, lactating women and children the groups most at risk. Deficiencies in nutrients can occur in several ways (Table 7.1).

An inadequate food intake was considered to be the main cause of micronutrient deficiencies in a community based survey carried out in rural India [3]. The intake of foods rich in micronutrients was found to be infrequent. Their survey revealed that the concomitant prevalence of between two and five micronutrient deficiencies was common.

Table 7.1. Causes of nutrient deficiency

Inadequate food intake
Food deficient in the nutrient
Conditions causing malabsorption
Increased requirement
Increased elimination through excessive diarrhoea

Conditions Affected by Nutrients

Conditions for which some nutrients are claimed to have a preventative effect on hearing loss are; deficiency diseases, otitis media, age associated hearing loss, noise induced hearing loss, sudden hearing loss and ototoxicity.

Deficiency Diseases

These include deficiency of one or more micronutrients through environmental causes e.g. iodine deficiency, or genetic conditions e.g. an autosomal recessive biotinadase deficiency.

Otitis Media (OM)

This condition may start acutely but persist as chronic otitis media if untreated or inadequately treated. Chronic otitis media (COM) is the main cause of hearing impairment in developing countries. Some nutrients, eg. zinc and vitamin A, have been effective in reducing the incidence and severity of acute and chronic otitis media particularly in infants and children [4]. This could be due to their role as antioxidants. Yarikdas et al. demonstrated in a controlled study that middle ear inflammation increases the levels of free oxygen radicals in erythrocytes and they suggested that this could contribute to the development of otitis media [5].

Age Associated Hearing Loss (AHL, Presbyacusis)

Hearing loss here is sensorineural, progressive and most marked in the higher frequencies. It has been estimated that 30-35% of those aged 65-74 and 40-50% of those 75 and older suffer from presbyacusis [6]. With people surviving to old age the incidence of disability as a result of this condition is increasing. Nutrients which can reduce the impairment co-incident with the aging process, and which are cheap, non-toxic and readily available could have major benefits in both developing and developed economies.

Noise Induced Hearing Loss (NIHL)

Exposure to loud noise is increasing in industrial and urban environments and is one of the main causes of hearing impairment in adults. It can cause a temporary or permanent loss of hearing. Oxidative stress is now being seen as an important factor in the causation of NIHL. Several micronutrients, e.g. magnesium and vitamin E, act as antioxidant scavengers and so are factors in preventing the effects of oxidative-stress [1].

Ototoxic Medication

A number of drugs in clinical usage can have deleterious effects upon the auditory and vestibular systems and need to be monitored in usage e.g. gentamycin and cisplatin. Nutrients can be used to prevent or reduce hearing impairment as a result of antibiotic medication for infection [7] and cisplatin, an anti-cancer drug [8].

Sudden Sensorineural Hearing Loss (SSNHL)

This has a number of different causations including vascular compromise and auto-immune disorders, and is uncommon. The hearing loss may or may not improve subsequently. Nutrients have been shown to reduce the residual severity of hearing loss [9].

Nutrients Linked to Hearing Impairment

Nutrients which are reported to affect hearing are listed in Table 7.2 and are mainly micronutrients. The list comprises both essential and non-essential nutrients.

Table 7.2. Nutrients linked to hearing impairment

Minerals:	Iodine, Magnesium, Selenium, Zinc
Vitamins:	A B5, B6, B7, B9, B12, C, D, E
Amino acids:	Methionine, Cysteine, Taurine
Co-enzymes:	Q10
Fatty acids:	Alpha – lipoic acid

Minerals

Iodine

Iodine is essential for the production of thyroid hormones thyroxine (T4) and triiodothyronine (T3), which are important for growth and development and regulate metabolic processes in body cells. Iodine is present in the human body in minute amounts. It is ingested as iodine and converted in the body to the iodide form in which it is taken up by the thyroid gland and used in hormone synthesis. Iodine is also a powerful antioxidant.

The main concentration of iodine in the world is found in the oceans, a consequence of rain, snow, flooding and glaciation on land. Soils on landlocked mountainous areas tend to be deficient in iodine and hence also the crops which grow upon them. Dietary sources of iodine include seafood and to a lesser extent foods such as dairy products and some vegetables e.g. potatoes and asparagus.

The iodine status of a population can be determined by measuring the size of the thyroid, urinary iodine (UI) or by measuring serum thyroid stimulating hormone (TSH) and thyrotropin and thyroglobulin [10]. Goitres are detected by palpation and ultrasound whereas the severity of iodine deprivation can be assessed by the measurement of IU. (Table 7.3)

Serum measures of thyroid hormones have been obtained using a heel prick but this is not now thought to be sufficiently accurate and umbilical cord serum has been proposed instead [11].

Inadequate iodine uptake (<100µ/l) has been reported in all WHO regions with the highest proportion in Europe, 56.9% of the population, with 39.8% in SE Asia and 42.6% in Africa [12]. In 47 countries iodine deficiency remains a public health problem [13].

Table 7.3. Levels of severity of iodine deficiency used in epidemiological studies

UI(ug/1)	Degree of deficiency
<20	Severe
20-49	Moderate
50-99	Mild
100-199	None
	(de Benoist et al. [10])

A recent survey of 810 schoolgirls aged 14-15years in Britain who gave urine samples, showed that 379(51%) had mild iodine deficiency 120(16%)a moderate deficiency and 8 (1%) severe deficiency, using the criteria for mild, moderate and severe described in Table 7. 3 [14].

Iodine Deficiency and Effects on Hearing

The main cause of iodine deficiency is a low dietary content and the presence of a goitre is the most visible sign of a deficiency. Low serum levels of iodine, and consequently low levels of thyroid hormones, results in the pituitary gland increasing production of thyroid stimulating hormone(TSH) causing the thyroid gland to increase in size in order to trap more iodine, with the result that a goitre develops.

An adequate intake of iodine is particularly important in pregnancy and in the first 2-3 years of infancy. In pregnancy, iodine deficiency occurring during the 1st trimester, which is a critical period for the foetal brain, can lead to defective neurological development and cretinism. Sensorineural hearing loss is frequently a feature of iodine deficiency but the pathology involved has still to be determined.

The RDAs for different ages and for pregnancy and lactation are published [2].

Association with Hearing Loss

The association of cretinism and hearing loss has long been recognised. Gosling et al. carried out a controlled investigation of hearing in 34 out of 41 patients of ages 5-20 years with cretinism, 92 normal subjects living in the same endemic area and 54 subjects from a nearby control area in which iodine deficiency was not endemic[15]. The hearing loss found in those with cretinism was greater in the higher frequencies than in lower frequencies. Five were recorded as being "deaf-mute", 8 had a hearing loss >60dB and 10 a hearing loss of 40-60dB. Hearing in those who were not cretins but who lived in the same endemic area, was also reported to be poorer than for those in a nearby control area without endemic goitre. A hearing loss averaging 20-30 dB was found in 2% living in the endemic area and 1.8% in the control area.

Hearing loss is associated with iodine deficiency in the absence of cretinism. Valeix et al. found hearing loss associated with iodine deficiency and confirmed that it was sensorineural [16]. These researchers examined UI excretion in 122 healthy children 10mth-4yrs living in France and with 45% coming from Africa, the West Indies and Southeast Asia. Hearing impairment at 4kHz and the average hearing loss at the speech frequencies of 500Hz,1kHz and 2kHz were found to be more severe in those with UI secretion < $10\mu g/100ml$, who were at risk for mild to moderate iodine deficiency, than those with UI excretions> $10\mu g/100ml$.

In 1998, the results of an examination in 1995-6 of the iodine content of table salt and in the hairs of 381 children with sensorineural hearing loss from Jiangsu province of China were compared to those of normal hearing children by Gao and Wang [17]. The iodine content in the hairs of the deaf children were much lower than that of the control children ($P < 0.01$); there was also a below standard level of iodine in table salt in that region than had been officially published. They postulated that, iodine deficiency (ID) in these regions may be one of the major factors causing the hearing loss in the children.

Hearing impairment is not always recognised where iodine deficiency is not severe [18, 19]. The association of iodine deficiency with hearing impairment in apparently normal children was found in an 11 month randomised double-blind placebo-controlled investigation carried out in an iodine-deficient area of Benin [19]. The effects of mild as opposed to severe iodine deficiency were determined in a study involving 197 school children 7-11years. 97 children were given iodised oil and 100 others were given a placebo. Both sets were given iodised salt 6-7 months into the study. Both groups had thyrotropin, free thyroxine, thyroglobulin and UI measured at the beginning and end of the investigation. Children with higher serum thyroglobulin concentrations had significantly worse hearing thresholds in frequencies $\geq 2000Hz$ when compared to those with lower concentrations.

Supplementation and Fortification

Various methods have been employed to introduce iodine into the diet using such iodine preparations as potassium iodide, potassium iodate and sodium iodide. Food has been targeted directly or iodine has been introduced indirectly.

Iodisation of salt has been the most widespread method employed as salt is commonly used around the world. By the year 2000, 70% of households in the world used iodised salt [20]. WHO/UNESCO/ICCIDD have recommended that 20-40 mg of iodine added per kg of salt depending on local conditions [21].

Fortification of salt with iodine has significantly reduced iodine deficiency in those countries implementing this programme. Iodine supplementation, especially using iodised oil, has been shown to be an effective means of improving iodine status in children. Bread, sugar, milk and tea are among the substances which have been used as vehicles for introducing iodine into the diet. Iodine supplementation has also been achieved indirectly through iodophor sanitising solutions being used in the dairy industry and by means of the food chain through irrigation water and animal fodder.

Vitamin A deficiency reduces the uptake of iodine into the thyroid gland and often co-exists with iodine deficiency. Zimmermann et al. found that a high supplementary dose of vitamin A could modify indicators of iodine deficiency such as thyroglobulin and goitre, independent of an alteration in iodine nutrition [22]. They stated that in areas where goitre is endemic, vitamin A supplementation may decrease excess TSH stimulation of the thyroid through suppression of transcription of the pituitary TSHß gene, and so reduce the risk of goitre. There was no significant decrease in thyroid hormone concentrations in the children they studied.

Effect of long term supplementation with iodised oil and iodised salt was investigated in Iran by Azizi et al. [23]. Pure tone audiometry was used to test the hearing of school children in an iodine deficient area and the size of goitre and serum thyroid hormone measurements were taken 3 years after injections of iodised oil and 7 years after consumption of iodised salt. They concluded that not only was there a decrease in the prevalence and severity of goitre, a decrease in thyroid stimulation hormone and an increase in thyroxine levels, but there was an improvement in the auditory thresholds of iodine deficient children. Before iodine supplementation, hearing was abnormal in 44% of schoolchildren, the mean hearing threshold was 15.8±5.9 HL and in all children was >10 dB HL. The mean hearing threshold decreased to 10.2±4.6dB HL and 10.0±5.9 dB HL, 3 and 10 years after intervention (p<0.001) and 47% and 62% of children had thresholds <10 dB HL respectively.

There have been some problems with national programmes introduced [20, 24]. The available salt is sometimes poor, iodisation of salt has not always been performed correctly, and even correctly iodised salt may deteriorate if it is exposed over a long period to light, heat or moisture. In some countries insufficient control of iodisation has led to excessive iodine intakes [24]. In some countries, with mild to moderate iodine deficiency, there have been instances of hyperthyroidism and the development of a nodular goitre.

More recently the practice of iodisation of salt has been brought into question. Concern about the risks of hypertension has resulted in some people restricting the use of salt in their diet. Efforts aimed at reducing dietary salt consumption will need to take into account the effect this could have on iodine intake and alternative foods identified as vehicles for iodine supplementation in countries currently using salt.

Magnesium

Magnesium is found in a variety of food but green vegetables, whole grains, nuts and seeds are particularly good sources of this mineral [25]. It is absorbed from the small intestine and absorption is aided by vitamin D. In the body magnesium is required for bone, muscle and nerve function, normal cardiac rhythm and the immune system. It is involved in energy metabolism and protein synthesis [26]. Magnesium is also involved in neural transmission and in enzyme systems requiring ATP.

Magnesium deficiency is signaled by hypocalcaemia and symptoms include muscle weakness and neuromuscular dysfunction [26]. A deficiency can occur in the elderly through lack of sufficient magnesium in the diet. Others may experience deficiencies as a result of poor absorption through the presence of gastro-intestinal diseases or depletion as a consequence of chronic diarrhoea. Certain medications eg diuretics and some antibiotics can result in a reduction in body stores [25].

Magnesium supplements can be given in various forms including magnesium oxide, magnesium citrate, magnesium chloride or magnesium lactate or aspartate. They are usually given in conjunction with another substance such as salt. The efficacy of these magnesium compounds differs with the chloride and the lactate having the highest bioavailablity [27].

Effects on Hearing of the Use of Supplements

In animal experiments and also in investigations on humans, magnesium supplements have been shown to be effective in ameliorating the effect on hearing of noise exposure, ototoxic substances and sudden hearing loss.

Noise-Induced Hearing Loss

Magnesium has been shown to reduce the incidence of temporary and permanent NIHL. It crosses the blood barrier and enters the cochlea where it has vasodilatory and neuroprotective effects [28]. It has few side effects and has been used to prevent acoustic trauma and to treat it.

The value of magnesium in the prophylaxis of noise-induced hearing loss was examined in a double blind study using a placebo-control [29]. 320 normal hearing subjects were examined after two months of military training in which they were exposed to firearms (420 shots: mean peak level 164 dBA) and wearing ear plugs. A week after the last exposure audiograms were obtained and compared with those obtained before the start of the study. The percentage of ears with permanent threshold shifts > 25db was found to be twice as high in the placebo group than in the magnesium treated group.

More recently, in a double-blind study using 20 subjects (16-37 years), Temporary Threshold Shift (TTS) was examined in the same subjects tested in three conditions, - magnesium, placebo, no drug. The TTS was significantly lower in subjects given magnesium [30].

Animal studies have allowed the cochlea to be examined microscopically. Haupt et al. investigated two groups of guinea pigs, one group given magnesium supplements and the other a placebo immediately after exposure to impulse noise [31]. They were then tested using auditory brainstem responses (ABR). Distortion product otoacoustic emissions (DPOAE) and compound action potentials (CAP) were measured one week after exposure. The permanent threshold shifts were smaller in the group given magnesium than in the control group. Scanning electron microscopy revealed less damage to hair cell stereocilia in the magnesium treated group.

Ototoxicity

It has also been demonstrated in rats that magnesium ions protect ganglion cells from quinolinic acid, a metabolite of the essential amino acid tryptophan. Quinolinic acid is neurotoxic and could be implicated in neurodegenerative conditions. It injures ganglionic cells by over-activation of N-methyl-D-aspartate receptors on the cell membrane [32].

Sudden Sensorineural Hearing Loss

The use of magnesium as therapy for patients with sudden hearing loss was trialed by Nageris et al. in patients with sudden hearing loss [9]. A group of 28 men with idiopathic acute onset hearing loss were either given oral magnesium and steroids or placebo and steroids. The group receiving magnesium had a significant improvement in their hearing (>10dB HL) compared to the control group. The improvement was across all frequencies.

There is a suggestion that magnesium supplements could reduce blood pressure levels and have a role in diabetic control [25]. This raises the possibility that supplementation could also indirectly reduce the prevalence or degree of hearing loss associated with these conditions.

Selenium

Selenium is mainly found in plant food, especially nuts, but can also be found in cereals and mushrooms. Some meats are a source of selenium through the animals grazing. The amount of selenium varies in soils and parts of Russia and China have low levels of selenium [33]. This leads to a lower dietary intake. Selenium is an essential trace element and is involved in the production of the selenoprotein enzymes which are powerful antioxidants. Selenium has a role in every gland and tissue using thyroid hormone and is involved in the activation and deactivation of thyroid hormones e.g. thyroxine to triiodothyronine.

Deficiency Diseases

Deficiencies are uncommon but can be found in some areas e.g. in parts of China, and also in some patient groups e.g. those with gastrointestinal disease and those fed by intravenous infusion. Selenium deficiency is thought to predispose to Keshin -Beck Disease, which affects growth and joints. An adequate intake of selenium is reported to protect against the neurological effects of iodine deficiency [33].

Ototoxicity

The role of selenium in protecting the ear was investigated in a case control study by Chuang et al. who measured lead, manganese, arsenic and selenium blood concentrations in 121 subjects with a hearing loss and 173 normal hearing controls [34]. They found that hearing thresholds were significantly associated with lead and selenium concentrations. In their study serum selenium levels were inversely proportional to hearing thresholds. Selenium appeared to protect against lead toxicity. and, in addition, may have a protective effect on auditory function.

Zinc

Zinc is an essential mineral and is found in meat and poultry, nuts and grains and certain seafoods such as oysters and crab. It is an important component of some proteins, enzymes and nucleic acids. It is a component of Cu/Zn superoxide dismutase, an enzyme which is anti-inflammatory and antioxidant and which prevents the tissue damage resulting from superoxide, a free radical. It has a role in DNA synthesis and in the immune system. Zinc is a cofactor in many of the enzymes influencing organ functions and which have a secondary effect on the immune system. Zinc also has direct effects on the production, maturation and function of leucocytes [35].

An insufficiency of zinc can result in a deficient immune system and growth retardation and is associated with an increased susceptibility to infections and the high rates of mortality due to these in developing countries. Those most at risk include pregnant and lactating women, older breast fed infants, vegetarians, and those with sickle cell disease.

Zinc interacts with the quinolone antibiotics and tetracyclines in the intestinal tract and this affects the absorption on both, Thiazide diuretics also increase the renal excretion of zinc, and zinc deficiency can result from prolonged use of these diuretics [36]. Zinc status should be monitored in those patients receiving such long-term therapy. However, zinc status is difficult to measure. Whereas serum and plasma levels can be measured these do not necessarily indicate zinc status within body cells.

Zinc has been shown to have a beneficial effect on hearing threshold in OM and SSNHL.

Otitis Media

Recent studies have revealed an association between zinc deficiency and hearing loss resulting from otitis media [4]. Otitis media affects both adults and children but is particularly prevalent in childhood. It accounts for considerable morbidity particularly in developing countries. The value of zinc supplements in reducing the incidence of otitis media was examined in a study involving 12 randomised placebo-controlled investigations [37]. They concluded that the evidence for benefit in children<5 years living in low-middle income countries was mixed.

Sudden Hearing Loss

Zinc supplements have also been found to be effective in enhancing the recovery of hearing thresholds of 66 subjects who experienced sudden idiopathic sensorineural hearing loss in a controlled study reported by Yang et al. [38]. In their randomized control study the 66 patients with a sudden sensorineural hearing loss were given corticosteroids with half being given zinc gluconate additionally. Serum zinc levels were measured before and after treatment in both groups. The group given zinc had a significantly larger hearing gain, an increased percentage of recovery, and an increased rate of successful recovery compared to the control group ($p < 0.05$). Yang et al. attributed the results to the antioxidant and anti-inflammatory effects of zinc. Zinc supplements can take such forms as the sulphate, gluconate or acetate administered in tablets, capsules and lozenges or as a nasal spray. The disadvantage of the use of nasal sprays is that some recipients develop anosmia.

Vitamins

Vitamins have been associated with hearing threshold improvement if, AHL, NIHL and SSNHL.

Vitamin A

This essential vitamin is important for scotopic vision and colour vision. It helps to regulate the immune system and is necessary for gene transcription and haematopoiesis. It is derived from animal or plant sources. In animal food it exists as retinol and is converted in the body to retinal and retinoic acid, its active forms. It may also be derived from plant sources. β carotene is the main carotenoid source of vitamin A and is converted in the body to retinol. The carotenoids are found in pigmented vegetables such as carrots. Vitamin A is toxic when ingested in excess.

Otitis Media

Vitamin A deficiency is a major public health problem reported to affect an estimated 127 million schoolchildren [39]. A role for vitamin A deficiency in the aetiology of acute otitis media (AOM) and COM has been indicated in an investigation by Lasisi et al. [39]. These investigators followed up patients with AOM in Nigeria by measuring serum retinol using liquid chromatography. At six months follow-up there were 358 subjects and 52 control subjects. 116 had persistence of otorrhoea (COM) whereas in the rest it had resolved. The mean serum retinol levels were significantly lower in the AOM group compared to the controls and in the resolved AOM group when compared to the COM group. The small number of controls in this study could have influenced the results.

Further evidence in support of the role of vitamin A deficiency in the development of acute otitis media (AOM) and lower respiratory tract infections (LRTIs) came from Cameron et al.'s investigation of Inuit neonates. Vitamin A concentrations were determined from umbilical cord sera of 305 neonates and the incidence rates of AOM were obtained. The children were subsequently followed up for 5 years and risk ratios for AOM were calculated. They concluded that vitamin A deficiency was a significant risk factor for AOM and LRTIs in the population studied [40].

B Complex

Several vitamins within the B complex have been associated with hearing loss – in particular vitamins, B5, B6, B7, B9 and B12.

Vitamin B5 (Pantothenic Acid)

This is a water soluble vitamin, found mainly in meat but also present in whole grains. It is required for the synthesis of Co-enzyme A which is needed for metabolic processes in the body and the synthesis of cholesterol and acetylcholine.

Ciges et al. have reported that pantothenic acid (PA) prevents deafness induced by cisplatin (CP) in the guinea pig if both drugs are administered together [41]. When given afterwards recovery did not necessarily take place. Their study indicated that pantothenic acid was effective through the production of Co-enzyme A.

Vitamin B6

This vitamin is found in grains, cereals, nuts and vegetables. This vitamin has a role in glycogen metabolism and also has a metabolic role as a co-enzyme in amino acid metabolism.

Additionally, B6 is involved in glucose and carbohydrate metabolism as well as the synthesis of haemoglobin.

Buckmaster et al. investigated the effects of B6 deficiency on cats using ABR and found that interpeak latencies I-5 were significantly increased [42]. The increase was found between waves 3-5 but not between waves 1-3. They observed that their findings were consistent with slow axonal conduction velocity as a result of defective myelination.

Vitamin B7 (Biotin, Vitamin H)

This vitamin is found in food in a free or protein-bound form. It is involved in the metabolism of fatty acids,, amino acids and gluconeogenesis and is important for the citric acid cycle (Krebs cycle) which is involved in energy production through aerobic respiration. Deficiencies are rare but can occur during pregnancy and also when there is absence of one of the enzymes involved in maintaining biotin homeostasis. An autosomal recessive condition in which biotidinase is deficient is associated with sensorineural hearing loss.

Biotidinase is one of the enzymes which help maintain biotin homeostasis. It is present in cochlear hair cells and ganglion cells as well as in the cochlear nucleus and is involved in the early development of the ear. Early detection of this condition and treatment with biotin can result in a reversal of some of the symptoms of biotidinase deficiency but hearing does not improve [43].

Vitamin B9 (Folate)

Vitamin B9 is a water soluble B complex vitamin and is involved in the synthesis of purines, pyramidases, methionine and glycine and also in the synthesis of thymine a fundamental part of DNA. Folate is its natural form and folic acid the synthetic form. It occurs naturally in liver, spinach and other green vegetables and nuts.

A deficiency of folic acid causes an increased accumulation of homocysteine which affects neurological development in the foetus and affects the endothelial lining of blood vessels [44]. A deficiency is most readily seen in tissues with a rapid turnover e.g. red blood corpuscles, and is a cause of megaloblastic anaemia. Folic acid deficiency in early pregnancy is associated with neural tube defects in the foetus.

Sudden Sensorineural Hearing Loss

The association between folate and hearing thresholds has been explored with varying results. An early study reported no association between folate and hearing levels [45]. A later study, however, linked low serum folate levels and high homocysteine levels to sudden sensorineural hearing loss [46].

Age Associated Hearing Loss

An investigation by Cadoni et al. of healthy adults >60 years, which examined the correlation between serum folic acid and hearing impairment, indicated that low serum folate was significantly related to higher hearing thresholds at high frequencies [47]. A study by Houston et al. in which both vitamin12 and folate levels were examined also found a relationship with age associated hearing loss [48].

Supplementation with Folic Acid

Supplementation with folate has been shown to reduce AHL. A three year study of 728 men and women in their 50s and 60s with elevated homocysteine levels found that a daily supplement of 800 μg of folic acid may help slow age associated hearing loss. During this placebo-controlled study, half of the participants received a folic acid supplement. Those getting the supplemental folic acid experienced less hearing loss over time than those getting the placebo. The difference in hearing loss in the study was slight, but the authors suggest that the benefit could be significant by age 70, as hearing loss generally accelerates with age [49].

Vitamin B12 (Cobalamin)

Vitamin B12 is involved in DNA synthesis in the body, fatty acid synthesis and blood formation. It is found in foods derived from animal sources e.g. meat especially liver, eggs, milk, and is also found in fish. It can be produced synthetically in the form of cyanocobalmin. A deficiency in vitamin B12 results in pernicious anaemia. Some of the effects of a deficiency in vitamin B12 can be corrected with folic acid, including pernicious anaemia.

A relationship has been found between vitamin 12 deficiencyand auditory dysfunction [50]. Poor vitamin B12 or folate nutrition might impair the vascular and nervous system of the auditory system through direct or indirect effects or both; the effect being on cellular metabolism, vascular perfusion, and myelin synthesis.

The prevalence of vitamin B12 deficiency is greatest in the elderly population. This is mainly due to atrophic gastritis which results in a reduction in gastric acid production and digestive enzymes which release the vitamin from proteins and food particles. More than twenty percent of older adults have marginal or frank vitamin B12 deficiency [51].

Noise Induced Hearing Loss

The effects of vitamin B12 administration on the TTS resulting from narrow band noise exposure was investigated by Quaranta et al. on 20 healthy young volunteers with normal hearing in a placebo-controlled study [52]. The group given cyanocobalamin had a significantly lower TTS at the test frequencies (3 and 4kHz) than the control group indicating a protective function of raised cyanocobalamin plasma levels on auditory function.

Age Associated Hearing Loss

The association of vitamin B12 and folate with hearing thresholds was examined by Houston et al. in 55 healthy women aged 60–71 years mean 65 years. Their hearing thresholds were determined using pure tone audiometry and they calculated the average threshold over 0.5, 1, 2, and 4 kHz. Two groups were identified for analysis 1) normal hearing (<20 dB hearing level; $n = 44$) and 2) impaired hearing (20 dB hearing level; $n = 11$). Women with impaired hearing were to found to have 38% lower serum vitamin B12 and 31% a lower red cell count than women with normal hearing. Among those participants who did not take supplements containing vitamin B12 or folate, women with impaired hearing had 48% lower serum vitamin B12 and 43% a lower red cell count than women with normal hearing. Those with normal hearing were 3 times more likely to meet the RDA for vitamin B12 and 8 times more likely to meet the RDA for folate than those with impaired hearing. One suggestion made to explain the association was that higher levels of homocysteine associated with low B12 and low folate could affect the blood flow to the cochlea [48].

Vitamin C (Ascorbic Acid)

An essential vitamin found in green vegetables and fruits, with citrus fruits being a particularly rich source. It is an essential vitamin which is important for formation of collagen and is involved in growth and tissue repair. A deficiency in vitamin C leads to scurvy a disease in which gums bleed and in which anaemia, swollen joints, dry skin and hair feature among the symptoms.

Vitamin C depletion has been studied in mice and the findings indicated that AHL could be accelerated by insufficient vitamin C but that supplementation may not increase levels of the vitamin in the inner ear or slow down AHL [53].

Vitamin D

This vitamin is not present in many foods but can be found in salmon, tuna, mackerel and fish oils. It is manufactured in the body as a consequence of ultraviolet stimulation of the skin, but in this form it is biologically inert and has to be converted to an active form in the body. Vitamin D promotes the absorption of calcium and helps maintain adequate levels of calcium and phosphate in the serum. A deficiency of this vitamin caused rickets in which bones are weakened.

Research into the relationship of vitamin D with hearing has produced variable results. Some have found vitamin D to be a cause of sensorineural hearing loss [54] whilst others have found no relationship [55]. Its involvement with calcium metabolism could be a factor in the causation of a hearing loss. Ikeda et al. suggested that hearing loss in vitamin D deficiency is mainly attributable to the depression of the Ca2+ (calcium ions) concentration in the perilymph [56].

Vitamin E

Vitamin E is a generic term for a group of lipid soluble compounds classified as tocopherols or tocotrienols. Alpha-tocopherol is the most biologically active and is found in such foods as cereals, nuts, olives and asparagus. It is important for the formation of blood vessels and it helps in the utilisation of vitamin K. Vitamin E is a powerful antioxidant in the body.

Ototoxicity

It has been demonstrated that vitamin E has a role in protecting the ear against ototoxic medication. Fetoni et al. examined the role of vitamin E (tocopherol) in a four groups of guinea pigs fed for 14 days with corn oil (Group1), corn oil plus gentamicin (Group 2), gentamicin alone (Group 3), and gentamicin plus alpha- tocopherol (Group 4) [56]. CAP were measured up to 18 days afterwards. A gentamicin induced progressive high-frequency hearing loss of 50-60 dB SPL (sound pressure level) was discovered with those fed alpha-tocopherol having a slower progression of hearing loss. The cochleae of animals protected with alpha-tocopherol did not show the significant loss of outer hair cells (OHC) in the cochlear basal turn found in gentamicin-only treated animals. They suggested that alpha-tocopherol interferes with gentamicin-induced free radical formation so that it may be useful in protecting OHC function from aminoglycoside ototoxicity.

Antioxidants such as alpha-tocopherol interfere with gentamicin and cisplatin damage and this suggests that they may be useful in preventing oto-vestibulotoxicity [57]. They pointed out that it is important to develop protective strategies that permit the avoidance of the toxic side effects of these drugs without interfering with their therapeutic effects.

Amino Acids

Methionine

This an essential amino acid which is a source of sulphur in the body. It gives rise to homocysteine and cysteine, is involved in the breakdown of fats, and is an antioxidant. Campbell et al. have drawn attention to the number of animal studies which have shown that methionine has an otoprotective effect against cisplatin and amikacin otoxicity as well as against permanent noise-induced hearing loss when given one hour after noise exposure [58].

Cysteine

This is a non-essential or semi-essential amino acid which is found in a variety of foods including poultry, eggs, broccoli and onions. It is conditionally essential as it is only deficient in certain groups of the population e.g. infants, because they lack the enzyme needed to produce it in sufficient quantities. In the body cysteine is biosynthesised from homocysteine which is itself derived from methionine an essential amino acid. Cysteine is required by the body for the production of the tripeptide, glutathione. This non-essential amino acid is formed from L-cysteine, glycine and L-glutamic acid and is a powerful antioxidant. The "thio" group (SH) in its structure, derived from cysteine, is believed to be responsible for its biological properties. Cysteine, in the form of N-acetyl cysteine (NAC), has been shown to be effective in reducing the effects of noise exposure. In a prospective double blind crossover study 53 male workers were randomised into two groups both of which were exposed to noise ranging from 88.4-89.4dB , peaking at 4kHz. One group was given NAC for 14 days and the other group was given a placebo instead of NAC. After a two week period free of noise the groups were reversed. NAC was found to reduce TTS significantly [59].

Taurine

This is an organic acid but is sometimes classed as an amino acid. It is found in meat and seafoods and is involved in conjugating bile acid and so aids lipid absorption. It can be deficient in premature babies.

Taurine has been shown to affect the transmission of electrical signals along auditory pathways in the brain. Supplementation of the diet with taurine has been demonstrated to result in a decrease in auditory brainstem wave latency and therefore faster transmission [60].

An investigation of three groups of neonates, fed with breast milk, taurine supplemented formula and formula without taurine supplementation respectively were examined using ABR and transient evoked otoacoustic emissions (TEOAE). The latency of the waveforms was significantly shorter in the non-supplemented group with wave V showing the most marked effect. Taurine is therefore involved in maturation of the auditory system [61].

Ototoxicity

A protective effect of taurine supplementation has been by Liu et al. who showed that guinea pigs given taurine prior to IV dosage with gentamycin and furosemide did not develop hearing damage as opposed to those not given taurine who developed a profound hearing loss [62]. It was suggested that taurine could provide protection by down-regulating nitric oxide synthase expression in the cochlea.

Coenzymes

CoQ10

Coenzymes are proteins which transport chemical groups from one enzyme to another and are essential for some enzymes to function. CoQ10 (also known as Q10) is present in meat, fish and vegetable oils. In the body it is found in cell membranes and is particularly abundant in the heart, lungs, kidneys, liver, spleen and pancreas. It is present in mitochondria and is involved in the oxygen transport system. As well as being involved in energy generation in the body and is also a powerful antioxidant.

Age Associated Hearing Loss

Q10 is reported to improve hearing in patients with presbyacusis. In an investigation by Guastini et al. 60 patients were divided into three treatment groups; one group received 60mg Q-TERN (which contains Q10) daily for 30 days, the second vitamin E (50mg), and the third a placebo for the same period [63]. Audiological testing was conducted before and after the 30 day period and six months later using pure tone audiometry, TEOAE and DPOAE tests, ABR and speech audiometry. Pure tone audiometric thresholds at 1, 2, 4 and 8 kHz were improved significantly in the Q10 treated group compared to the group taking vitamin E and this was confirmed by speech audiometric results. There were no other significant changes found in the investigation.

Noise Induced Hearing Loss

Animal studies have also shown a reduction in cochlear oxidative stress induced by noise exposure. In a controlled experiment by Hirose et al. guinea pigs were exposed to 130dB noise for 3 hours after being given coenzyme Q [64]. Seven days later ABR threshold shift and cochlear hair cell damage were assessed. ABR threshold shift was significantly less in the coenzyme Q10 group than in the control group. In addition, the percentage of missing outer hair cells was lower in the coenzyme Q10 group than in the control group when measured by analysis of hydroxy radical scavenging activity by electron spin resonance. CoQ10 may be helpful in delaying the progression of hearing loss in patients with the 7445A-->G mitochondrial mutation [65]. It has also been suggested that it may be beneficial in SSNHL [66]. Ahn et al.'s study showed a significant improvement in speech discrimination after treatment although the improvement in hearing thresholds was not significantly different to that found in patients not given this substance in treatment [66].

Fatty Acids

Alpha-Lipoic Acid

This substance is found in such foods as kidney liver, spinach, broccoli and sprouts but can also be synthesised in the body. It is a potent antioxidant and, as it is both lipid soluble and water soluble has a role in many body tissues. The hearing threshold of mice fed with alpha- lipoic acid fed 2, 4, 8 weeks after birth were compared with those of a control group in a study by Ahn et al. [67]. Hearing thresholds were found to be significantly better at all frequencies in the alpha-lipoic acid-fed group than the group not given this supplement. The levels of hypoxia-inducible factor were found to be lower in the group fed with alpha-lipoic acid leading the researchers to suggest that it prevented early onset deafness in the group to which it was fed.

Multiple Micronutrient Supplements

Many studies into the effectiveness of nutrients in protecting against hearing impairment have used multiple supplementation. These include a study by Weijl et al. on patients with cancer receiving treatment with cisplatin [8]. They found that patients given supplementation with vitamin C, vitamin E and selenium who produced the highest plasma concentration levels had less loss of high frequency hearing than subjects treated with a placebo.

There is some evidence of synergism so that several antioxidants are more effective than any one alone. This was the conclusion from an investigation by Le Prell et al. [68]. They discovered that the antioxidants vitamins A, C, and E acted in synergy with magnesium to prevent noise-induced trauma effectively but not when administered alone. Together they were highly effective in reducing both hearing loss and cell death even when therapy was introduced one hour before noise exposure. The advantages of combination nutrient supplementation is that different antioxidants are effective against different free radicals and are distributed differently in tissues [69]. Which of the aforementioned studies have shown a beneficial effect on hearing thresholds in OM, AHL, NIHL, Otoxicity and SSNHL is shown in Table 7.4.

Supplementation and Fortification

Supplementation and food fortification have been used to reduce or eliminate micronutrient deficiencies. Supplementation programmes are usually short term and target particular groups within the population.

Table 7.4. A summary of the hearing conditions for which those studies reviewed have found some nutrients to be beneficial

	Mag	Sel	ZN	Vit. A	B 5	B 9	B 12	Vit. C	Vit. E	Meth	Cyst	Taur	Q10	Reference Nos.
OM			+	+										[5,37,39, 40]
AHL						+	+	+					+	[47,48,49, 53,63]
NIHL	+						+			+	+		+	[29,30,52, 58,59,64]
Otot	+	+			+				+	+		+		[7,8,31,32,34, 41,56,57, 58,62]
SSNHL	+		+			+								[9,38,46]

+ indicates a beneficial effect; reference numbers marked in red are human studies.

Food fortification is a public health initiative which is widely practised and has been successful in the near elimination of many micronutrient deficiencies in high economic industrialised countries.

The food to be fortified has to be appropriate for the population concerned. It must be a staple part of the diet and consumed most of the year round. Milk, bread, salt and sugar are commonly used vehicles.

Many countries have fortification programmes for the public at large to improve dietary intake of nutrients to prevent deficiencies. Multiple nutrients may need to be administered in areas where the standard of nutrition is generally poor as several deficiencies may co-exist.

It is more cost effective than single element supplementation and is acceptable to populations at risk.

Giving multiple micronutrient supplementation to pregnant women in Mali was found to be acceptable and the programme adhered to when certain elements were there within the programme [70].

These were 1) a guarantee of supplement provision, 2) this being accompanied by straightforward, easily understandable, relevant and consistent information, 3) counselling. Care needs to be taken however as the effect of some micronutrients on the absorption and utilisation of others needs to be considered when planning supplementation in a population [71].

An example is the negative effect of iron supplementation on zinc and copper status reported in some studies and zinc on iron and copper status. National fortification programmes are not directly aimed at preventing hearing loss but may do so indirectly. The use of supplementation to prevent hearing loss in specific conditions is mainly limited to research studies at present, but realisation of the protective role of some nutrients suggests that there may be a wider clinical usage in the future, especially where the nutrient concerned is cheap and where overdosage is not a medical problem.

In spite of the efforts to eliminate nutrient deficiencies these still occur worldwide and are a particular problem in developing countries where multiple micronutrient deficiencies frequently occur concomitantly. Governments considering the economic cost of introducing programmes to remedy the effects of deficiencies, need to better appreciate the high cost in terms of morbidity and mortality of failing to do so.

Targeting those most at risk would be a first step towards ensuring less disability within the population and, in terms of hearing impairment, less need for more expensive schooling, and less equipment and rehabilitative services being required over a lifetime.

Conclusion

A number of the studies referred to in this chapter are based upon animal research and there have been no corresponding studies in humans. Human studies have tended to involve small numbers and so should be interpreted with caution.

There is, however, sufficient evidential support for further large scale research into the potential use of some nutrients in the prevention of hearing impairment.

References

[1] Haase, G. M., Prasad, K. N., Cole, W. C., Baggett-Strehlau, J. M., Wyatt, S. E. (2011). Antioxidant micronutrient impact on hearing disorders: concept, rationale, and evidence. *American Journal of Otolaryngology,* 32, 55-61.

[2] Recommended Dietary Intake Tables. Available from: http://www.iom.edu/Activities /Nutrition/SummaryDRIs/~/media/Files/Activity%20Files/Nutrition/DRIs/New%20Mat erial/5DRI%20Values%20SummaryTables%2014.(Accessed 15 June 2011).

[3] Pathak, P., Kapil, U., Kapoor, S. K., Saxena, R., Kumar, A., Gupta, N., Dwivedi, S. N., Singh, R., Singh, P. (2004). Prevalence of multiple micronutrient deficiencies amongst pregnant women in a rural area of Haryana. *Indian Journal of Pediatrics,* 71, 1007-1014.

[4] Elemraid, M. A., Mackenzie, I. J., Fraser, W. D., Brabin, B. J. (2010).Nutritional factors in the pathogenesis of ear disease in children: a systematic review. *Annals of Tropical Paediatrics,* 29, 85-99.

[5] Yariktas, M., Doner, F., Dogru, H., Yasan, H., Delibas, N. (2004). The role of free radicals on the development of otitis media with effusion. *International Journal of Pediatric Otorhinolaryngology,* 68, 889-894.

[6] National Institute on Deafness and Other Communication Disorders. Presbycusis. Available from: http://www.nidcd.nih.gov/staticresources/health/healthyhearing/tools /pdf/presbycusis.pdf (Accessed 5 May 2011).

[7] Sergi, B., Fetoni, A. R., Ferraresi, A., Troiani, D., Azzena, G. B., Paludetti, G., Maurizi, M. (2004). The role of antioxidants in protection from ototoxic drugs. *Acta Otolaryngologica Supplement,* 552, 42-45.

[8] Weijl, N. I., Elsendoorn, T. J., Lentjes, E. G., Hopman, G. D., Wipkink-Bakker, A., Zwinderman, A. H., Cleton, F. J., Osanto, S. (2004). Supplementation with antioxidant micronutrients and chemotherapy-induced toxicity in cancer patients treated with cisplatin-based chemotherapy: a randomized, double-blind, placebo-controlled study. *European Journal of Cancer,* 40, 1713-1723.

[9] Nageris, B. I, Ulanovski, D., Attias, J. (2004). Magnesium treatment for sudden hearing loss. *Annals of Otology Rhinology and Laryngology,* 113, 672-675.

[10] De Benoist, B., Andersson, M., Egli, I., Takkouche, B., Allen, H. (2004). Iodine status worldwide. Global Database on Iodine Deficiency. Department of Nutrition for Health and Development. World Health Organisation. Geneva.

[11] Rajatabavin, R. (2007). Iodine deficiency in pregnant women and neonates in Thailand. *Public Health Nutrition,* 10, 1602-1605.

[12] Andersson, M., De Benoist, B., Darnton-Hill, I., Delange, F. (2007). Iodine Deficiency in Europe. Geneva: World Health Organisation.

[13] WHO, UNICEF, ICCIDD. (2001) Assessment of the iodine deficiency disorders and monitoring their elimination. Geneva: World Health Organisation.

[14] Vanderpump, M. P., Lazarus, J. H., Smyth, P. P., Laurberg, P., Holder, R. L., Boelaert, K., Franklyn, J. A. on behalf of the British Thyroid Association UK Iodine Survey Group.(2011). Iodine status of UK schoolgirls: a cross-sectional survey. *Lancet,* 377, 2007- 2012.

[15] Goslings, B. M., Djokomoeljanto, R., Hoedijono, R., Soepardjo, H., Querido, A.(1975) Studies on hearing loss in a community with endemic cretinism in Central Java, Indonesia. ,*Acta Endocrinologica,* (Copenh.), 78, 705- 713.

[16] Valeix, P., Preziosi, P., Rossignol, C., Farnier, M. A., Hercberg, S. (1994).Relationship between urinary iodine concentration and haring capacity in children. *European Journal of Clinical Nutrition,* 48, 54-59.

[17] Gao, H., Li, J., Wang, E. (1998). Iodine deficiency and perceptive nerve deafness. *Lin Chuang Er Bi Yan Hou Ke Za Zhi,* 12, 228-230.

[18] Wang, Y. Y, Yang, S. H. (1985). Improvement in hearing among otherwise normal schoolchildren in iodine-deficient areas of Guizhou, China, following use of iodized salt. *Lancet,* 2, 518-520.

[19] Den Briel, T., West, C. E., Hautvast, J. G., Ategbo, E. A. (2001). Mild iodine deficiency is associated with elevated hearing thresholds in children in Benin. *European Journal of Clinical Nutrition,* 55, 763-768.

[20] Maberly, G. F., Haxton, D. P., Van der Haar, F. (2003). Iodine deficiency: consequences and progress towards elimination. *Food and Nutrition Bulletin,* 24(Suppl. 4), S91-98.

[21] Zimmermann, M. B., Jooste, P. L., Pandav, C. S. (2008). Iodine-deficiency disorders. *Lancet,* 72, 1251-1262.

[22] Zimmerman, M. B., Jooste, P. L., Mabapa, N. S., Schoeman, S., Biebinger, R., Mushaphi, L. F., Mbhenyane, X. (2007). Vitamin A supplementation in iodine – deficient African children decreases thyrotropin stimulation of the thyroid and reduces the goiter rate. *American Journal of Clinical Nutrition,* 86, 1040-1044.

[23] Azizi, F., Mirmiran, P., Hedayati, M., Salarkia, N., Noohi, S., Rostamian, D. (2005). Effect of 10yr iodine supplementation on the hearing threshold of iodine deficient schoolchildren. *Journal of Endocrinological Investigation,* 28, 595-598.

[24] Andersson, M., De Benoist, B., Rogers, L. (2010). Epidemiology of iodine deficiency: Salt iodisation and iodine status. *Best Practice and Research in Clinical Endocrinology and Metabolism,* 24, 1-11.

[25] Office of Dietary Supplements Fact Sheet. Magnesium, National Institutes of Health. Available from http:/ods.od.nih.gov/factsheets/magnesium.asp (Accessed 6 June 2011).

[26] Barasi, M. (2003). Minerals, electrolytes and fluids. In: *Human Nutrition. A Health Perspective.* (2nd Ed. pp. 194-226). London: Edward Arnold.

[27] Fine, K. D., Santa Ana, C. A., Porter, J. L., Fordtran, J. S. (1991). Intestinal absorption of magnesium from food and supplements. *Journal of Clinical Investigation,*88, 396-402.

[28] Sendowski, I. (2006). Magnesium therapy in acoustic trauma. *Magnesium Research,* 19, 244--54.

[29] Joachims, Z., Netzer, A., Ising, H., Rebentisch, E., Attias, J., Weisz, G., Gunther, T. (1993). Oral magnesium supplementation as prophylaxis for noise-induced hearing loss: results of a double blind field study. *Schriftenr Ver Wasser Boden Lufthyg,* 88, 503-516.

[30] Attias, J., Sapir, S., Bresloff, I., Reshef-Haran, I., Ising, H. (2004). Reduction in noise-induced temporary threshold shift in humans following oral magnesium intake. *Clinical Otolaryngology and Allied Sciences,* 29, 635-641.

[31] Haupt, H., Acheibe, F., Mazurek, B. (2003).Therapeutic efficiency of magnesium in acoustic trauma in the guinea pig. *ORL Journal of Otorhinolaryngology and Related Species,* 65, 134-139.

[32] Xiao, H., Yang, C., He, Y., Zheng, N. (2010). Neurotoxicity of quinoloic acid to spiral ganglion cells in rats. *Journal of Huazhong University of Science and Technology and Medical Science,* 30, 397-402.

[33] Office of Dietary Supplements, National Institutes of Health, NIH, Selenium. Available from: http://ods.od.nih.gov/factsheets/selenium.asp (Accessed 2 February 2011).

[34] Chuang, H. Y., Kuo, C. H., Chiu, Y. W., Ho, C. K., Chen, C. J., Wu, T. N. (2007). A case-control study on the relationship of hearing function and blood concentrations of *Nutrition Society.* 59, 541-552.

[35] Rink, L., Gabriel, P. (2000). Zinc and the immune system. *Proceedings of the Nutrition Society,* 59, 541-552.

[36] Office of Dietary Supplements, National Institutes of Health, NIH, Zinc. Available from: http://ods.od.nih.gov/factsheets/zinc.asp (Accesses 18 April 2011).

[37] Abba, K., Gulani, A., Sachdev, H. S. (2010). Zinc supplements for preventing otitis media. Cochrane Database of Systematic Reviews.lead, manganese, arsenic and selenium. *The Science of the Total Environment,* 387, 79-85.

[38] Yang, C. H., Ko, M. T., Peng, J. P., Hwang, C. F. (2011). Zinc in the treatment of idiopathic sudden sensorineural hearing loss. *Laryngoscope,* 121, 617-621.

[39] Lasisi, A. O. (2009).The role of retinol in the aetiology and outcome of suppurative otitis media. *European Archives of Otorhinolaryngology,* 266, 647-652.

[40] Cameron, C., Dallaire, F., Vezina, C., Muckle, G., Bruneau, S., Ayotte, P., Dewailly, E. (2008). Neonatal vitamin A deficiency and its impact on acute respiratory infections among preschool Inuit children. *Canadian Journal of Public Health,* 99, 102-106.

[41] Ciges, M., Fernández-Cervilla, F., Crespo, P. V., Campos, A. (1996). Pantothenic acid and coenzyme A in experimental cisplatin-induced ototoxia. *Acta Otolaryngologica,*116, 263-268.

[42] Buckmaster, P. S., Holliday, T. A., Bai, S. C., Rogers, Q. R.(1993). Brainstem auditory evoked potential interwave intervals are prolonged in vitamin B-6-deficient cats. *Journal of Nutrition,* 123, 20-26.

[43] Brumwell, C. L., Hossain, W. A., Morest, D. K, Wolf, B. (2005). Biotinidase reveals the morphogenetic sequence in cochlea and cochlear nucleus of mice. *Hearing Research,* 209, 104-121.

[44] Best, B. (2009). Miscellaneous nutrient supplements. Available from: www.benbest.com/nutrceut/MiscSupp.html (Accessed 2 March 2011).

[45] Berner, B., Odum, L., Parving. A. (2000). Age-related hearing impairment and B vitamin status. *Acta Otolaryngologica,*120, 633-637.

[46] Cadoni, G., Agostino, S., Scipione, S., Galli, J. (2004). Low serum folate levels: a risk factor for sudden sensorineural hearing loss? *Acta Otolaryngologica,* 124, 608-611.

[47] Lasisi, A. O., Fehintola, F. A., Yusuf, O. B. (2010). Age-related hearing loss, vitamin B12, and folate in the elderly. *Otolaryngology Head and Neck Surgery,* 143, 826-830.

[48] Houston, D. K., Johnson, M. A., Nozza, R. J., Gunter, E. W., Shea, K. J., Cutler, G. M., Edmonds, J. T. (1999). Age-related hearing loss, vitamin B-12, and folate in elderly women. *American Journal of Clinical Nutrition,* 69, 564-571.

[49] Durga, J., Verhoef, P., Anteunis, L. J, Schouten, E., Kok, F. J. (2007). Effects of folic acid supplementation on hearing in older adults: a randomised, controlled trial. *Annals of Internal Medicine,* 1461, 1-9.

[50] Shemesh, Z., Attias, J., Ornan, M., Shapira, N., Shahar, A. (1993).Vitamin B12 deficiency in patients with chronic tinnitus and noise-induced hearing loss. *American Journal of Otolaryngology,* 14, 94-99.

[51] Park, S., Johnson, M. A. (2006). What is an adequate dose of oral vitamin B12 in older people with poor vitamin B12 status? *Nutrition Review,* 64, 373-378.

[52] Quaranta, A., Scaringi, A., Bartoli, R., Margarito, M. A., Quaranta, N. (2004). The effects of "supra-physiological" vitamin B12 administration on temporary threshold shift. *International Journal of Audiology,* 43, 162-165.

[53] Kashio, A., Amano, A., Kondo, Y., Sakamoto, T., Iwamura, H., Suzuki, M., Ishigami, A., Yamasoba, T. (2009). Effect of vitamin C depletion on age-related hearing loss in SMP30/GNL knockout mice. *Biochemical and Biophysical Research Communications,* 390, 394-398.

[54] Ikeda, K., Kobayashi, T., Itoh, Z., Kusakari, J., Takasaka, T. (1989). Evaluation of vitamin D metabolism in patients with bilateral sensorineural hearing loss. *American Journal of Otology,* 10, 11-13.

[55] Irwin, J. J. (1986) Hearing-loss and calciferol deficiency. *Journal of Laryngology and Otology,* 100, 1245-1247.

[56] Fetoni, A. R., Sergi, B., Ferraresi, A., Paludetti, G., Troiani, D. (2004). Alpha-Tocopherol protective effects on gentamicin ototoxicity: an experimental study. *International Journal of Audiology,* 43, 166-171.

[57] Sergi, B, Fetoni, A. R., Ferraresi, A., Troiani, D., Azzena, G. B., Paludetti, G., Maurizi, M. (2004).The role of antioxidants in protection from ototoxic drugs. *Acta Otolaryngologica Suppl.,* 552, 42-45.

[58] Campbell, K. C., Meech, R. P., Klemens, J. J., Gerberi, M. T., Dyrstad, S. S., Larsen, D. L., Mitchell, D. L., El-Azizi, M., Verhulst, S. J., Hughes, L. F. (2007). Prevention of noise- and drug-induced hearing loss with D-methionine. *Hearing Research,* 226, 92-103.

[59] Lin, C. Y., Wu, J. L., Shih, T. S., Tsai, P. J., Sun, Y. M., Ma, M. C., Guo, Y. L. (2010). N-Acetyl-cysteine against noise-induced temporary threshold shift in male workers. *Hearing Research,* 269, 42-47.

[60] Gaull, G. E. (1989).Taurine in pediatric nutrition: review and update. *Pediatrics,* 83, 433-442.

[61] Dhillon, S. K, Davies, W. E., Hopkins, P. C., Rose, S. J. (1998). Effects of dietary taurine on auditory function in full-term infants. *Advances in Experimental Medicine and Biology,* 442, 507-514.

[62] Liu, H. Y., Chi, F. L., Gao, W. Y. (2008). Taurine attenuates aminoglycoside ototoxicity by inhibiting inducible nitric oxide synthase expression in the cochlea. *Neuroreport,* 19, 117-120.

[63] Guastini, L., Mora, R., Dellepiane, M., Santomauro, V., Giorgio, M., Salami, A. (2011).Water-soluble coenzyme Q10 formulation in presbycusis: long-term effects. *Acta Otolaryngologica,* 131, 512-517.

[64] Hirose, Y., Sugahara, K., Mikuriya, T., Hashimoto, M., Shimogori, H., Yamashita, H. (2008). Effect of water-soluble coenzyme Q10 on noise-induced hearing loss in guinea pigs. *Acta Otolaryngologica,* 128, 1071-1076.

[65] Angeli, S. I., Liu, X. Z., Yan, D., Balkany, T., Telischi, F. (2005). Coenzyme Q-10 treatment of patients with a 7445A--->G mitochondrial DNA mutation stops the progression of hearing loss. *Acta Otolaryngologica,* 125, 10-12.

[66] Ahn, J. H., Yoo, M. H., Lee, H. J, Chung, J. W., Yoon, T. H. (2010). Coenzyme Q10 in combination with steroid therapy for treatment of sudden sensorineural hearing loss: a controlled prospective study. *Clinical Otolaryngology,* 35, 486-489.

[67] Ahn, J. H., Kang, H. H., Kim, T. Y., Shin, J. E., Chung, J. W. (2008). Lipoic acid rescues DBA mice from early-onset age-related hearing impairment. *Neuroreport,* 19, 1265-1269.

[68] Le Prell, C. G., Hughes, L. F., Miller, J. M. (2007). Free radical scavengers vitamins A, C, and E plus magnesium reduce noise trauma. *Free Radical Biology and Medicine,* 42, 1454-1463.

[69] Heman-Ackah, S. E., Juhn, S. K., Huang, T. C., Wiedmann, T. S. (2010). A combination antioxidant therapy prevents age-related hearing loss in C57BL/6 mice. *Otolaryngology Head and Neck Surgery,*143, 429-434.

[70] Aguayo, V. M., Kone, D., Bamba, S. I., Diallo, B., Sidebe, Y., Traore, D., Signé, P., Baker, S. K. (2005). Acceptability of multiple micronutrient supplements by pregnant and lactating women in Mali. *Public Health Nutrition,* 8, 33-37.

[71] Sandstrom, B. (2001). Micronutrient interactions: effects on absorption and bioavailability. *British Journal of Nutrition.* 85(Suppl.2), S181-5.

In: Prevention of Hearing Loss
Editors: V. Newton, P. Alberti and A. Smith

ISBN: 978-1-61942-745-7
© 2012 Nova Science Publishers, Inc.

Chapter VIII

Genetic Counselling

Katherine Dewes Rutledge and Nathaniel H. Robin[*]

Abstract

Hearing impairment (HI) is a complex disorder, requiring a number of healthcare professions working together. The role of the genetics professional, either a medical geneticist or genetic counselor, is to identify the genetic aetiology of the hearing impairment-distinguishing non-genetic from genetic as well as syndromic from non-syndromic forms of genetic hearing impairment. The past decade has seen tremendous advances in understanding the genetic basis of non-syndromic HI, which has resulted in the clinical availability of several genetic tests. These have important implications for patients and family members as well as the healthcare team, as the results impact medical management. However, the benefits of such testing are not realized without proper pre- and post- test genetic counseling. Such counseling can provide not only accurate recurrence risk assessment but also guide medical management and provide some prognostic information.

Introduction

Hearing impairment (HI) is a complex disorder at many levels. Clinically, for individuals with HI to maximize their potential, they should be managed by an array of specially trained healthcare professions working together. Included in that group should be a genetics professional, either a medical geneticist or genetic counselor, whose role is to identify the genetic aetiology of the hearing impairment- distinguishing non-genetic from genetic as well as syndromic from non-syndromic forms of genetic hearing impairment. Once a specific diagnosis is made, prognostic, management, recurrence risk, and treatment information are subsequently available to the individual and family. HI is an incredibly aetiologically

[*] Corresponding author: nrobin@uab.edu.

heterogeneous disorder, with over a hundred different genes involved in hearing, as well as numerous non-genetic causes as well.

Within the last decade remarkable advances in the understanding of the genetic basis of HI have been made and hundreds of genes have been identified in association with both syndromic and non-syndromic forms of hearing loss. These gene discoveries have led to a greater understanding of the disorders of hearing, and have generated new tests for several genetic forms of HI. Such testing has very important implications for the patient and family members as well as the healthcare team, as the results have implications for medical management. However, as previous studies have shown, the benefits of such testing are not realized without proper pre- and post- test genetic counseling. Brunger et al. [1] surveyed a large group of parents who themselves had normal hearing but had a child with HI. Their study is reviewed in detail later in this chapter, but ultimately concluded that parents are less like to be able to accurately interpret their genetic testing results or determine a modified recurrence risk after genetic testing in the absence of pre- and post- test genetic counselling. As current genetic research uncovers more and more genetic factors involved in HI, the degree of complexity will only increase in the coming years, which also increases the need for genetic counseling.

Why Is a Genetics Evaluation Important?

Establishing a specific aetiology for an individual's diagnosis of HI provides many benefits to the affected individual, their family, and their healthcare providers. Thanks to rapid progress, this is a time when genetics research is changing how we view many diseases, including isolated HI as well as the genetic syndromes that can be associated with HI. This increased knowledge, including the advances in genetic testing, makes it more likely that we will be able to make a genetic diagnosis. In other words, it means that a genetics evaluation will be able to explain why a child has HI in many cases. It is worthwhile to point out that many question the benefit of knowing that answer. It is true that knowing the cause of the HI will not change that the child has HI, nor will it lead (in 2012) to an immediate cure. However, making a genetic diagnosis is far more than an academic exercise. It does have many clear benefits for the person with HI, their family, and the medical team caring for the child. Some of the most obvious reasons include:

Prognosis and Management

A genetic diagnosis allows for accurate prognostic information to be provided, as well as for help guiding management decisions. For example, a child with HI due to Down syndrome has many more medical issues that need to be screened for than a child with isolated HI.

This is an extreme example, as most healthcare providers would recognize a child with Down syndrome, but many genetic syndromes are far more subtle in their presentation. They require a trained expert to identify the condition and provide accurate counseling. The same is true for isolated HI as well, as the prognosis varies for different genetic subtypes.

Recurrence Risk

At some point, parents will ask what their chances are of having another child with HI. Such information cannot be provided unless an accurate diagnosis has been made. For a child with isolated HI born to healthy parents with no family history, the likelihood that a subsequent child will have HI is 1 in 6 (Table 8.1). This estimate varies if there are other family members with HI. However, that figure may be drastically different if the genetic cause is identified, or if HI is part of a syndrome. In such cases, depending on the genetic inheritance pattern, the likelihood of a future child having HI ranges from as high as 50% to as low as <1%.

Table 8.1. *Empiric* **recurrence risk for profound childhood sensorineural hearing impairment of unknown cause**

	Risk
affected child	1/6
1 child, consanguinity	1/4
1 child, 2+ normal sibs	1/10
2 affected children	1/4
1 parent, 1 child	1/2
1 parent	1/20
parent + parent's sibs	1/100
sibs of parent, parent normal	<1/100

Adapted from Harper PS. *Practical genetic counselling.* Bristol: Wright, 1984.

Why?

Parents will also wonder what caused their child to be born with a HI. Many will incorrectly attribute it to prenatal exposures that have no contributing role, such as a medical X-ray or a glass of beer, resulting in parental guilt. It is hoped that by discussing the origin of the birth defect at a scientific level, such feeling can be mitigated at least to some degree. It is important to recognize that this is true not only for genetic syndromes, but for non-syndromic instances as well. However, the discussions are obviously very different if the environmental exposure did contribute to the HI, and any other birth defect.

Access to Support Groups

This aspect of making a genetic diagnosis is underappreciated, but is very important. While they can provide excellent medical care, most healthcare professionals do not know what it is like to be a parent of a child with a HI, syndromic or isolated. While many issues are common to all with a disability, others are specific to a particular disorder. Furthermore, there are opportunities for children with a particular disorder. However, to take advantage of these opportunities one must have an accurate and correct diagnosis.

Reduction of Cost

Last, but by no means the least important, is the cost of medical care. Not only does making a correct genetic diagnosis improve medical management by permitting more targeted testing and evaluations, it also obviates the need for unnecessary diagnostic tests. In this manner, a correct genetic diagnosis saves both money and inconvenience to patients and their families. For example, one study found that the cost of the evaluation of children with Williams syndrome, a particular disorder that features developmental delay and other medical complications including the risk for progressive sensorineural hearing loss, was significantly lower once a geneticist was consulted, owing to fewer unnecessary diagnostic tests being undertaken.

Genetics Evaluation

A comprehensive genetics evaluation is needed to reach a genetic diagnosis. The first goal of a genetics evaluation for a patient with HI is to make the determination if the HI is isolated, or part of a genetic syndrome. As discussed above in the context of Down syndrome, many genetic syndromes are readily apparent. The audiologist or otolaryngologist may not recognize that a child has HI as part of, for example, oto-palatal-digital syndrome, but they can recognize that the child has more than just HI, and therefore would benefit from a genetics evaluation. A genetic evaluation is warranted not only for the children with multiple anomalies but also for children with isolated hearing loss. Excluding an underlying genetic syndrome and diagnosing isolated HI is also important. Not only does this eliminate the need to screen for (and worry about) other problems, it also defines a different type of genetic testing, namely, for non-syndromic HI genes (see section on Non-syndromic Hearing Impairment below). Just as the other healthcare providers actively involved in the care of children with HI, genetics professionals have specific tasks and goals, the first being to determine if the HI is syndromic or isolated. Further evaluation and counseling is provided for syndromic cases, while for non-syndromic cases, the next goal is to determine the inheritance pattern and, if possible through genetic testing, the genetic subtype, and provide appropriate counseling. However, for each, the first step is the genetics evaluation. For this reason all individuals with HI deserve at least an initial genetics evaluation, be they isolated or associated with other findings. Parents will often ask what is involved in a genetics evaluation. While it sounds daunting, it is in fact similar in to a standard medical evaluation, as it includes a history and physical examination, and it is supplemented by appropriate laboratory testing. The genetics evaluation is, however, different in its execution and emphasis. First, for obvious reasons, there is a greater focus on the family history.

Personal and Family Medical History

Like any standard medical evaluation, a genetics evaluation includes a medical and developmental history, a family history, and a physical examination. In obtaining a medical history, such information as the age of onset, laterality, and the degree of HI is ascertained. It also allows the genetics professional to elucidate other medical problems unassociated with the HI. A developmental history addresses the age-appropriate completion of early milestones such as gross motor control, fine motor control, and speech. All of this information assists the genetics professional in determining the potential aetiology of the HI. For example, unilateral HI with an age of onset of 5 years old is unlikely to be associated with DFNB1 hearing loss. Likewise, a child with bilateral profound congenital sensorineural hearing loss with significant developmental delays is less likely to have a non-syndromic form of HI.

A detailed three generation family history can also reveal information that may suggest a diagnosis of one specific genetic disorder. This is true for both non-syndromic as well as syndromic forms of HI. For example, in the case of an individual with syndromic hearing loss, clues to a patient's diagnosis may be found in the family history. A family history suspicious for Waardenburg syndrome may include a proband with bilateral sensorineural HI who has relatives reported to exhibit such features as premature graying and heterochromia. A complete family history may also be able to identify family members who are at-risk for the genetic disorder in question or provide recurrence risk estimates for the affected individual and their family members. In some forms of congenital HI, a family history lacking other individuals with HI in addition to an otherwise non-contributory health history and normal physical examination may support the diagnosis of an isolated, non-syndromic form of HI.

Lastly, a family history can also identify consanguinity (the existence of a close biological relationship between parents). This is a valuable clue, as consanguineous unions carry an increased risk for producing offspring with autosomal recessive conditions due to the increased amount of shared genes between parents. For an individual with unexplained HI born to parents who are biologically related, it would be reasonable to assume that the HI is autosomal recessive, and their risk for future children to have a similar HI would be 1 in 4, or 25%, with each pregnancy.

A family history is the compilation of the medical, developmental, and mental health of an individual's family, and a pedigree is the figure that records this information. An accurate, detailed family history can prove an invaluable diagnostic tool as it can provide assistance with establishing the inheritance pattern and familial manifestations of a specific disorder or trait. Specific nomenclature in the form of specific symbols and abbreviations has been established as a measure of conformity for obtaining a family history [2]. Determining the pattern of inheritance of a specific disorder or trait within a family can also assist in determining whether an individual has a syndromic or non-syndromic form of HI.

Genetics Physical Examination

The genetics physical examination is also different than that performed by other physicians. It is mostly done by inspection and involves little actual palpation. There is greater emphasis placed on morphology, including body proportions and the form of structures, such as the external ear, nose, and mouth. Subtle variations of anatomic structures are termed "minor anomalies". A minor anomaly is by definition a variation in a structure that has no medical importance, but are most valuable in making a genetic diagnosis.

Minor anomalies are most often noted in the facial appearance, and such individuals with an unusual facial appearance are commonly referred to being "dysmorphic". While such determinations may seem arbitrary, there are in fact normal values for those structures that can be measured, such as eye spacing and ear length. Others, such as the contour of the eyes or the shape of the nose, are based on the viewer's experience, and are therefore somewhat subjective (see Figure 8.1). But it is through cataloguing of these subtle findings in a given patient that the diagnosis of a genetic syndrome can be reached.

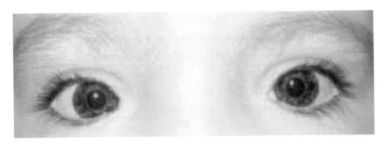

Figure 8.1. Dystopia canthorum.

Genetic Testing

Depending on the clinical and family history information gleaned from the genetics evaluation, genetic testing may be recommended. A peripheral blood draw provides material for the test. Both cytogenetic and molecular genetic testing can be recommended to determine the genetic aetiology of HI, and the specific test ordered will depend on whether the HI is determined to be isolated or syndromic. If determined to be syndromic, the specific syndrome suspected will dictate which genetic test is ordered.

Cytogenetic Analysis

Chromosomes are the structures in each cell of an individual's body that contain the genetic information that ultimately determines an individual's growth, development, and appearance. Structural chromosome abnormalities can result in an individual's cells containing too much or too little of a specific sequence of genetic information. When an individual is suspected to have a syndromic form of HI, either one specific genetic syndrome or even in cases when a specific genetic syndrome is not readily apparent to the genetics clinician, cytogenetic analysis may be recommended. Many times cytogenetic imbalances such as those detectable by chromosome analysis will be identified in individuals suspected to have a syndromic form of HI.

Within the last decade, the advent of array comparative genomic hybridization (array CGH) has provided an alternative to traditional G-banded chromosome analysis. This cytogenetic technique accomplishes, with higher resolution than chromosome analysis, the detection of genomic copy number variants (or areas of genetic information that are missing or extra). Like chromosome analysis, when an individual with HI is suspected to have an underlying genetic syndrome, array CGH analysis can be a helpful diagnostic tool for clinicians.

Targeted, Single Gene Molecular Genetic Testing

In some cases, a specific genetic syndrome is suspected in an individual with HI. In these cases, [3] a general genetic test such as chromosome analysis or array CGH analysis is less useful than a molecular genetics test targeting the specific gene with which that syndrome has been associated. These are carried out through a simple blood test, but unlike most medical tests, genetic tests are done by a select few laboratories. For some tests, there may only be one lab in the US that does the test, and these tests can be expensive (some over $5000). As many insurance policies have restrictions, it is prudent to refer patients to a genetics professional for testing.

However, genetic testing is a very important component in the evaluation of the HI. For example, approximately 1 in 3 individuals with congenital bilateral sensorineural HI, no family history of HI, Northern European Caucasian ancestry, and a normal physical examination, are found to have mutations in the genes associated with Connexin 26 and 30. Another example is branchio-oto-renal (BOR) syndrome, a genetic condition characterized by HI, branchial fistulae and cysts, and renal malformations. Mutations in the *EYA1* gene are identified in over 40% of individuals with this specific syndrome. Therefore, molecular genetic analysis of the *EYA1* gene specifically would be recommended.

Future genetic testing for HI will involve the availability of HI panels. These panels will provide a low-cost method of analyzing multiple genes associated with HI with a single test and blood draw.

Importance of Pre- and Post- Test Genetic Counselling

Regardless of the specific genetic test that is recommended by the genetics clinician, pre- and post test genetic counseling is an important component of the genetics evaluation. Many studies have addressed the benefits of the involvement of a genetics professional in coordinating genetic testing for individuals with any potential genetic disorder, including HI. Brunger et al. [1] and Palmer et al. [3] both address the important role of a genetics professional facilitating both pre- and post-test genetic counseling. Approximately 90-95% of babies with HI are born into normal hearing families. Understanding the complexities of HI in general can be a challenge for most families. Combining this with the various possible genetic etiologies of HI can prove even more frustrating and confusing. In addition, these and other studies have shown that parents of children with HI have a strong desire to learn why their child has HI and the recurrence risk for other family members as well as to obtain information to help with their child's medical care. While parents of children with HI express general interest in genetic testing, the majority had a poor understanding of genetics and the inheritance of HI. Most inaccurately estimate their risk to have another child with HI, and most were unable to accurately interpret a normal genetic testing result.

Progress has been made with regards to the number of genetic tests for HI available. However, genetic testing is still confusing in certain situations. Inconclusive results such as a variant of unknown significance or the identification of only one pathogenic mutation when two are expected can cause extensive misunderstanding for individuals who have not been properly counseled regarding all of the possible outcomes of genetic testing. These authors conclude that the potential for misinterpretation of test results and misunderstanding of the inheritance of HI support the need of pre- and post- test genetic counseling. Genetic counseling ensures that families are provided with "appropriate and accurate information" so that an informed decision regarding genetic testing can be facilitated.[1] Post-test genetic counseling provides the family with an accurate interpretation of test results and the modified recurrence risk provided by genetic testing.

HI is a complex disorder, both with regards to clinical management, but also with regards to aetiology, both genetic and non-genetic. With the genetic complexity of an already complicated disorder increasing, the benefits of genetic counseling have become more and more apparent.

History of Genetic Counselling

The genetic counselling profession is still relatively young. While the term "genetic counselling" was introduced as early as 1947, the first recognized programme that honoured its graduates with a masters-level degree in genetic counselling began in 1969 at Sarah Lawrence College, USA.

The field of genetic counselling sprung from the recognition of the need for genetics healthcare professionals to contest the negative public view of genetics in the era of the eugenics movement and the atrocities carried out by scientists in Nazi Germany. In the United States today, there are currently 30 accredited genetic counselling programmes, and that number continues to grow as more and more programmes around the country are formed. The American Board of Genetic Counselling (ABGC), ensures that each programme is accredited and meets professional competence standards of training.

ABGC also serves as the governing body that issues certification and re-certification to genetic counsellors who have graduated from an accredited programme and passed the ABGC Board Examination. The National Society of Genetic Counsellors (NSGC) is a professional membership organization for members of the profession.

The mission of NSGC is to "promote the professional interests of genetic counsellors and provide a network for professional communication." (www.nsgc.org) Genetic counselling, as defined by the NSGC in 2005, is "the process of helping people understand and adapt to the medical, psychological, and familial implications of genetic contributions to disease."

Specialty Areas for Genetic Counsellors

Genetic counsellors work in multiple clinical settings serving patients referred for preconception, prenatal, pediatric, and adult genetic counselling. These patient populations can be further separated into more specific specialty clinics treating individuals with cleft and craniofacial disorders, metabolic diseases, connective tissue disorders, inherited cancer syndromes, and, of course, HI. Genetic counsellors can work independently or as a part of a multidisciplinary team. For example, in evaluating a HI patient, they routinely work with audiologists, speech and language pathologists, and otolaryngologists. Therefore, it is important for each of these other specialties to understand the role that a genetic counsellor plays in the care of their patients. Several underlying principles govern the genetic counselling professional, including the fact that pre- and post- test genetic counselling ensures that an individual is able to make an informed, independent decision regarding genetic testing. This concept of informed consent is an important principle. Another primary principle surrounds the concept of respect for patient autonomy. The NSGC code of ethics states that the duty of genetic counsellors is to "enable their clients to make informed independent decisions, free of coercion, by providing or illuminating the necessary facts and clarifying the alternatives and anticipated consequences." Members of the profession believe that each patient has the right to make his or her own decision with regards to their genetics evaluation and/or the option of genetic testing. This decision should be facilitated in the absence of coercion, influence, or persuasion from a source of bias. Bias can take the form of a healthcare professional, a family member, societal influence, and concern for finances. It is of course almost impossible to remove all forms of bias from a medical evaluation, so a genetic counsellor strives to limit these influences by providing accurate, balanced, and complete information to each patient during a genetics evaluation. "Non-directive" genetic counselling is the term used to describe the process of guiding a patient through the complexities of the genetic and medical issues they face in an unbalanced, evenhanded way, while allowing them full autonomy to make decisions regarding their medical care.

Addressing Cultural Differences

While healthcare professionals tend to address HI as a medical condition, to be treated, cured, and prevented, it is important to remember that some deaf individuals consider HI as part of their cultural identity and not an affliction. While the term "deaf" (lower case d) refers to individuals who may have congenital, early-onset, or late-onset HI, the term "Deaf" (with a capital D) is used in reference to the Deaf community, a vibrant cultural group with specific traditions, beliefs, and customs whose members communicate by sign language. Most individuals in the Deaf community have congenital HI, and often times they were born to parents who are also deaf. Members of the Deaf community do not view HI as a condition requiring treatment or a cure. Instead, individuals who self-identify as a member of the Deaf community feel that HI should be conserved and recognized as a culture or population subgroup with a unique culture and a language that differs from English. Unfortunately, traditionally individuals who identify themselves as a member of the Deaf community have been wary about the field and study of the genetics of HI. Their particular fears tend to surround the belief that genetic testing and counselling aims to or will lead to prevention of deafness or a reduction in the number of individuals in their community. In contrast, "deaf" individuals do not necessary self-identify with the Deaf community. While previous studies have indicated that some deaf individuals are hesitant to embrace the concept of genetic testing and genetic counselling for HI, they tend to be less distrustful than individuals who identify themselves as part of the Deaf community [4]. These individuals also tend to harbour fewer concerns regarding the implications of genetic testing and counselling on the Deaf culture. A genetics professional working with deaf and Deaf individuals must be aware of and sensitive to the specific views of their clients and their families. It is important for genetic counsellors to be aware of the cultural issues surrounding HI while also understanding and accurately relaying the complex genetics of HI to their patients.

Examples of Genetic Syndromes Associated with HI

About 30% of hearing impairment is 'syndromic', meaning it is one of several findings in a child with multiple abnormalities. There are several hundred genetic syndromes that have hearing impairment as one component. An abbreviated list is provided in Table 8.2, and a more complete list may be found in reference [1]. Included in this list are many syndromes that are readily apparent, presenting with easily recognizable findings such as facial dysmorphia, developmental delay, or other birth defects, while other syndromes are far more subtle. For this reason, the evaluation for a possible genetic syndrome of a seemingly normal individual with a hearing impairment must be carried out in a careful and systematic manner, and additional specific questions should also be asked to try to identify particular findings in the individual and other family members that might suggest the presence of one of these underlying syndromes. Below is a brief review of several of the more common genetic syndromes associated with HI, including several that may present with very subtle findings.

- *Hunter syndrome* is an X-linked disorder, so it is only seen in boys. It is caused by deficiency of the enzyme iduronate-2-sulfatase. This leads to a toxic accumulation of mucopolysaccharides in various organs and tissues of the body, including the brain. Affected boys manifest coarse facial characteristics, enlargement of the liver and spleen, and significant developmental delay.
- *Cleidocranial dysplasia* is an autosomal dominant syndrome that has hearing impairment as a common component. It is caused by mutations in the *RUNX2* gene. While the craniofacial appearance is less dramatic than that of Hunter syndrome, the associated findings are striking. These include absent clavicles, which allow affected individuals to touch their shoulders in the midline, and supernumerary teeth, as many as several dozen extra.
- Hearing impairment can also be a component of many syndromes, such as *MELAS* and *Refsum disease*. These metabolic disorders typically cause significant neurological and other organ dysfunction, including mental retardation. Other mutations in the mitochondrial genome may cause non-syndromic hearing loss, such as the A1555G mutation that is associated with aminoglycoside toxicity (see section on non-syndromic hearing impairment).
- *Jervell-Lange Neilson syndrome (JLNS)* is an important HI-related disorder to know, as affected individuals also manifest long QT syndrome (LQTS), a disorder of cardiac conduction that predisposes affected individuals to sudden death. JLNS is associated with a normal physical appearance, and is inherited as an autosomal recessive trait, caused by mutations in the gene *KCNQ1*.
- *Waardenburg syndrome* is a group of disorders that share the common finding of HI and segmental hypopigmentation that involves the skin, hair select, or eye color. There are several different sub-types that are distinguished by the presence of

additional findings. Due to the clinical variability between and within subtypes, an affected individual may be very noticeable, with a white forelock and distinct facial appearance, while in others the absence of other findings makes it a very difficult disorder to detect.

- *Pendred syndrome* is an autosomal recessive disorder characterized by congenital non-progressive hearing impairment that is typically severe to profound, but can be late onset. It is accompanied later in life by goiter (enlargement of the thyroid gland) that is often or bilateral dilated vestibular aqueducts, with or without cochlear hypoplasia. Pendred syndrome is caused by mutations in the gene *SLC26A4*.

Table 8.2. Select syndromes with hearing impairment

Abruzzo-Erickson	Nager
Achondroplasia	oculo-auticulo-veterbral spectrum
Adelaide/FGFR3	oral-facial-digital II
Apert	osteogenesis imperfecta I-IV
branchio-oto-renal	osteopetrosis
campomelic dysplasia	otopalatodigital I and II
cervico-oculo-acoustic	Pallister-Killian
CHARGE	premature aging and multiple nevi
cleidocranial dysplasia	sclerosteosis
craniodiaphyseal dysplasia	Stickler
Crouzon	symphalangism-brachydactyly syndrome
EEC	Townes-Brocks
hyperphosphatasemia	velocardiofacial
hypertelorism-microtia-clefting	Waardenburg
Kartagener	Wildervanck
Klippel-Feil	Adapted from Smith's Recognizable Patterns of Human Malformations, 6th Ed.Philadelphia,USA: Saunders
Kniest	
LADD	
dysotosis	
Marshall-Stickler	
MPS I, II, IV, VI	

Non-Syndromic Hearing Impairment

Non-syndromic hearing impairment refers to hearing impairment that occurs without other medical problems. As discussed above, it is characterized by age of onset, severity, and anatomic location. It is among the most genetically heterogeneous disorders. For a current figure on HI-related genes the reader is referred to the hereditary hearing loss home page at http://webhost.ua.ac.be/hhh/. There are several important issues to recognize when considering the genetics of non-syndromic hearing impairment. First is nomenclature (Table 8.3).

Table 8.3. Designation for genetic loci associated with non-syndromic (isolated) hearing impairment*

Autosomal dominant forms: **DFNA**

~22%, DFNA1-54

Autosomal recessive forms: **DFNB**

~77%, DFNB1-67

X-linked forms: **DFN**

~1%, DFN1-8

Y-linked forms: **DFNY**

<1%, DFNY1

Maternal (mitochondrial) inheritance

~1% 7 known mutations

*as of Dec 2009; see the Hereditary Hearing Loss homepage (http://webhost.ua.ac.be/hhh/) for more details.

DFNA refers to a genetic locus that causes autosomal dominant hearing impairment; DFNB refers to autosomal recessive; and DFN and refers to an X-linked locus. There is no designation for mitochondrial inherited hearing impairment. While there are over several dozen genes known to be involved in prelingual non-syndromic hearing impairment, the most common by far is *GJB2,* the gene that codes for Connexin 26, at the locus DFNB1. Mutations in *GJB2* account for about 30% of non-syndromic prelingual hearing impairment in individuals of northern European descent, over 50% if the family history suggests autosomal recessive inheritance. It is also common in Israel, parts of Asia and Latin America as well. The carrier rate for a *GJB2* mutation in Caucasians is about 3%, with one mutation, 35delG, accounting for almost 2/3rds of cases. Different mutations are more common in other ethnic groups. There are several dozen additional HI-genes known, some of which can be tested for through commercial labs.

These include both autosomal recessive, autosomal dominant, X-linked, and even mitochondrial forms. However, none are individually nearly as common as *GJB2*, and for most testing is available only on a research basis (Table 8.4). It is expected that advancing genetic testing technology will permit screening of multiple genes simultaneously and relatively inexpensively. So, in the near future we will likely have technology that can test many genes at once for a given profile – eg, autosomal dominant high frequency HI.

Table 8.4. Deafness-related genes for which clinical genetic testing is available*

> While there are over 70 known genes involved in hearing impairment, clinical testing is available only for a small number. Below is a list adopted from the Molecular Otolaryngology Laboratory at the Molecular Otolaryngology Research Laboratories at the University of Iowa (http://www.medicine.uiowa.edu/otolaryngology/MorlLab/).
> Autosomal Dominant
>
> *EYA1* encodes the protein Eyes Absent 1. Mutations or deletions in *EYA1* cause Branchio-oto-renal (BOR) syndrome. However, *EYA1* mutations are found in only 30% of BOR patients, so negative tests does not exclude BOR syndrome.
> WFS1 (DFNA6/14) encodes the protein Wolframin. Mutations in *WFS1* cause a familial low-frequency hearing loss that can progress over time to involve all frequencies.
> *KCNQ4* (DFNA2) encodes voltage-gated potassium channels that regulate electrical signaling and the ionic composition of biologic fluids in the inner ear.
> *COCH* (DFNA9) encodes an inner ear protein. Mutations in COCH cause an autosomal dominant hearing loss that can be associated with variable vestibular malfunction in some patients. Onset of hearing loss patients with DFNA9 occurred between 20 and 30 years of age, is initially more profound at high frequencies, and displayed variable progression to anacusis by 40 to 50 years of age.
>
> *Autosomal Recessive*
> GJB2 (DFNB1) encodes the Connexin 26 protein. Mutations in *GJB2* is the most common genetic cause of congenital hearing impairment. Testing should be done for any patient with congenital hearing impairment of any degree with a negative family history, or a history that suggests autosomal recessive inheritance. Testing for *GJB2* typically includes screening for the associated deletion of the neighboring gene, *GJB6*.
> *SLC26A4* (DFNB4) encodes the protein Pendrin. Mutations in *SLC26A4* cause Pendred syndrome, as well as a subset of hearing loss associated with either Mondini dysplasia or dilated vestibular aqueduct syndrome.
>
> *X-linked*
> *POU3F4* (DFN3) encodes a transcription factor, a gene whose product regulates the expression of other genes. Mutations in or near the POU3F4 gene cause deafness that can be conductive (due to impaired stapes mobility), and/or mixed with a superimposed sensorineural component that can be progressive.
>
> *Mitochondrial*
> *MTRNR1* encodes the mitochondrial 12S ribosomal RNA protein. Two different mutations in this gene, C1494T and A1555G, have been associated with hearing loss as a result of aminoglycoside exposure.
> *MTTS1* encodes the mitochondrial transfer RNA-Serine protein. The A7445G mutation has been found in several families with maternally inherited, progressive, non-syndromic sensorineural hearing loss.
> *MTTL1* encodes the mitochondrial transfer RNA-Leucine protein. The A3243G mutation has been found in several families segregating maternally inherited diabetes mellitus and sensorineural hearing loss. The A3243G mutation also is found in MELAS (Myopathy, Encephalopathy, Lactic Acidosis, Stroke-Like Episodes), and in a small percentage of diabetics.

*This list represents a very small percentage of known hearing-related genetic loci and genes. For a complete list please, and for more details, see the Hereditary Hearing Loss homepage (http://webhost.ua.ac.be/hhh/).

Mitochondrial Deafness and Aminoglycoside Ototoxicity

In studying a large family that segregated maternally inherited HI, a mutation in the mitochondrial genome, called A1555G, was identified. This mutation caused a very variable type of HI – some carriers would lose their hearing slowly, beginning at any age, while other did not develop any hearing loss. Interestingly, it was found that exposure to an aminoglycoside antibiotic hastened the onset of the HI. Aminoglycoside are a class of antibiotics that have a well-known ototoxic effect. However, the ototoxic effect is somewhat idiosyncratic; while high levels are clearly toxic to hearing, not everyone exposed to even very high levels of these antibiotics lose their hearing. This and other mitochondrial gene mutations are one explanation for this susceptibility. Importantly, as these mutations have as a maternal inheritance pattern, anyone at risk individual in a family should avoid aminoglycoside antibiotics.

The Hearing Impaired Adult

There are several scenarios for the adult with HI. First is an adult with prelingual onset of hearing impairment who has never had a genetics evaluation in an effort to investigate the aetiology for their HI. These individuals can be evaluated as one would evaluate a pediatric HI patient, knowing that the prelingual age of onset is more indicative of an autosomal recessively inherited form of HI. Therefore, these individuals have a relatively low risk of having a child with a hearing impairment. Of course, these individuals may have a partner who also has HI. In this case, their risk to have a child with HI may be as high as 100% if their hearing impairment is due to the same autosomal recessive factor; it may be zero if due to a different autosomal recessive factor or something in between. This can only be determined through genetic evaluation.

A second scenario would be that the individual lost their hearing at a young age. While this is characteristic of some genetic forms of HI, typically autosomal dominant forms, it is also consistent with an infectious aetiology. This can be difficult to differentiate, and again requires a genetic evaluation.

Lastly, one may see individuals with adult-onset hearing impairment. This category of hearing impairment is very heterogeneous with most cases having a multifactorial aetiology. This presents a significant challenge for the genetics professional in providing recurrence risk counselling. It is anticipated that, as more discoveries are made into the genetic causes of HI, more information will become available in the future.

Conclusion

A genetic evaluation is an important part of the assessment of any individual with a hearing impairment (HI). The goal of this is to determine whether the HI is syndromic versus isolated and provide testing and counselling recommendations based on that assessment.

Today, genetic testing is carried out in a stepwise manner, guided by findings on family history and physical examination. In the future, newer technologies may permit more comprehensive testing. However, genetic counselling is vital if patients are to completely understand their genetic evaluation and test results.

References

[1]   Brunger, J.W., Murray, G.S., O'Riordan, M., Matthews, A.L., Smith, R.J., Robin, N.H. (2000). Parental attitudes toward genetic testing for pediatric deafness. *American Journal of Human Genetics, 67*, 1621-1625.

[2]   Bennett, R.L., French, K.S., Resta, R.G., Doyle, D.L. (2008). Standardized human pedigree nomenclature: update and assessment of the recommendations of the National Society of Genetic Counsellors. *Journal of Genetic Counselling, 17*, 424-433.

[3]   Middleton, A., Hewison, J., Mueller, R.F. (1998). Attitudes of deaf adults toward genetic testing for hereditary deafness. *American Journal of Human Genetics, 63*, 1175-1180.

[4]   Palmer C.G., Lueddeke, J.T., Zhou, J. (2009). Factors influencing parental decision about genetics evaluation for their deaf or hard of hearing child. *Genetic Medicine, 11*, 248-255.

Recommended Reading

Hereditary Hearing Loss Homepage (http://webh01.ua.ac.be/hhh/). This website is intended for researchers and clinicians are involved in hearing impairment. It provides an up-to-date catalogue of genes and genetic loci involved in hearing impairment.

Robin, N.H., Prucka, S.K., Woolley, A., Smith, R.H.J. (2005). Genetic testing as a component of the evaluation of the child with hearing impairment. *Current Opinion in Pediatrics 17*:709-712. This paper proposes a cost-effective method for evaluating newborns with sensorineural hearing impairment.

Genetics Evaluation Guidelines for the Etiologic Diagnosis of Congenital Hearing Loss. Genetic Evaluation of Congenital Hearing Loss Expert Panel. (2002)American College of Medical Genetics position statement. *Genetic Medicine, 4,* 162-171. This position statement put forth by an expert panel convened by the American College of Medical Genetics, the largest society for clinical genetics. It reviews the role of genetics evaluation and genetic testing for the child with hearing impairment.

Smith, R.J., Bale, J.F Jr., White, K.R. (2005). Sensorineural hearing loss in children. *Lancet, 365*:879-890. An excellent overview of sensorineural hearing impairment.

Hilgert, N., Smith, R.J.H., Van Camp, G. (2009). *Mutation Research 681*:189-196. Forty six genes causing non-syndromic hearing impairment: Which ones should be analyzed in DNA diagnostics? A thorough review of the current state of the art for genetic testing for non-syndromic hearing impairment.

In: Prevention of Hearing Loss
Editors: V. Newton, P. Alberti and A. Smith

ISBN: 978-1-61942-745-7
© 2012 Nova Science Publishers, Inc.

Chapter IX

Screening and Surveillance

Bolajoko Olusanya[*]

Abstract

Routine screening and surveillance for medical disorders are essential components of public health care delivery worldwide. These services facilitate the early detection of persons who require prompt treatment or rehabilitation to prevent or minimize the immediate and long-term burden of the underlying disorders. This chapter examines screening programmes for permanent hearing impairment among population groups of newborns and young infants, school children, workers engaged in high-risk formal/informal occupation, as well as the military and the elderly. It outlines the ethical rationale for hearing screening in newborns and young infants as well as the range of options available for implementing hearing screening programmes. It also highlights possible surveillance programmes that may be set-up to support the various screening programmes given the variability in the onset and pattern of hearing disorders in all age groups.

Introduction

Hearing impairment is the most prevalent sensory disability in humans affecting all age-groups [1]. The importance and disabling effects of this health condition is often masked by its hidden nature. The underlying causes of hearing impairment can be categorized into those which are preventable and non-preventable across the various age-groups, namely neonates and infants, school-age children, the elderly and high-risk workers including the military. It is estimated that about 50% of the burden of hearing loss can be prevented [1]. However, in some populations about half of the incidence of hearing loss may be idiopathic [2]. Reducing the incidence of hearing loss through the prevention of known causes (primary prevention) may be inadequate or ineffective. Secondary prevention initiatives through screening are

---

[*] E-mail: boolusanya@aol.com.

necessary to reduce the impact of the life-long consequences of hearing loss on social participation and overall daily life functioning. A successful early detection initiative will also lead to effective early intervention programmes for non-preventable causes of hearing loss as well as provide a safety net for individuals who may not benefit from these.

The onset of hearing loss is variable from in-utero to birth and throughout life. An essential component of any prevention programme entails the prevention, close monitoring and management of risk factors for hearing loss. Some hearing loss may have delayed-onset or manifest progressively. It is therefore necessary for screening programmes to be complemented by on-going surveillance programmes with the overall aim of preventing the occurrence of hearing loss or minimising the time-lag between the onset and appropriate intervention.

This chapter will discuss hearing screening among population groups of newborns and young infants, school children, workers engaged in high-risk formal/informal occupation, as well as the military and the elderly. It will also examine possible surveillance programmes that may be set-up to support screening programmes and facilitate early detection of hearing loss. Considering that distinction may sometimes be made among the three related objects of screening: "hearing disorders", "hearing impairment or loss" and "hearing disability"; the term hearing screening in this chapter refers to hearing loss except otherwise specified.

Criteria for Hearing Screening

Screening is the proactive or systematic application of a test or enquiry by the health service provider to identify individuals at sufficient risk of a specific disorder that will benefit from direct preventive action or further investigations among individuals who have not sought medical attention because of symptoms of that disorder [3]. There are numerous guidelines for setting up screening programmes with slight variations across target conditions but mostly adapted from the pioneering work of Wilson & Jungner which consisted of 10 requirements (see Box 9.1 A) [4]. These adaptations are often justified on the grounds of a few concerns with the original screening criteria by Wilson & Jungner [5]. Firstly, the criteria were presented as discrete interests with no clear indications of what constitutes part or full satisfaction of the individual criteria or what combination of part satisfaction would justify the commencement of screening for any specific condition. Secondly, the contribution of critical or sensitive-period to early detection and optimal intervention for developmental conditions was not envisaged. Thirdly, the evidence from randomised-controlled trials was not specified or mandatory. Fourthly, the importance of non-technical influences particularly from advocacy groups was not recognised. However, the Wilson & Jungner criteria are universally accepted as the foundation for setting appropriate guidelines for screening across various specialties and health conditions.

A list of requirements that typically could be considered for any hearing screening programme based on the current criteria by the UK National Screening Committee (NSC) [6] and practices in a number of developed countries where mass hearing screening has been implemented is presented in Box 9.1B.

Box 9.1. Screening Criteria

A: The Wilson-Jungner criteria for a screening programme [Reference 4]
<ul><li>The condition being screened for should be an important health problem</li><li>The natural history of the condition should be well-understood</li><li>There should be a detectable early stage</li><li>Treatment at an early stage should be of more benefit than at a later stage</li><li>A suitable test should be devised for the early stage</li><li>The test should be acceptable</li><li>Intervals for repeating the test should be determined</li><li>Adequate health service provision should be made for the extra clinical workload resulting from screening</li><li>The risks, both physical and psychological, should be less than the benefits</li><li>The costs should be balanced against the benefits</li></ul>
B: Typical requirements for hearing screening programmes*

The Condition

- Evidence that hearing loss by the case definition is frequent and severe enough to be of public health concern.
- The natural history of the condition is well-known and understood.
- There are detectable risk factors, disease markers as well as a recognisable latent period or early asymptomatic stage.
- Evidence that cost-effective primary prevention interventions have been implemented as far as practicable and found to be inadequate.

The Screening Test(s)

- Suitable screening tests which may be subjective or objective, in terms of a requirement for a response from the testee, are currently available for all age groups.
- The screening tests are safe, simple, reliable, easy to perform and acceptable to the target population.
- There is an agreed policy on the further diagnostic investigation required by individuals with a positive test result and on the choices available to those individuals.

The Treatment

- There is effective treatment or intervention for patients identified through early detection, with evidence of early treatment leading to better outcomes than late treatment.
- There is agreed evidence-based policies covering which individuals should be offered treatment and the appropriate treatment to be offered.
- The treatment and procedures are acceptable to both the health authorities and the patients.

The Screening Programme

- The benefit from the screening programme should outweigh the physical and psychological harm (caused by the test, diagnostic procedures and treatment).
- The opportunity cost of the screening programme (including testing, diagnosis and treatment, administration, training and quality assurance) should be economically balanced in relation to expenditure on medical care as a whole (i.e. value for money).
- There should be a plan for managing and monitoring the screening programme and an agreed set of quality assurance standards
- Adequate staffing and facilities for testing, diagnosis, treatment and programme management should be available preferably prior to the commencement of the screening programme or a capacity-building roadmap clearly identified and implemented.
- There should be equitable access to all services offered under the screening programme

*Adapted from the UK National Screening Committee. Criteria for appraising the viability, effectiveness and appropriateness of a screening programme. March 2003. http://www.screening.nhs.uk/criteria.

Evidence from developed countries have demonstrated that public policy regarding screening programmes in general is a subject of continuing debate among various interest groups as to what constitutes acceptable thresholds for the various criteria. The decision on the minimum requirements to be met in any country will be determined by appropriate bodies appointed by the health authorities. For example, the U.S. Preventive Services Task Force (USPSTF) makes recommendations on preventive healthcare services such as routine screening for patients without recognised signs or symptoms of the target condition based on a systematic review of the available scientific evidence of the benefits and harms and an assessment of the net benefit of the service [7]. The most recent USPSTF review regarding hearing loss found that there is "moderate certainty that the net benefit of screening all newborn infants for hearing loss is moderate" [8] and therefore endorsed universal newborn hearing screening in USA. Similar evaluation in a growing number of countries, particularly in the developed world, has resulted in the introduction of national/state-wide programmes for universal newborn hearing screening [9,10]. A major observation with all existing mass newborn screening programmes is the recognition of inadequate facilities and personnel at commencement to provide all the range of services required by those identified with hearing loss [11,12]. Strategic plans towards addressing these essential criteria were often initiated in parallel with the screening programmes as rigidly waiting for all follow-up services to be in place before embarking on screening may prove counter-productive. It is therefore not unusual that some developed countries still have shortage of requisite professionals with skills and expertise in both paediatrics and hearing loss to support the programme years after implementing NHS programmes, underscoring the magnitude of the tasks of achieving an ideal situation as required under the principles of screening [13].

Ethical Issues for Hearing Screening Programmes

The subject of ethics in screening is complex involving moral, socio-cultural, philosophical and legal dimensions beyond the scope of this chapter. The range of ethical considerations including consent and confidentiality regarding genetic screening for inborn errors of metabolism or HIV/AIDS would differ from those for non-invasive tests like hearing screening. Beauchamp proposed four broad moral principles at the level of the individual and society that may be applied to hearing screening [14]. These are, 1) respect for autonomy (the obligation to respect the decision making capacities of autonomous persons); 2) non-maleficence (the obligation to avoid causing harm); 3) beneficence (obligations to provide benefits and to balance benefits against risks), and 4) distributive justice (obligations of fairness in the distribution of benefits and risks). These principles have been adapted for newborn hearing screening particularly within the context of the developing world [15].

Respect for Autonomy

Every individual offered screening must be given the freedom to decide to freely accept or reject this healthcare service. Such decision must be informed by adequate disclosure from the service provider of the goal of the screening programme, the cost (if any) as well as the potential risks and benefits of this intervention before screening is conducted. The medium of communication and language of communication must be fully understood by the patient themselves with or without the assistance of an interpreter. Simple and culturally appropriate educational materials including audio-visual aids may be used. Consent must be in writing or by thumb-printing for non-literate patients. In occupational screening major concerns such as fear of losing employment or certain benefits should be recognised and handled with sensitivity.

In the case of newborn screening, consent must be sought from at least one of the parents or legal guardians. Sufficient time must be given to allow for a decision to be made. The disclosure of a permanent abnormality in an apparently normal baby must be handled with sensitivity [16]. Evidence from various newborn hearing screening programmes shows that parental consent is readily given especially if screening is presented within the context of the routine neonatal examinations, which parents expect shortly after delivery or before hospital discharge. Parents are also likely to accept current hearing screening tests because they are, painless, non-invasive and quick to administer.

Benefits and Harms of Screening

Understanding the benefits and potential risks of hearing screening is imperative for service providers as it forms the basis of any informed decision by the patient. Striking the right balance between not exaggerating the benefits and understating the potential harms requires skill and confidence building. It may be useful to have some information leaflets to ensure consistency in the level of disclosure to each patient. Providing opportunity for questions about any aspects of the screening programme should be seen as a moral duty.

The primary goal and the principal benefit of a hearing screening programme is to facilitate the early detection of a disorder which has irreversible life-long adverse consequences on communication, psycho-social, academic, vocational and economic attainment. The burden imposed by these consequences depends on the nature or type (affecting one or both ears) and severity (slight, mild, moderate, severe or profound) of the hearing loss. The burden may be moderated by whether the onset of hearing loss is pre-lingual or post-lingual. With early detection comes the increased prospect for timely intervention to minimise rather than eliminate the potential consequences of the condition. The benefits of hearing screening are perhaps greatest for newborns and young infants before the development of speech and language as it allows the condition, to be detected for timely intervention. In contrast, the benefit of screening may be minimal in children and adults with severe-to-profound hearing loss as they are more likely to be detected by an obvious communication difficulty or recognisable symptoms. Hearing screening also provides assurance that an individual does not have a hearing loss.

Infant hearing screening offers the parents of a hearing-impaired child the knowledge of their baby's special needs as early as possible. In the absence of screening, hearing impairment is unlikely to be detected until the parents or caregivers observe a child's inability to respond to sound, inappropriate behaviours or speech and language defects. During this process, suspecting parents are often anxious, confused, and make false assumptions about the nature, degree and full effects of the condition until they receive appropriate professional attention. This process may often entail making futile consultations with a variety of both orthodox and traditional "service providers".

Screening is associated with false-positive and false-negative outcomes. The principal harm of false positive results is psychological and emotional in the form of anxiety about the consequences of a life-long condition that is actually not present. This may be exacerbated in communities where hearing loss and other disabilities are viewed as culturally and socially unfavourable. It is an ethical requirement that this period of uncertainty is not unduly prolonged by the service provider. Heightened anxiety is also common in occupational screening either pre-employment or routine health checks for workers exposed to noise because of the fear of a potential financial loss of a detected hearing disorder. At the programme level, false-positives place a lot of burden on screening resources and undermine efficiency and cost-effectiveness.

False-negatives give the patient or the parent false-assurance which only brings temporary relief and may later damage trust between the patient and the service provider. This outcome undermines the very essence of a screening programme for timely intervention. This is because a confirmation test is more commonly delayed, as those who passed the first-stage of the screening test are often not required to undergo any further testing.

Distributive Justice in Screening

The principle of distributive justice essentially demands equitable rationing of resources to meet often competing societal needs. Limitation in resources available to cater for all identified needs necessitates priority setting across all sectors. The most prominent and recent approach to setting health care priorities especially at the global level is based on the concept of the "burden of disease" and "cost-effectiveness analysis" [17].

For many years, mortality was used as sole measure of the burden of disease and efforts to curtail mortality was seen as reducing disparity in global burden of disease and by so doing reflected a measure of equity in global health. However, the exclusive use of mortality as an index for disease burden while providing an "objective" measure failed to reflect the full spectrum of the consequences of a disease on individuals or the society and thus undermines equity in global health. For instance, most communicable and chronic non-communicable diseases that are life-threatening are equally associated with significant life-long physical and functional disabilities. Summary measures such as quality-adjusted life years (QALYs) and disability-adjusted life years (DALYs) were therefore introduced to address this "inequality" or "inequity" in population health assessment.

The use of either burden of disease or cost-effectiveness in gauging the importance of health conditions is still subject to concerns. An approach that combines cost-effectiveness and burden of disease in order to compensate for their individual limitations in these two concepts to provide a level-playing-field among diverse health conditions has been explored in Figure 9.1 [18].

Conditions in the HH (high disease burden with highly cost-effective intervention) category would be expected to rank highest and deserving of priority attention and typically may include vaccine preventable fatal diseases such as polio, tuberculosis and measles. In contrast, cosmetic surgery to conceal aging for instance will fall into the LL category and would rightly be overlooked. However, ranking conditions such as hearing loss and many chronic diseases that fall into HL/LH categories pose the greatest challenge. Some would argue that the more cost-effective interventions should take precedence in resource-poor settings. But there are occasions when this process may be legitimately modified by the "rule of rescue" - the "moral or psychological imperative" to provide an effective intervention for an identified health need that is time-bound regardless of the opportunity costs [19]. For example, when an individual's life is threatened cost-effectiveness is downplayed. Similarly, when life is not endangered but effective intervention is time-bound as with permanent hearing loss in infants, the rule of rescue may be the overriding consideration for introducing a screening programme.

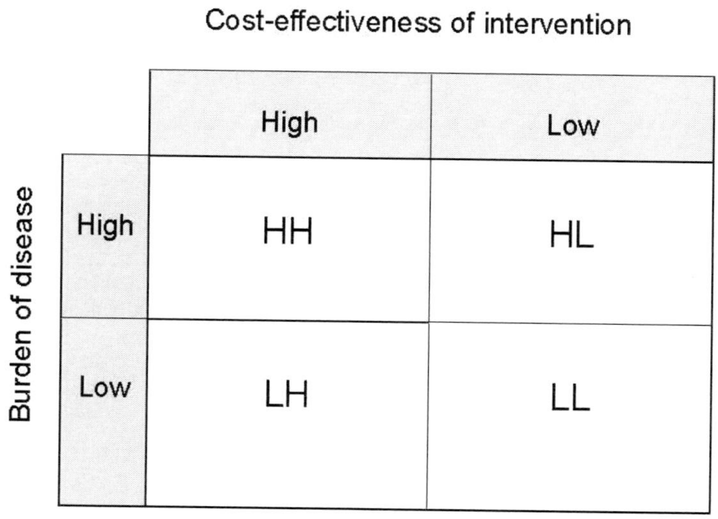

Cost-effectiveness of intervention

		High	Low
Burden of disease	**High**	HH	HL
	Low	LH	LL

Figure 9.1. Model for equitable rationing in health care.

Effectiveness Measures for Hearing Screening Tests

In practice, the process of screening should identify individuals with hearing impairment for whom further action is warranted (Test-positives) and individuals without hearing loss for whom no further action is warranted (Test-negatives). A failed hearing screening would necessarily require confirmation by further testing. A hearing screening test usually results in four main outcomes:

1. Individuals with hearing loss accurately identified (True-Positives)
2. Individuals without hearing loss not accurately identified and classified as having abnormal hearing (False-Positives)
3. Individuals with hearing loss not accurately identified and classified as having normal hearing (False-Negatives)
4. Individuals without hearing loss accurately identified (True-Negatives)

The commonly used parameters for evaluating the performance of hearing screening tests are summarised in Box 9.2.

An ideal hearing screening test would be simple to apply, safe, reliable and valid. It is reliable if it provides consistent results and valid if it detects the majority of individuals with hearing loss (high sensitivity); does not pick most individuals without hearing loss as failing the test (high specificity) or the percentage of individuals without hearing loss among those with positive test results is very low (low FPR); and if the percentage of those with hearing loss among those with positive test results is high (high PPV).

In practice there may be a trade-off between high sensitivity and high specificity, and it is always better to go for high sensitivity in the initial screening test and tolerate higher numbers of false-positives who can be picked up at the second stage.

Box 9.2. Parameters for evaluating the performance of hearing screening tests

	Parameter	Description
1	Sensitivity	Probability of a positive test in individuals with hearing loss or the percentage of individuals with hearing loss correctly detected.
2	Specificity	Probability of a negative test in individuals without hearing loss or the percentage of individuals without hearing loss correctly detected as having normal hearing.
3	False-Positive Rate [FPR] = 1 – Specificity	Probability of an individual without hearing loss testing positive or the percentage of individuals without hearing loss who had positive test results.
4	False-Negative Rate [FNR] = 1 – Specificity	Probability of an individual with hearing loss testing negative or the percentage of individuals with hearing loss who had negative test results.
5	Positive Predictive Value [PPV]	Probability of an individual having hearing loss when the test is positive or the percentage of those with positive test results who actually have hearing loss.
6	Negative Predictive Value [NPV]	Probability of an individual not having hearing loss when the test is negative or the percentage of those with negative test results who actually have no hearing loss.
7	Positive Likelihood Ratio [PLR] = Sensitivity/1 – Specificity	The likelihood that a positive test result will be found in individuals with hearing loss compared to individuals without hearing loss. In effect, PLR tells us how much more likely a positive test is to be found in patients with hearing loss as opposed to patients without hearing loss.
8	Negative Likelihood Ratio [NLR] = 1 – Sensitivity/Specificity	The likelihood that a negative test result will be found in individuals without hearing loss compared to individuals with hearing loss. In effect, NLR tells us how much more likely a negative test is to be found in patients without hearing loss as opposed to patients with hearing loss.

Tools for Hearing Screening

All hearing tests measure an individual's level of response to sound. Current techniques for hearing screening in all age groups can be classified into objective and subjective (or behavioural) tests.

Objective tests are those that do not require the patient to respond to sound or auditory stimuli externally such as automated otoacoustic emissions (OAE) and auditory brainstem response (AABR). In contrast, subjective tests such as pure tone audiometry and tone-emitting otoscope ("Audioscope") require a visible response by the patient. Another form of subjective test which does not require response to sound at the time of testing is a screening questionnaire based on a set of predetermined items that are indicative of the presence of a hearing loss. Although they do not test for hearing loss per se, otoscopy and impedance audiometry or tympanometry can be very valuable as complementary tests to hearing screening. The main features of these tests are described briefly in this section.

Otoacoustic Emissions (OAE)

Otoacoustic emissions are low intensity sounds generated from the outer hair cells of the cochlea in response to audible sounds. Two kinds of otoacoustic emissions are used for hearing screening - Transient-evoked otoacoustic emissions (TEOAE) and Distortion Product otoacoustic emissions (DPOAE).

The TEOAE test is a physiological test for the specific measure of the integrity of the outer hair cells in the cochlea and can be elicited in response to clicks or tone bursts presented to the ear. One disadvantage with this test in newborns is that it is sensitive to peripheral hearing impairment such as mild conductive hearing loss resulting from debris associated with vernix caseosa and amniotic fluid in the external ear canal in the first day of life [20]. The test is sensitive to excessive internal noise from patient or ambient noise in the test environment and will not detect any retro-cochlear dysfunction of the inner hair cells and beyond such as auditory neuropathy/dys-synchrony.

Distortion-product otoacoustic emissions (DPOAE) differs from TEOAE because they are generated by two continuous pure tones introduced to the ear simultaneously and result from the normal nonlinear amplifying process within the inner ear. A good but imperfect correspondence may be observed between DPOAE amplitude and pure-tone audiograms usually in the frequency region above 1,500Hz.

Automated Auditory Brainstem Response (AABR)

The ABR is an electro-physiological measure of the function of the auditory pathway from the eighth cranial nerve through the brainstem. The major advantage of this test which is the electrical recording from three surface scalp electrodes to auditory stimuli is the fact that it is not state-dependent as recordings can be obtained when the subject is sleeping or sedated. In addition, the response is significantly correlated with the degree of hearing loss. An automated version of ABR (AABR) has been designed for screening purposes.

Pure-Tone Audiometry

Pure-tone screening audiometry, usually with a portable audiometer, requires that the individual undergoing the test signifies every time a tone is heard. Test stimuli are presented to alternate ears to determine response to each tone at the various intensities (usually between

15 dB HL to 25 dB HL) and frequencies (typically 500, 1000, 2000, and 4000 Hz),. It is therefore not suitable for testing babies and young infants.

Otoscopy

This is the process of examining the external ear, the tympanic membrane and the middle ear with an otoscope to detect any foreign body or abnormalities that could interfere with hearing. It could be valuable for detecting abnormalities that can cause temporary hearing loss such as impacted cerumen, perforated tympanic membranes, otitis media and otitis external.

Tympanometry

Tympanometry is an objective, rapid and reliable means of evaluating the status of the tympanic membrane and the middle ear. It is not a hearing test but is useful for detecting perforations including latency/dysfunction of the Eustachian tube, glue ear, acoustic neuroma as well as middle ear effusion which can cause hearing loss. The test measures the sound reflected from the ear drum while the pressure of the external canal is varied by the operator.

Questionnaire-Based Instruments

Questionnaire-based screening uses a set of questions to elicit symptoms or indicators of possible hearing loss directly in individuals being tested or indirectly through proxies like parents, teachers or care-givers. Its major attraction is that it is the cheapest form of mass screening tool especially in resource-poor settings. Like any health-related questionnaire, the value is usually enhanced if it is quick and simple to administer and has been properly validated. The evidence on the effectiveness of questionnaire-based tools is being examined. In one comprehensive systematic review, the performance of parental questionnaires was highly variable with reported sensitivity of 34-71% and specificity of 52-95% from a comparison of three studies from Nigeria, Brazil and Australia [21]. Questionnaires may therefore be cost-ineffective for mass screening programmes.

Types of Hearing Screening Programmes

Neonatal and Infant Hearing Screening

The development of objective, rapid, reliable, non-invasive and simple-to-use hearing screening technologies such as automated OAE and AABR has facilitated the widespread introduction of neonatal and infant hearing screening (NHS) as an essential component of neonatal care globally. The primary goal is to allow the prompt detection of infants with congenital or early-onset sensorineural hearing loss. Such early detection provides an opportunity for timely enrolment into appropriate intervention services for optimal speech and language development in early childhood.

Quality benchmarks for newborn hearing screening programmes commonly include high coverage (≥95% of eligible infants), low referral rates (≤4%), short time-frame (screening completed by 1 month) and low follow-up default rate (≤30% for diagnostic evaluation). However, vital context-specific choices are needed on a variety of aspects of the programme to facilitate the attainment of these quality indicators. Some of these issues are briefly examined as follows.

Case Definition

Some NHS programmes may choose to exclude all cases of unilateral hearing loss. Thus any infant failing only one ear is exited. Others may decide to focus on hearing loss at least of moderate (40 dB HL) degree. However, in an attempt to justify such exclusions efforts must be made to ensure that the infants affected are not portrayed as having no significant hearing problem.

Choice of Screening Technology/Protocol

There is no hard and fast rule about the choice of technology or the protocol to be used. However, a two-stage screening with an initial TEOAE followed by AABR for all TEOAE referrals has several advantages over a single or two-stage screening protocol with either TEOAE or AABR. For example, while TEOAE is commonly preferred for the initial screening, the referrals can be excessive especially in busy hospitals where the discharge policy is less than 48 hours. Introducing AABR will reduce the pre-discharge referral rates substantially thus minimising the burden on follow-up services. The combination of TEOAE and AABR in a screening protocol also facilitates the identification of infants with auditory neuropathy.

Universal versus Targeted Screening

Hearing screening is universal when it is directed at the whole population and it is targeted when a sub-group or high-risk fraction of the community is selected for screening. Universal screening is more ideal but may be forestalled by lack of requisite resources much more in developing countries which account for a disproportionate burden of infant hearing loss. Selecting those to screen based on the presence of established risk factors for hearing loss helps to curtail the quantum of resources required and potentially provides a better alternative than no screening. Risk factors used for screening of babies in resource-limited or rural settings typically include [22]:

1. Family history of sensorineural hearing loss
2. In-utero infections such as rubella, cytomegalovirus, syphilis, toxoplasmosis and herpes
3. Cranio-facial anomalies
4. Birth weight less than 1,500g (3.3lbs)

5. Hyperbilirubinaemia at levels requiring exchange transfusion
6. Ototoxic medications including but not limited to aminoglycosides
7. Bacterial meningitis
8. Birth asphyxia with Apgar score 0-4 at 1 minute or 0-6 at 5 minutes
9. Mechanical ventilation lasting five days or more
10. Stigmata or other findings associated with a syndrome known to include a sensorineural and/or conductive hearing loss

Hospital-Based or Community-Based Screening

In order to achieve good coverage among eligible infants at the population level, newborn screening must be implemented shortly after birth. While hospitals provide the most convenient location for screening, hospital-based screening cannot cater for infants born outside hospitals that are in the majority in many low-income countries and will miss a significant proportion of infants with acquired, delayed-onset or progressive hearing loss. One approach is to have a community-based programme to complement the hospital-based programme in such settings.

Alternatively, community-based platform such as provided by routine immunisation in the first weeks of life can be considered for infant hearing screening as has been demonstrated in a number of countries in sub-Saharan Africa [23-25]. Community-based programmes also have disadvantages. They will miss infants that are presented late or not presented at all for immunisation. Facilities for conducting newborn screening may not be readily available such as a suitable test site with tolerable ambient noise levels.

Tracking and Follow-Up

The vast majority of infants with hearing loss are likely to be tested more than once. Incomplete screening or lack of confirmatory evaluation after screening failure confers no benefit for the affected infant. It compromises the (cost) effectiveness of screening programmes. Effective tracking and follow-up after the initial or pre-discharge screening is therefore a critical element of an efficient NHS programme.

Screening Personnel

A critical requirement of a mass screening as distinct from diagnostic service is that it must be simple and quick to administer within a primary care setting. The available automated hearing screening technologies (e.g. TEOAE/DPOAE, AABR and Audioscope) have these qualities and only require few days of training to operate by non-specialists. However, the screening programme must be supervised and monitored by ear care specialists such as audiologists and otolaryngologists or audio-vestibular physicians where these are available.

NHS programmes ideally should be managed by paediatricians with the context of the overall developmental trajectory of infants detected with hearing loss with or without other medical conditions requiring specialist attention.

School-Based Hearing Screening

School screening is perhaps the commonest hearing screening programme worldwide with a history dating back to mid-20th century. It is conducted in mainstream schools as those with severe-to-profound hearing loss are likely to be enrolled in special schools for the deaf. The detrimental effects of the apparently "less severe" hearing impairments including mild and unilateral hearing loss on academic achievements and linguistic skills among school children are well documented [26]. For example, Bess et al investigated the functional status of school children with minimal hearing loss (16 – 40 dB HL) and found that they exhibited greater dysfunction than their normal hearing peers. The burden placed on vocational attainment in adulthood has also been reported [27].

Various studies worldwide have substantiated the preventive and epidemiological value of audiometric screening of school children [28,29]. While the benefits of school screening are well-established, the impetus for this programme seems to be weakened by the current drive towards infant hearing screening worldwide. A recent survey in the UK shows that despite many years of implementing school screening programmes in that country there were still some unresolved challenges resulting from lack of national guidelines on best practices including quality standards, variations in protocol especially pass/fail criteria although coverage of over 90% was reported [21]. It is therefore important to recognise the role of school screening in an era of NHS. This section will briefly examine some key issues related to school screening as a guide towards implementing such a programme especially in developing countries.

Historically, the major route to identification of infant hearing loss worldwide was parental or professional concern, followed by the school entry screening [21]. Parental and professional concern remains a steady source of identification post-natally, but still, at school entry 34% of bilateral (16% moderate or greater and 18% mild) and 17% of unilateral permanent hearing impairments remained to be identified based on data from the UK [21].

The primary benefit provided by school screening is the unique opportunity it provides for the prompt identification of children whose academic performance is likely to be compromised by hearing loss that will otherwise go unnoticed. It also provides evidence that the affected child required appropriate support in order to function optimally. Consequently, school screening is an essential complement to NHS programmes to ensure that regardless of the onset of hearing loss in early childhood opportunities exist for timely intervention. Routine identification of hearing disorders should also be considered in any hearing screening programme for school children. Where universal screening is not practicable it may be useful to consider targeting children with risk factors based on identified hearing disorders.

Majority of hearing screening in schools is conducted at school entry which also provides the opportunity to ascertain if the degree of hearing loss would permit enrolment into a mainstream school. However, it is necessary to conduct additional screening at some point to allow for the timely detection of any hearing loss that may result during school years. For instance, children with recurrent otitis media should receive hearing screening more frequently. Children treated for severe illness or infections particularly with the use of ototoxic medications should be tested immediately after recovery. Routine screening beyond school entry may also be required in schools located in noisy neighbourhood or close to an airport or busy freeway [30].

Prior to screening parental consent must be obtained in writing or by thumb printing. A suitably quiet location in the school premises where the tests can be conducted must be decided in advance as this could be quite a challenge in schools in urban areas or big cities. Although pure-tone audiometry is the commonest screening technique especially in developing countries, an increasing number of studies have demonstrated the usefulness of physiological tests like TEOAE [28,31].

School screening is not an alternative for infant hearing screening considering that optimal intervention for pre-lingual hearing loss must be initiated within the first year of life [32]. Neither is it able to fully reverse the consequences of late detection of pre-lingual hearing loss. Secondly, school screening will miss all infants with profound hearing loss not enrolled into mainstream schools. Unlike newborn screening programmes, there are currently no uniform quality benchmarks for evaluating the school screening programmes. Some children may need to be seen by an ear care specialists for an existing disorder before they can be screened which entail extra logistical support.

Hearing Screening in the Elderly

Hearing impairment is one of the age-related chronic conditions in elderly persons (usually aged 65 years or more)..Hearing impairment assumes greater importance than some other conditions because of its unique ability to sever previously established communication links with family members, friends and associates. The aging process is linked with degenerative changes in the outer hair cells from the apical to the basal regions of the cochlea. Changes have also been described in the inner hair cells as well as atrophy of spiral ganglion and the eighth nerve but these are generally confined to the basal area while the central auditory system is not completely spared from the widespread changes associated with this condition. Age-related hearing loss known as presbycusis often has a devastating effect on the social life of many elderly people with breakdown of existing social ties that consequently leads to loneliness, isolation and depression.

The auditory effects of presbycusis are more pronounced on the frequencies above 1000 Hz producing a sloping sensorineural high frequency hearing loss even as low frequency hearing is preserved. The overall effect is that speech perception/audibility will be spared relative to speech understanding especially in the presence of background noise. Because of its insidious nature, presbycusis may take several years to develop and at the same time the individual may be unaware of the impairment. In view of the fact that the ability to respond to low frequency sounds in speech remains fairly well preserved, family and caregivers may in turn attribute misunderstanding to confusion, forgetfulness or inattention. This in turn prevents effective communication with the elderly that may culminate into subsequent, physical, emotional, cognitive, behavioural and social functioning difficulties.

Systematic review of evidence in developed countries [33,34] has confirmed that hearing screening programme in the elderly is justified on the following criteria:

- The burden of the hearing loss in this population is significant enough to warrant screening effort.
- The natural history of the disease (presbycusis) allows time for intervention.
- Accurate, practical and convenient screening tests exist.
- Efficacious treatment is available for those detected with hearing loss.

Otoscopy is necessary before the commencement of a screening test as impacted cerumen is highly prevalent in the elderly and may substantially account for hearing loss in the affected persons. Screening should only commence when the ear canal is free and the tympanic membrane is clearly visible.

A self-administered questionnaire and audioscope are perhaps the two least expensive and complicated tests that have been found quite valuable for hearing screening for the elderly. Perhaps the most popular self-reported questionnaire worldwide is the Hearing Handicap Inventory for the Elderly—Screening version (HHIE–S) and its various adaptations [35,36]. This instrument consists of 10 questions designed to assess perceived emotional and social problems associated with impaired hearing (e.g. frustration, embarrassment or difficulty in certain situations). There is evidence that the value of a self-reported questionnaire is enhanced when complemented with either an objective screening test like OAE [37], pure-tone audiometry [38] or the Audioscope [39]. The combination of both a questionnaire and pure-tone screening has been found quite helpful because of possible denial of a hearing problem [37]. In addition, while pure-tone audiometry is a physiological measure of hearing sensitivity, self-assessment questionnaires identify a disability due to a hearing impairment. It has been argued that using both measures may identify those individuals who have a hearing loss and a disability and are thus more likely to follow up on recommendations for further testing [37,38]. This is corroborated by the report of Davis et al who found a two-stage screen using a five-question questionnaire and a simple audiological screen at 35 dB HL with a 3 KHz pure tone as the most efficient in the UK [34].

Other commonly administered screening tests in the elderly are whispered voice, tuning fork and finger-rub tests.

The whispered voice test at a set distance of 6 inches to 2 feet from the test ear is administered by whispering six test words out of field of vision, and asking the patient to repeat the words. Sensitivity for detecting hearing impairment is between 80% to 100%, and specificity around 82-89%. Although recommended routinely in Canada, the difficulty in standardizing the "loudness" of the whisper and eliminating background noises are practical issues that may affect the reliability as well as the utility of this test [40]. Failure to hear a vibrating 512 Hz fork at a distance of one foot has a reported sensitivity and specificity of 80% and 82% respectively.

However, the tuning fork test, because it is a low frequency test, is not suitable for screening the elderly who are more likely to have the characteristic high frequency loss from presbycusis. The finger-rub test is carried out by rubbing thumb and forefinger together and failure to hear this at a distance of 6-8 inches from the ear has a reported sensitivity of 80% and a specificity of 49%. At 3 inches, the sensitivity is reported to be 90%, and the specificity 85%.

Most studies on hearing screening in the elderly are from developed countries. Among the limited studies from developing countries a combination questionnaire and pure-tone audiometry was reported in Brazil [41,42]. In Nigeria, hearing loss in a cohort of adults aged 65 years or more was identified based solely on whether or not the respondent indicated that they had hearing difficulty [43]. However, self-reported hearing based solely on this single question as has been suggested in some developed countries [44,45] has not yet been validated within the socio-cultural settings in many developing countries including Nigeria.

Although the use of OAEs has been demonstrated as a tool for adult screening, it is still relatively poorly applied routinely [34]. However, it has the unique advantage of being able to detect any deterioration in cochlear function due to aging far ahead of conventional pure-tone audiometry [46].

Unlike NHS or school screening there is presently no organised platform for undertaking mass screening in the elderly. However, in the USA, routine screening is generally recommended "periodically" based on the discretion of primary care physicians or during other clinical visits [40]. In contrast, ASHA recommends screening every 3 years. In practice, an adult showing obvious signs of communication difficulties such as not being able to hear except with a shout should be screened for hearing loss as soon as possible. Other issues related to frequency of screening are discussed in the section on surveillance programme for the elderly.

Industrial Hearing Screening

Worldwide, it is estimated that 16% of disabling hearing loss (>40 dB HL) in adults (over 4 million DALYs) is attributable to occupational noise ranging from 7% in Western Pacific A sub-region (comprising countries such as Japan, Australia, New Zealand and Singapore) to 21% in Western Pacific B sub-region, (predominantly China and Philippines) [47]. About 18% is estimated for South Asia and Africa. Excessive noise from industrial equipment such as heavy machinery and power generators is a significant cause of hearing loss besides other adverse outcomes such as physical and psychological stress, reduction in productivity, communication difficulties and failure to hear warning signals resulting in accidents and injuries. The range of industries or occupations where such equipment are used include but not limited to construction, mining, aviation, metal fabrication, bottling, textiles, woodworking, foundries, agriculture and entertainment. Noise-induced hearing loss (NIHL) is one of the most prevalent occupational diseases. It is often cumulative, insidious and bilateral but preventable with appropriate actions to identify and protect those at risk. NIHL could result from an acoustic trauma when the ears are exposed to impulsive or single sound in excess of 140 dBA or from prolonged exposure to noise above 85 dBA, though not necessarily permanent depending on the duration of exposure. Prolonged exposure to noise usually begins with a temporary blunting of hearing sensitivity which causes a temporary threshold shift (TTS) that reverses when the noise exposure ceases. It is usually an early warning sign of NIHL. The effects of noise on hearing sensitivity occur predominantly in the higher frequencies (3.0-6.0 kHz). The largest impact occurs at 4.0 kHz with the likelihood of extending to lower frequencies.

In many countries employers are mandated by regulations to identify individuals who are affected by high level noise exposure and arrange for their hearing to be tested. Thus, periodic noise-level measurements with an integrated sound level meter are required to establish when hearing screening is warranted. Notwithstanding, workers who experience symptoms of a hearing loss regardless of whether noise levels have been measured may demand a hearing test routinely. Usually, while people have to speak very loudly to be able to communicate when noise levels are over 80 dBA, they are likely to have to shout when the noise levels are around 90 dBA. More recent OSHA regulations require pre-placement or baseline hearing test within 6 months of exposure at or above 85 dBA and annually thereafter [48].

A major challenge in many developing countries is the lack of enforcement of any standards, thus resulting in lack of a routine hearing test. Generally, although hearing loss due to presbycusis may have distinguishable patterns until 60-70 years, presbycusis often exacerbates NIHL in workers older than 60 years thus making hearing screening of high priority in this group of workers. Industrial screening may also be expanded to include routine hearing test for all employees as part of pre-employment medical examination or for patients who may be at risk of hearing loss unrelated to the nature of their work. Industrial screening is also warranted rather than merely determining excessive noise levels because not all persons exposed to noise are likely to have NIHL more so as individuals vary in their susceptibility to noise.

Pure-tone audiometry is the commonest technique for occupational hearing screening and may be accompanied by a hearing handicap questionnaire such as the HHIE-S questionnaire or a 10-item self-administered questionnaire developed by the National Institute of Deafness and Communication Disorders (NIDCD) in USA. Otoscopy routinely must precede any hearing test to detect any abnormalities in the external ear or tympanic membrane. Physiological tests such as OAE tests are also valuable because of their greater sensitivity to cochlear dysfunction. In fact several studies have demonstrated that DPOAE is quicker and more sensitive than pure-tone audiometry thresholds in detecting the early stages of NIHL often characterised by normal or near normal hearing sensitivity but absent or poor OAEs [49,50]. One study found that low-level OAEs were predictive of an increased risk of future hearing loss from an impulsive noise by almost nine fold compared to pure-tone audiometry [50]. However, TEOAE is less predictive of NIHL than DPOAE as it is associated with a greater false-positive rate [49].

A major hurdle to industrial screening in developing countries is that most workers are reluctant to undergo hearing test for fear of unfavourable actions by the employers even where NIHL can be established for which the employers are by regulation responsible. The rights of such workers have to be assured and protected as a necessary step towards facilitating routine hearing screening particularly among the most vulnerable groups who often can barely survive on their wages and cannot afford the requisite services to address the life-time consequences of NIHL.

Hearing Screening in the Military

The term "military" refers to members of the core Armed Forces such as the Army, Navy, Air Force and the Marine Corps and excludes the Police and Para-Military units such as Customs, Immigration, Road Traffic and Civil Defence Corps. The sources of potentially damaging noise include weapons systems (e.g. handguns, rifles, artillery pieces or rockets), wheeled and tracked vehicles, fixed- and rotary-wing aircraft, ships, and communications devices [51]. Service members may encounter these noise sources through training, standard military operations, and combat. Exposure to combat-related noise may be unpredictable in onset and duration. Service members may also be exposed to hazardous noise through activities that are not unique to the military environment, including various engineering, industrial, construction, or maintenance tasks.

A recent study on the epidemiology of hearing impairment and NIHL in the US Army estimated that about 22.2 per 1000 active-duty personnel had NIHL-medical related encounters totalling 88,285 visits between year 2003 and 2005, with men accounting for 88% [52]. Another study from the UK reported an annual incidence of work-related NIHL among British military of 28.3 per 100,000 personnel compared with 1.94-1.23 per 100,000 in the general working population [53].

Perhaps the most definitive report on NIHL in the military commissioned by the US Congress was published by the Institute of Medicine in 2006 [51]. Among its key findings was that there was sufficient evidence that certain military personnel while in active service exhibited hearing thresholds typical of NIHL but that in the absence of audiograms obtained at the beginning and end of military service, it was difficult or impossible to determine with certainty how much of a specific individual's hearing loss was attributable to service in the military. Such a conclusion makes routine hearing screening imperative and serves as a motivation by those at risk of NIHL to seek routine hearing test provided of course that the pre-employment hearing status had been documented.

The screening methods commonly employed in military hearing screening are identical to those used in industrial screening. DPOAE should be of unique advantage for the simple reason that many of the personnel are unlikely to have an 8-hour per day prolonged exposure at the action level of 85 dBA that except during vocational military training.

However, the risk of impulsive noise may be prominent necessitating accurate identification of a potential acoustic trauma without immediate evidence of a shift in hearing thresholds.

Surveillance Programmes for Hearing Loss

Generically, health surveillance is the ongoing, systematic collection, collation, analysis and interpretation of data to identify exposure or risk factor essential to the planning, implementation and evaluation of practices closely integrated with the timely dissemination of such information to those who need timely prevention and control [54].

The key goals of surveillance programmes are: 1) to identify those who are likely to be at risk of an asymptomatic disease or health condition, and 2) to minimise the period between the onset of the condition and its detection with a view to facilitating timely management. As related to hearing loss, a surveillance programme should ideally be directed towards the following goals:

- Identifying potential risk factors for hearing loss that could serve as basis for selective intervention (screening, diagnosis and treatment).
- Maximising screening coverage by tracking those who did not participate in or complete the screening protocol.
- Compliance with all post-screening follow-up services.

- Prompt detection of those with false screening outcomes.
- Evaluation of screening programme performance.

Thus every screening programme must be complemented with a surveillance programme to optimise the benefits of early detection. The four most prominent surveillance programmes for hearing loss are examined in this section.

Infant Surveillance Programme

A major challenge in NHS programmes is ensuring that all eligible infants complete the specified screening protocol. For example, in NHS programmes in busy hospitals with early discharge policy of 24 hours for well babies following delivery screening coverage is not only likely to be compromised but depending on the screening technology a large proportion of those tested (if at all possible) may have inaccurate results.

Surveillance programmes also can be designed to target infants born outside hospitals to facilitate provision of hearing screening for eligible infants. This is particularly applicable to developing countries in Africa and Asia where a high proportion of births occur outside hospitals.

A typical surveillance programme for infants will require that any baby that was missed or failed the initial screening test before hospital discharge is given an appointment for screening at the first routine post-natal check-up at 6 weeks. In some countries this first visit coincides with routine immunisation for the first dose of diphtheria, pertussis and tetanus (DPT).

Subsequent visits within the first three months after delivery provide opportunity to screen any infant that has not completed the required screening protocol. In some countries there may be services for home visits by social/health workers which may also incorporate hearing screening for missed babies. As much as possible, the surveillance programme should be integrated with existing child health services to ensure their effectiveness.

Infants detected with hearing loss may have multiple health problems requiring services from a range of professionals. These services need to be properly coordinated to enhance the overall benefit of the screening programme.

Since hearing loss may just be one of the developmental or medical problems facing the child, it is necessary that hearing screening be placed within the context of the developmental needs of the infant to ensure timely delivery of support for the child and family.

For this reason, as far as practicable the surveillance programme should be managed or coordinated preferably by a paediatrician. Moreover, an effective surveillance programme will require the active participation of the family who are more likely to consult a paediatrician on all health issues affecting the child.

School Surveillance Programme

Most school screening takes place at school entry whereas the risk of hearing loss persists throughout the school years. The primary goal of surveillance programme is to prevent, control or promptly detect any adventitious hearing loss especially associated with common risk factors such as otitis media and impacted cerumen. As previously noted, the ease of concealing the handicapping effect of mild or unilateral hearing loss may be at the risk of poor educational achievement. A good surveillance system allows children to be promptly detected and helped before the consequences of this invisible handicap become apparent.

The surveillance programme can be designed to identify children who may require further screening following an episode of otitis media, serious illness or consistently poor performance in class tests. In countries where routine school health checks are conducted hearing screening should necessarily be incorporated, including otoscopic examination. Teachers should be instructed in the signs of hearing impairment so that they can identify those children having difficulties as soon as possible.

Surveillance Programme for the Elderly

Mass hearing screening programmes for the elderly are currently not implemented in any country. And as such there is presently no platform for organised surveillance programme for this group. However, for those in residential homes hearing screening may be routinely offered as part of the overall medical check-up. Surveillance programmes for the elderly where practicable can be targeted at providing prompt hearing screening for those with known risk factors for hearing loss. Since the onset of hearing loss is unpredictable at any age, routine hearing screening should also be offered routinely after bouts of severe illnesses including stroke. Hearing screening needs to be considered following the use of ototoxic medications such as antibiotics for common infections including otitis media; antineoplastics; loop diuretics; and anti-inflammatory drugs including aspirin. Routine ear examination to detect and manage impacted cerumen which may be found in up to 30% of elderly patients with hearing loss is essential [40]. Even after cerumen has been removed a hearing test should be done. Those with chronic conditions such as diabetes and hypertension should be equally tested and closely monitored.

Occupational Surveillance Programme

The hearing surveillance programmes for both industrial and military NIHL are identical and are often integrated into an overall hearing conservation programme (HCP). The primary goal of HCP is to eliminate or curtail the risk of NIHL in all workers exposed to noise. This begins by identifying sources of excessive noise through environmental surveillance of the work area including noise level survey with a view to reducing noise exposure to injurious impulsive noise as well as chronic excessive noise as far as practicable. Options for possible administrative and engineering control of the noise source including diagnostics to eliminate causes such as loose or worn out parts or outright replacement of the equipment are then explored. Administrative control may require that management ensures that no employee is exposed to as much as 8 hours per day in areas where the noise levels persist beyond the action level. In the event that all possible options for reducing the noise significantly from the source fail, then an audiometric surveillance is required for all the affected staff which entails periodic hearing screening/evaluation in addition to use of personal protective devices. A detailed description of the components of a hearing conservation can be found in many of the existing publications by occupational health and safety bodies [55,56]. The benefit of well-executed HCP on reducing the burden of NHIL has been demonstrated in many countries [57]. However, in the vast majority of industries including the military excessive exposure to either prolonged or impulsive noise cannot be completely eliminated in the foreseeable future especially in the developing world thus underscoring the critical role of audiometric surveillance.

Since audiometric surveillance is likely to be part of an HCP, the responsibility for coordinating the entire programme may reside with the human resources department or contracted to professional hearing conservationists. A key element of a successful programme is effective monitoring to ensure compliance from both the employer and the employee on their specific responsibilities.

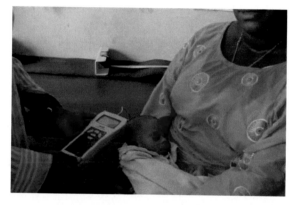

TEOAE screening at a community health centre with baby in mother's arms.

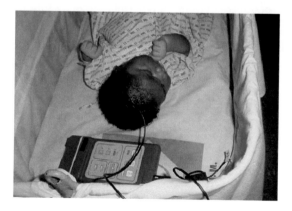

TEOAE screening in a well-baby nursery of a maternity hospital with baby in a cradle.

Conclusion

Several practical options now exist for the early detection of permanent hearing impairment in all age groups and in different birth, socio-demographic or vocational settings through routine hearing screening and surveillance programmes. The opportunity to provide a continuum of care from birth to adulthood to curtail the burden of this life-long disorder using objective and reliable screening technologies is now available to all the regions of the world. However, systematic and sustainable investment would be required in resource-poor countries to develop requisite capacity to provide effective hearing screening and surveillance services at all levels of public health care delivery.

References

[1]   World Health Organisation. (2006). Primary Ear & Hearing Care Training Resource. Advanced Level. Geneva: World Health Organisation.

[2]   Morzaria, S., Westerberg, B.D., Kozak, K. (2004). Systematic review of the aetiology of bilateral sensorineural hearing loss in children. *International Journal of Pediatric Otorhinolaryngology, 67*, 1193 –1198.

[3]   Strong, K., Wald, N., Miller, A., Alwan, A. (2005). Current concepts in screening for non-communicable disease: World Health Organisation Consultation Group Report on methodology of non-communicable disease screening. *Journal of Medical Screening, 12*, 12-19.

[4]   Wilson, J.M.G., & Jungner, G. (1968). *Principles and practice of screening for disease.* Public Health Paper Number 34. Geneva: World Health Organisation.

[5]   Bailey, D.B. Jr, Skinner, D., Warren, S.F. (2005). Newborn screening for developmental disabilities: reframing presumptive benefit. *American Journal of Public Health, 95*, 1889-1893.

[6]   National Screening Committee, U.K. (2003). *Criteria for appraising the viability, effectiveness and appropriateness of a screening programme.* London: National Screening Committee, London Department of Health.

[7]   Harris, R.P., Helfand, M., Woolf, S.H., Lohr, K.N., Mulrow, C.D., Teutsch, S.M., Atkins, D. Methods Work Group, Third US Preventive Services Task Force. (2001). Current methods of the US Preventive Services Task Force: a review of the process. *American Journal of Preventive Medicine, 20(3 Suppl)*, 21-35.

[8]   US Preventive Services Task Force. (2008). Universal screening for hearing loss in newborns: US Preventive Services Task Force recommendation statement. *Pediatrics, 122*, 143-148.

[9]   Davis, A., Bamford, J., Wilson, I., Ramkalawan, T., Forshaw, M., Wright, S. (1997). A critical review of the role of neonatal hearing screening in the detection of congenital hearing impairment. *Health Technology Assessment, 1*, 1-176.

[10] Wolff, R., Hommerich, J., Riemsma, R., Antes, G., Lange, S., Kleijnen, J. (2010). Hearing screening in newborns: systematic review of accuracy, effectiveness, and effects of interventions after screening. *Archives of Disease in Childhood, 95*, 130-135.

[11] Uus, K., Bamford, J., Young, A., McCracken, W. (2005). Readiness of paediatric audiology services for newborn hearing screening: findings and implications from the programme in England. *International Journal of Audiology, 44*, 712-720.

[12] White, K.R., Forsman, I., Eichwald, J., Munoz, K. (2010). The evolution of early hearing detection and intervention programs in the United States. *Seminars in Perinatology, 34*, 170-179.

[13] Joint Committee on Infant Hearing (JCIH). (2007). Year 2007 Position Statement: Principles and guidelines for early hearing detection and intervention programs. *Pediatrics, 120,* 898-921.

[14] Beauchamp, T.L. (2003). Methods and principles in biomedical ethics. *Journal of Medical Ethics, 29,* 269–274.

[15] Olusanya, B.O, Luxon, L.M., Wirz, S.L. (2006). Ethical issues in screening for hearing impairment in newborns in developing countries. *Journal of Medical Ethics, 32,* 588-591.

[16] Gilbey, P. (2010). Qualitative analysis of parents' experience with receiving the news of the detection of their child's hearing loss. *International Journal of Pediatric Otorhinolaryngology, 74,* 265-270.

[17] Jamison, D.T., Breman, J.G., Measham, A.R., Alleyne, G., Claeson, M., Evans, D.B. (2006). *Disease control priorities in developing countries.* 2nd edn. New York: Oxford University Press.

[18] Olusanya, B.O. (2008). Global health priorities for developing countries: some equity and ethical considerations. *Journal of National Medical Association, 100,* 1212-1217.

[19] McKie, J., & Richard, J. (2003). The rule of rescue. *Social Science and Medicine, 56,* 2407-2419.

[20] Doyle, K.J., Rodgers, P., Fujikawa, S., Newman, E. (2000). External and middle ear effects on infant hearing screening test results. *Otolaryngology Head & Neck Surgery, 122,* 477-481.

[21] Bamford, J., Fortnum, H., Bristow, K., Smith, J., Vamvakas, G., Davies, L., Taylor, R., Watkin, P., Fonseca, S., Davis, A., Hind, S. (2007). Current practice, accuracy, effectiveness and cost-effectiveness of the school entry hearing screen. *Health Technology Assessment, 11,* 1-168.

[22] American Academy of Pediatrics. (1995). Joint Committee on Infant Hearing 1994 Position Statement. *Pediatrics, 95,* 152–156.

[23] Swanepoel, D.W., Hugo, R., Louw, B. (2006). Infant hearing screening at immunization clinics in South Africa. *International Journal of Pediatric Otorhinolaryngology, 70,* 1241-1249.

[24] Olusanya, B.O., Wirz, S.L., Luxon, L.M. (2008). Community-based infant hearing screening for early detection of permanent hearing loss in Lagos, Nigeria: a cross-sectional study. *Bulletin of the World Health Organisation, 86,* 956-963.

[25] Tanon-Anoh, M.J., Sanogo-Gone, D., Kouassi, K.B. (2010). Newborn hearing screening in a developing country: results of a pilot study in Abidjan, Côte d'ivoire. *International Journal of Pediatric Otorhinolaryngology, 74,* 188-191.

[26] Bess, F.H., Dodd-Murphy, J., Parker, R.A. (1998). Children with minimal sensorineural hearing loss: prevalence, educational performance and functional status. *Ear and Hearing, 19,* 339-354.

[27] Jarvelin, M.R., Maki-Torkko, E., Sorri, M.J., Rantakallio, P.T. (1997). Effect of hearing impairment on educational outcomes and employment up to the age of 25 years in northern Finland. *British Journal of Audiology, 31,* 165-175.

[28] McPherson, B., & Olusanya, B. (2008). Screening for hearing loss in developing countries. In: B. McPherson, R. Brouillette (Eds). *Audiology in developing countries.* (pp 75–105). New York: Nova Science Publishers Inc.

[29] Pascolini, D., & Smith, A. (2009). Hearing Impairment in 2008: a compilation of available epidemiological studies. *International Journal of Audiology*, *48*, 473-485.

[30] Chen, T.J., & Chen, S.S. (1993). Effects of aircraft noise on hearing and auditory pathway function of school-age children. *International Archives of Occupational and Environmental Health, 65*:107-111.

[31] Clark, J.L. (2008). Hearing loss in Mozambique: current data from Inhambane Province. *International Journal of Audiology*, *47(Suppl 1)*, S49-56.

[32] Yoshinaga–Itano, C., Sedey, A.L., Coulter, D.K., Mehl, A.L. (1998). Language of early and later–identified children with hearing loss. *Pediatrics*, *102*, 1161-1171.

[33] US Preventive Services Task Force. Screening for hearing impairment. (1995). (2nd ed., pp 393-405). Baltimore, MD; Williams & Wilkins.

[34] Davis, A., Smith, P., Ferguson, M., Stephens, D., Gianopoulos, I. (2007). Acceptability, benefit and costs of early screening for hearing disability: a study of potential screening tests and models. *Health Technology Assessment*, *11*, 1-294.

[35] López-Torres Hidalgo, J., Boix Gras, C., Téllez Lapeira, J., López Verdejo, M.A., del Campo del Campo, J.M., Escobar Rabadán, F. (2009). Functional status of elderly people with hearing loss. *Archives of Gerontology and Geriatrics*, *49*, 88-92.

[36] Saito, H., Nishiwaki, Y., Michikawa, T., Kikuchi, Y., Mizutari, K., Takebayashi, T., Ogawa, K. (2010). Hearing handicap predicts the development of depressive symptoms after 3 years in older community-dwelling Japanese. *Journal of American Geriatric Society*, *58*, 93-97.

[37] Jupiter, T. (2009). Screening for hearing loss in the elderly using distortion product otoacoustic emissions, pure tones, and a self-assessment tool. *American Journal of Audiology*, *18*, 99-107.

[38] Ventry, I.M., & Weinstein, B.E. (1982). The hearing handicap inventory for the elderly: a new tool. *Ear and Hearing*, *3*, 128-134.

[39] Lichtenstein, M.J., & Hazuda, H.P. (1998). Cross-cultural adaptation of the hearing handicap inventory for the Elderly-Screening Version (HHIE-S) for use with Spanish-speaking Mexican Americans. *Journal of American Geriatric Society*, *46*, 492-498.

[40] Yueh, B., Shapiro, N., MacLean, C.H., Shekelle, P.G. (2003). Screening and management of adult hearing loss in primary care: scientific review. *Journal of American Medical Association*, *289*, 1976-1985.

[41] Calviti, K.C., & Pereira, L.D. (2009). Sensitivity, specificity and predictive values of hearing loss to different audiometric mean values. *Brazilian Journal of Otorhinolaryngology*, *75*, 794-800.

[42] Chang, H.P., Ho, C.Y., Chou, P. (2009).The factors associated with a self-perceived hearing handicap in elderly people with hearing impairment--results from a community-based study. *Ear and Hearing*, *30*, 576-583.

[43] Lasisi, A.O., Abiona, T., Gureje, O. (2010). The prevalence and correlates of self-reported hearing impairment in the Ibadan study of ageing. *Transactions of the Royal Society of Tropical Medicine and Hygiene*, *104*, 518-523.

[44] Sindhusake, D., Mitchell, P., Smith, W., Golding, M., Newall, P., Hartley, D., Rubin, G. (2001). Validation of self-reported hearing loss. The Blue Mountains Hearing Study. *International Journal of Epidemiology*, *30*, 1371-1378.

[45] Gates, G.A., Murphy, M., Rees, T.S., Fraher, A. (2003). Screening for handicapping hearing loss in the elderly. *Journal of Family Practice*, *52*, 56–62.

[46] Uchida, Y., Ando, F., Shimokata, H., Sugiura, S., Ueda, H., Nakashima, T. (2008). The effects of aging on distortion-product otoacoustic emissions in adults with normal hearing. *Ear and Hearing*, *29*, 176-184.

[47] Nelson, D.I., Nelson, R.Y., Concha-Barrientos, M., Fingerhut, M. (2005). The global burden of occupational noise-induced hearing loss. *American Journal of Industrial Medicine*, *48*, 446-458.

[48] Occupational Safety and Health Administration (OSHA). (2009). Screening and surveillance: a guide to OSHA standards. OSHA, 3162-12R.

[49] Shupak, A., Tal, D., Sharoni, Z., Oren, M., Ravid, A., Pratt, H. (2007). Otoacoustic emissions in early noise-induced hearing loss. *Otology and Neurotology*, *28*, 745-752.

[50] Marshall, L., Lapsley Miller, J.A., Heller, L.M., Wolgemuth, K.S., Hughes, L.M., Smith, S.D., Kopke, R.D. (2009). Detecting incipient inner-ear damage from impulse noise with otoacoustic emissions. *Journal of Acoustical Society of America*, *125*, 995-1013.

[51] Humes, L.M., Joellenbeck, L.M., Durch, J.S. (editors). (2006). Noise and military service: implications for hearing loss and tinnitus/Committee on Noise-Induced Hearing Loss and Tinnitus Associated with Military Service from World War II to the Present, Medical Follow-up Agency Institute of Medicine. Washington DC: National Academy Press.

[52] Helfer, T.M., Canham-Chervak, M., Canada, S., Mitchener, T.A. (2010). Epidemiology of hearing impairment and noise-induced hearing injury among U.S. military personnel, 2003-2005. *American Journal of Preventive Medicine*, *38*(1 Suppl), S71-77.

[53] Meyer, J.D., Chen, Y., McDonald, J.C., Cherry, N.M. (2002). Surveillance for work-related hearing loss in the UK: OSSA and OPRA 1997-2000. *Occupational Medicine*, *52*, 75-79.

[54] Last JM. (Ed.). (2001). A dictionary of epidemiology. Fourth Edition. New York: Oxford University Press.

[55] Concha-Barrientos, M., Campbell-Lendrum, D., Steenland, K. (2004). Occupational noise: assessing the burden of disease from work-related hearing impairment at national and local levels. Geneva: World Health Organisation.

[56] European Agency for Safety and Health at Work (EASHW). (2005). Reducing the risks from occupational noise. Belgium: EASHW.

[57] Davies, H., Marion, S., Teschke, K. (2008). The impact of hearing conservation programs on incidence of noise-induced hearing loss in Canadian workers. *American Journal of Industrial Medicine*, *51*, 923-931.

In: Prevention of Hearing Loss
Editors: V. Newton, P. Alberti and A. Smith

ISBN: 978-1-61942-745-7
© 2012 Nova Science Publishers, Inc.

Chapter X

Treatment: Surgical and Medical

Ulf Rosenhall*

Abstract

The cure of hearing impairments has been focussed on middle ear diseases, causing conductive hearing loss. Examples of diseases that can be treated surgically, with subsequent restoration of hearing, are otosclerosis and chronic otitis media. Even a minor surgical procedure, insertion of a tympanostomy tube, restores hearing. The situation is much more complicated regarding treatment of sensorineural hearing loss. The restoration of hearing in ears with severe deafness or profound hearing loss is achieved by cochlear implants, described in Chapter 11. Medical treatment of sensorineural hearing loss is currently based on prevention and intervention before permanent hearing loss has developed, and research to achieve this goal is in progress.

Introduction

The Roman medical encyclopedist Aulus Cornelius Celsus, who lived in the 1st century AD, has described the first known treatment of hearing loss. He softened ear wax and foreign bodies in the ear canal with hot oil, honey, grape juice and rose oil, for subsequent syringing and washing out. Since then, treatment of hearing loss has been a story of success as well as failure, but with possibilities. The success story is the surgical treatment of middle ear diseases with the establishment of modern surgical procedures for chronic otitis media, and otosclerosis in the 1950s and 60s. However, middle ear diseases causing conductive hearing loss, causes only a minority of hearing impairments, 17% or less, depending upon the communi. A majority of permanent hearing impairments are sensorineural, and the most common location of the causative lesion is the cochlea. Cochlear hearing impairments are caused by a variety of factors, intrinsic (like genetic factors) as well as extrinsic (like excessive noise and ototoxic substances). The complexity of cochlear anatomy, physiology,

---

* Corresponding author: ulf.rosenhall@karolinska.se.

and biochemistry has rendered it an area of inaccessibility for treatment procedures. Sensorineural hearing loss has, with great success, been managed by habilitation / rehabilitation including fitting of hearing aids, and, in cases of severe deafness, with cochlear implants. The possibility of restoring a permanently malfunctioning cochlea has been very limited, but this is now changing. Obviously, prevention of a lesion in the cochlea, before it has been established, is the most attractive alternative, but also treatment of an established cochlear lesion has become a realistic alternative in some instances, with good future potential.

Surgical Treatment of Hearing Loss

Introduction

Diseases, malformations, and lesions affecting the external ear canal, the tympanic membrane, and the middle ear, might interfere with the conduction of sound to the cochlea, resulting in conductive hearing loss. Sometimes, the inner ear is affected as well, resulting in combined hearing loss. There are some major causative groups of conductive hearing loss: chronic otitis media (COM), secretory otitis media (SOM), congenital malformations, stapes fixation with a hereditary trait (otosclerosis, and osteogenesis imperfecta), and traumatic middle ear lesions. The mechanisms causing conductive hearing loss vary. The external ear canal can be occluded by cerumen or by foreign bodies. Atresia of the external ear canal is often caused by a congenital malformation, but can occasionally be the result of a chronic infection causing an irritation of the skin and soft tissues of the external ear canal. Fixation of the ossicular chain can be caused by otosclerosis and related diseases, or by COM. Discontinuity or incomplete continuity of the ossicular chain can be caused by COM, trauma to the ear, or be the result of a congenital malformation.

The basic diagnostic programme of conductive hearing loss includes a thorough medical history, oto-microscopy, and pure tone audiometry with measurement of air- and bone conduction thresholds. Patient selection for restorative middle ear surgery is based on the preoperative audiogram. The potential to improve hearing and to regain serviceable hearing must be considered. For the best postoperative result, e.g. to obtain optimal binaural input to central auditory areas, the operated ear should be brought within 15 dB of the hearing of the contralateral, better ear.

Complementary preoperative audiological tests include impedance audiometry with tympanometry and stapedius reflex measurements, and speech audiometry. Imaging techniques, especially computerised tomography (CT), have an important diagnostic function in selected cases before middle ear surgery.

A "third window" to the inner ear (like a superior canal dehiscence, a large vestibular aqueduct syndrome, or X-linked deafness with stapes gusher) might mimic a conductive or a combined hearing loss [1]. It is very important to separate this kind of "inner ear conductive hearing loss" from a middle ear disorder, since surgery based on false premises, might result in profound deafness. A third window lesion should be suspected if the bone conduction thresholds are "abnormally" low, better than 0 dB HL. Stapedial reflexes are generally present. Vestibular evoked myogenic potentials (VEMP) are typically absent in middle ear disorders, but in third window lesions they are present with thresholds lower than normally seen. Otoacoustic emissions, normally absent in middle ear diseases, may be present in third window lesions. A CT scan should be performed if a third window lesion is suspected.

Patients with middle ear lesions and conductive or mixed hearing loss should be informed about aural rehabilitation including hearing aid fitting, counselling or group rehabilitation programmes, depending on the experiences and local traditions. Before a decision for otosurgery is made, it may be appropriate for the patient to be offered hearing aid amplification. If bilateral hearing loss remains after surgery it is very important to offer the patient the option of aural rehabilitation. Some of the most important causes of conductive hearing loss, that can be treated surgically, will now be described.

Otosclerosis

Otosclerosis is a metabolic bone disease affecting the otic capsule, a compact part of the temporal bone surrounding the inner ear. The otosclerotic focus is characterised by active metabolism including enzyme mediated bone formation, bone resorption, and vascularisation. The site of predilection of symptomatic otosclerotic foci is the region anterior to the oval window, close to the footplate of the stapes. The slow growth of an otosclerotic focus leads to a gradual immobilisation, and eventually to fixation, of the footplate (fenestral otosclerosis).

Otosclerosis is among the most common causes of adult-onset hearing loss. The first signs are usually apparent in young adult age, with an onset age often between 20 and 40 years. The disease usually starts in one ear, but eventually, in 70 -80% becomes bilateral. The prevalence of manifest symptoms (clinical otosclerosis) has been decreasing, and is now 0.3-0.4% in a population of European ancestry. The prevalence is lower in Asian populations, and still lower in populations of African ancestry. More women than men are affected. In postmortem studies otosclerosis is much more common, up to 10% (histological otosclerosis). A majority of those with histologic otosclerosis apparently have no symptoms.

The aetiology of this disease is largely unknown, but epidemiological studies suggest the involvement of both genetic and environmental factors. Otosclerosis is an autosomal dominant heritable disease. The inheritance is complex involving many genes and with variable penetrance and degree of expression. A variant in the RELN gene on chromosome 7, encodes for the glucoprotein reelin, which in a genome-wide association study has been shown to be highly associated with otosclerosis [2]. It has been proposed that otosclerosis is related to a disturbed bone metabolism due to persistent measles virus infection of the otic capsule. It has been shown that the incidence of otosclerosis has decreased in subjects vaccinated for measles, with a greater decline in men than in women [3]. This is an unexpected, positive effect of childhood vaccination programmes, and is one explanation for the decreasing prevalence of the disease in developed countries. It has been suggested that hormonal factors, like oestrogen or oral contraceptives are involved in the development of otosclerosis. However, there is no evidence of an adverse effect of contraceptives [4], and the course of otosclerosis is not influenced by a pregnancy [5].

The clinical course is a of gradually increasing hearing loss, usually starting in one ear, and eventually becoming bilateral . The audiological profile is of a conductive hearing loss, generally with elevated bone conduction thresholds around 1.5 kHz caused by the effect of middle ear resonance when one of the windows to the inner ear is immobile (Carhart's notch). After successful stapes surgery both air- and bone conduction thresholds may be lower than the pre-surgery bone conduction thresholds in this area. Combined hearing loss can occur in cases with both fenestral otosclerosis and otosclerotic foci situated in other parts of the otic capsule, cochlear otosclerosis. Preserved speech perception might indicate fenestral otosclerosis, while poor speech perception indicates cochlear otosclerosis. If there are diagnostic difficulties a CT scan can be recommended in selected cases. Impedance audiometry provides important pre-operative information. A conductive hearing loss with normal tympanometry or low compliance, in combination with absent stapedial reflexes in the affected ear, indicates otosclerosis.

The indications for stapes surgery in otosclerosis may vary. A rough rule of thumb is that bilateral conductive hearing loss with a better ear air conduction pure tone average (0.5 – 4 kHz) of ≥40 dB constitutes an indication for stapes surgery. Depending on the communicative needs of the patients surgery can be recommended in cases with less pronounced hearing loss, or for patients with unilateral otosclerosis. If the indication is doubtful, hearing aid fitting and a follow-up after 1 – 2 years can be recommended.

Surgical Treatment of Otosclerosis

Modern stapes surgery started in the 1950-ies when a method to mobilize the fixed stapes was developed. The method was replaced by stapedectomy, in which the entire stapes was removed and replaced by a prosthesis placed on a bed of fascia or vein in the oval window. The modern type of stapes surgery, stapedotomy, was developed in the 1980s. The joint between the stapes and the incus is divided, and the upper parts of the stapes (the crura and the stapes head) are removed. A small hole, with a diameter between 0.4-1 mm, is drilled in the stapes footplate using a microdrill or an argon laser. A prosthesis often consisting of a piston, a shaft and a clamp, is used to replace the stapes. The piston, with a diameter of 0.3 to 0.8 mm and a length of about 4 mm, is placed in the hole of the footplate, and the prosthesis is securely anchored to the long process of the incus with a clamp. Various materials have been used, earlier often stainless steel, and more recently platinum, titanium, and teflon [6].

Recent literature, including a review, shows that the success rates are between 85-95%, where success is defined as the improvement of air conduction thresholds and air-bone gap closure according to the American Academy of Otolaryngology, Head and Neck Surgery Committee on Hearing and Equilibrium guidelines, 1995 [7, 8]. It is also important to consider the patient's assessment of the benefit of surgery since it may not always be identical to the improvement measured with audiometry. Success rates, evaluated with questionnaires (e.g. the Glasgow Benefit Plot) of 64 to 79% have been reported [8, 9, 10].

Postoperative complications include deafness, loss of vestibular function, and tinnitus. Postoperative partial or total hearing loss is one of the most feared complications of stapedectomy, with an incidence that ranges from 0.6% to 3% with older techniques (for a review see, Bajaj et al. [11]). Other complications are displacement of the prosthesis (reported in 30-46% of failed cases), tympanic membrane perforation, perilymphatic leakage, and damage to the chorda tympani. Vertigo can be a manifestation of serous labyrinthitis, which usually subsides within a few days. The currently recommended, and commonly used, small fenestra stapedotomy, performed by experienced surgeons, has reduced the risk of intraoperative complications. Revision stapedectomy is associated with an increased risk of severe sensorineural hearing loss.

Medical Treatment of Otosclerosis

Since otosclerosis is a metabolic disease medical treatment trials have been attempted. The most common treatment of cochlear otosclerosis is peroral sodium fluoride administration, often used in combination with calcium carbonate and vitamin D. Fluoride treatment cannot reverse conductive hearing loss, but may slow the progression of otosclerotic hearing loss, both conductive and cochlear. A review of the literature have identified several case control studies that have found a hearing benefit, but only one double-blind, placebo controlled trial that showed that sodium fluoride reduces the deterioration of otosclerotic hearing loss. There is evidence of a benefit of fluoride regime in otosclerosis, but the evidence is low [12] and the issue is still controversial.

Otitis Media

Otitis media (OM) is an inflammation of the middle ear, or sequelae after an inflammation. There are many variations of OM depending on pathogenesis, duration, and sequelae.

Acute Otitis Media (AOM)

AOM is an acute viral or bacterial infection of the middle ear. It is most prevalent in childhood, and occurs often in conjunction with an upper respiratory infection (URI). The symptoms are earache, catarrhal symptoms with congestion, and fever. It is often self-limited within a few days. Complications affecting the mastoid process (mastoiditis), the inner ear (bacterial labyrinthitis), or CNS-infection, are extremely uncommon in developed countries but are prevalent in developing countries.

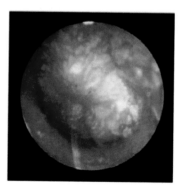

Figure 10.1. Acute otitis media (AOM) with bulging tympanic membrane.

Pathogens are respiratory syncytial virus (RSV), and the most common causative bacteria are *Streptococcus pneumoniae, Pseudomonas aeruginosa, Moraxella catarrhalis*, and *Haemophilus influenza*. A bacterial AOM may result in perforation of the tympanic membrane with suppurative discharge from the ear. About 10% of all children aged 6 months to two years, will have three or more episodes of AOM within half a year [13].

Treatment of AOM

The recommendations for the management of AOM vary considerably in different parts of the world. Because of the risk of development of antibiotic resistant bacteria, it is desirable that the use of antibiotics is restricted. In a majority of the cases AOM is self-limiting, and frequently no pharmaceutical treatment is needed. Some general principles regarding antibiotic treatment can be suggested; the following recommendation is based on a consensus conference arranged by the Swedish Medical Products Agency in 2010 [14].

Antibiotic treatment (penicillin V or amoxicillin, especially after therapeutic failure with penicillin V) should be restricted to the following indications.

All cases with perforated tympanic membrane should be treated. Infants under the age of one to two years, and juveniles over the age 12 years, and adults, with verified AOM, should also get antibiotic treatment. Children between 1-2 years, up to 12 years, should only get antibiotic treatment if complicating factors are present. Children with recurrent AOM have an increased risk to develop conductive or mixed hearing loss, and should be followed up. Paracetamol can be recommended to alleviate earache, fever, and symptoms from an upper respiratory infection.

Secretory Otitis Media (SOM)

SOM, or otitis media with effusion (OME) is a complication after AOM, or can arise spontaneously. In SOM the middle ear contains an effusion of variable viscosity and extent. In mild cases there is a retraction of the tympanic membrane with both effusion and air in the middle ear cavity. SOM is a typical childhood disease, it is very common, about 90% of all children have had SOM at some time before school age. It is most prevalent between 6 months and four years of age. During the first year of life half of the children have had OM, and at age 2 years the figure has increased to >60%. Most children have only had SOM occasionally, but >5% have episodes lasting for one year or longer [15, 16].

A predisposing factor is poor Eustachian tube function. Children at a special risk are those with craniofacial anomalies, like orofacial cleft malformations, and Down syndrome. In uncomplicated cases the condition is self-limiting within weeks or months. If the condition is persistent, the middle ear effusion thickens and becomes glue-like, glue ear. The hearing varies from normal hearing, to a mild conductive hearing loss in the low frequencies, to a moderate or even pronounced conductive hearing loss in glue ear cases. When present in adults, a causative factor like cancer of the nasopharynx, or an autoimmune disease (Wegener´s granulomatosis), should be considered.

The diagnosis of SOM is done with pneumatic otoscopy in combination with tympanometry, or otomicroscopy, preferably also combined with tympanometry. Follow-up hearing testing is important.

Treatment of SOM

Watchful waiting is recommended for a child with uncomplicated SOM, for up to three months. An episode of SOM exceeding three months might need surgical treatment. The preferred surgical procedure for is myringotomy and insertion of a tympanostomy drainage tube [15]. There is evidence that the hearing, as well as the quality of life, is improved after tube insertion, compared with no treatment [13].

Antihistamines and decongestants are ineffective for SOM, and antimicrobial therapy, with or without complementary steroids, has not been demonstrated to improve the prognosis in the long-term [15].

Chronic Suppurative Otitis Media (CSOM)

In (CSOM) there is a perforation of the tympanic membrane and a persistent discharge, otorrhea, from the middle ear. The mucous membrane in the middle ear is swollen, hyperemic, and polyps or granulation tissue may occur. There is a bacterial infection and the discharge is purulent. According to WHO [17] CSOM affects up to 330 million individuals, of whom 60% have hearing loss. Over 90% of the global burden of CSOM comes from countries in south-east Asia, the western Pacific region, Africa, and among circumpolar populations. In these areas the condition not only causes a heavy disease burden but also a significant mortality. In regions with the highest prevalence values >4% of the population have CSOM, and in regions with high prevalence values 2-4%. CSOM is uncommon in Europe, the Americas, the Middle East, and Australia (1% or <1%).

Many patients with CSOM can be managed by conservative, medical treatment. The infection must be eliminated, and the discharge be controlled. The treatment includes aural toilet, antibiotic treatment, antiseptic treatment and topical antibiotics. Notice that topical application of ototoxic drugs must be avoided! Surgical treatment is indicated if CSOM cannot be managed by medical treatment, complications are expected, and to close a perforation of the tympanic membrane.

Middle Ear Cholesteatoma

A cholesteatoma is a cyst-like growth (not neoplastic, tumor growth!) that has a tendency to expand and destroy surrounding tissues including the ossicles and the bone structures surrounding the inner ear. Histologically, it consists of keratinizing squamous epithelium. The most common form is acquired and is derived from squamous epithelium from the outer layer of the tympanic membrane. In many cases it is closely related to CSOM. It starts as retraction of the tympanic membrane (often the upper, thin part, the pars flaccida) or the mastoid antrum, in the upper – posterior part of the tympanic membrane. An important causative factor is decreased pressure in the middle ear, in connection to COM or Eustachian tube dysfunction. An uncommon type of cholesteatoma is congenital and is a form of an epidermoid cyst in the middle ear. The cholesteatoma sac contains debris of desquamated cells and white, cholesterol crystals, and it often becomes infected. The symptoms are in the initial stage often very discrete, a mucopurulent discharge and a mild hearing loss. When the cholesteatoma expands conductive hearing loss develops when the middle ear space is occupied, and especially when the ossicles are eroded and a discontinuity of the ossicular chain appears. At this stage most patients seek otological services and are treated. In countries with poor access to otological services the disease can progress, and severe complications might occur. Erosion to the inner ear causes deafness, vertigo, facial paralysis might occur, as well as serious, life-threatening CNS-complications like brain abscess and septicemia. A cholesteatoma should be treated with surgery.

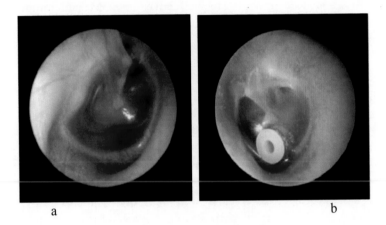

a   b

Figure 10.2. a) Secretory otitis media (SOM) with an effusion in the middle ear and beginning aeration. b) Transtympanic drainage tube on place in the tympanic membrane.

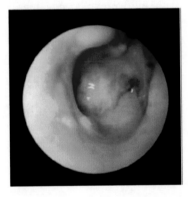

Figure 10.3. Chronic suppurative otitis media (CSOM) with a purulent discharge.

Surgical Treatment of CSOM and Cholesteatoma

Surgical treatment of a middle ear with discharge aims to remove infection and granulation tissue, to eradicate a cholesteatoma, and to stop the progress of a destructive process. The primary goal is to create a dry middle ear. A conductive hearing loss can be treated with reconstruction of the ossicular chain and the tympanic membrane at a later occasion, or in conjuncture with the primary operation. A number of surgical procedures have been available for many years to treat CSOM and cholesteatoma [18]. A disease limited to the attic and a symptomatic retraction pocket can be treated with anterior atticotomy. Inactive COM with simple mastoidectomy frequent reactivations can be treated with simple mastoidectomy or canal wall-up mastoidectomy, in which canalplasty is done. Extensive disease with poorly pneumatised mastoid can be treated with canal wall-down mastoidectomy.

Sequelae of Chronic Otitis Media (COM)

Tympanic membrane perforation is a sequel of CSOM, or of a traumatic perforation of the tympanic membrane. Prevalence values are coupled to those of CSOM, with highly variable frequencies in different countries and regions. A tympanic membrane perforation without otorrhea affects less than 1% (~0.5%) in developed countries. Conductive hearing loss may be present, with an air-bone (A-B) gap of ≤30 dB, provided that the middle ear including the ossicular chain is not affected. The ear is sensitive to water in the external ear canal, which can cause restrictions when swimming and bathing.

Surgical Treatment of a Dry Perforation of the Tympanic Membrane

Tympanoplasty is a common surgical procedure, which is often performed under local anaesthesia in adults. The perforation is sealed with a graft material, often a piece of prepared muscular fascia that is placed under the tympanic membrane on a cushion of absorbable material placed in the middle ear (medial grafting). In lateral grafting the graft material is placed on the tympanic membrane, after removal of squamous cell tissue around the perforation. The outcome of the operation is dependent on the function of the Eustachian tube, if this tube is functioning the result is excellent, if not there is a risk of recurrence.

Ossicular chain discontinuity and fixation. In more than 80% the cause of damage to the ossicular chain, both fixation and discontinuity, is CSOM or middle ear cholesteatoma. Most of the remaining cases are caused by trauma to the ear or congenital malformations. The weakest part of the ossicular chain is the long process of the incus and the incudo-stapedial joint. The long process has a diameter of less than one mm, and it is often corroded away by the CSOM. A total discontinuity of the ossicular chain results in a maximal conductive hearing loss with an A-B gap of about 60 dB over the entire frequency range. Sometimes the discontinuity is only partial with a defect transmission of sound over the affected part of the chain. The low frequency sound transmission less affected than the high frequency transmission. The pure tone audiometric pattern is a conductive hearing loss with a widening gap towards the high frequency regions (high frequency conductive hearing loss).

Ossicular fixation may also occur as an end result of CSOM, and is caused by fibrous tissue formation surrounding the ossicular chain, or calcification in the middle ear cavity (tympanosclerosis). The upper, epitympanic part of the ossicular chain, including the head of the malleus and the corpus of the incus, is often affected. The conductive hearing loss might be maximal (~60 dB A-B gap), or partial with the most pronounced A-B gap in the low- and mid frequencies. The audiogram resembles that of otosclerosis, but sometimes the A-B gap is less pronounced around 1-2 kHz, compared with that seen in the low frequencies, compared with otosclerosis. Carhart´s notch might, or might not, be present.

The preoperative investigation might include impedance audiometry (provided that the tympanic membrane is intact and not too scarred) and, sometimes a CT scan.

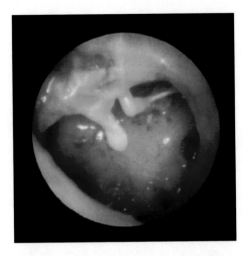

Figure 10.4. Subtotal perforation of the tympanic membrane. Part of the ossicular chain can be seen in the exposed middle ear.

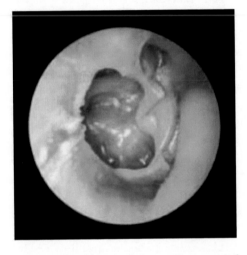

Figure 10.5. Adhesive otitis with the atelectatic tympanic membrane pasted on the middle ear ossicles, on the promontory, and in the round window niche.

In adhesive otitis media the tympanic membrane is severely retracted and is attached to the ossicles and medial wall of the middle ear. The condition is caused by chronic dysfunction of the Eustachian tube, often related to COM, or as an end stage of SOM. There is often fibrosis or even calcification in the middle ear. The hearing varies. Ears with air in the round and oval windows the hearing can be good, provided that the ossicular chain functions. In other cases there is a conductive hearing loss with maximum A-B gap.

Surgical Treatment of Ossicular Chain Discontinuity and Fixation

The missing part of the ossicular chain can be replaced in a surgical procedure, ossiculoplasty [19]. One possibility is to replace the defect with autograft material. This can be achieved by using the incus which is reshaped and rearranged to bridge the gap from the manubrium of the malleus to the stapes, either the head or the footplate of the stapes (interposition of the incus). Another option is to use cortical bone. Synthetic materials are used in allografts, often ceramic materials like hydroxylapatite, or titanium [20]. A malleus head fixation can also be operated with ossiculoplasty, where the malleus head is removed, and possibly also with the incus. A reconstruction is then performed by incus interposition or an allograft.

Traumatic Middle Ear Lesions

Discontinuity of the ossicular chain can be a solitary finding after an ear trauma, or in association with a temporal bone fracture. The incus is the most commonly affected ossicle, and there is often a luxation of the incudostapedial joint, or even a total displacement of the incus. Sometimes, the crura of the stapes are fractured. There is a conductive hearing loss with a maximal air-bone gap, or a partial disruption with a less pronounced hearing loss with mid- and high frequency conductive loss. The preoperative investigation should include impedance audiometry (provided that the tympanic membrane is intact and not too scarred). The tympanometric pattern of an ossicular discontinuity is very typical irrespective of which probe frequency that is used. Preserved stapedial reflexes indicate disruption of the crura of the stapes. A CT scan is suggested for a pre-operative analysis.

Congenital Ear Malformations of the External and Middle Ear

Congenital malformations of the ear are caused by defective embryogenesis. The auricle and the external auditory canal are developed from the first groove and the first and second branchial arches. The first and second branchial arches differentiate into the auditory ossicles. The first pharyngeal pouch develops into the middle ear cavity and the Eustachian tube. There are also connections with the otic vesicle and the anlage of the facial nerve. Due to the complex embryology, anomalies of the external and middle ear can vary enormously. Congenital abnormalities can be genetic or non-genetic. A malformation can be solitary, or associated with various syndromes, and a large number of syndromes that include conductive or mixed hearing impairments have been described. Further information can be provided by the Hereditary Hearing Loss Homepage: http://hereditaryhearingloss.org.

There are various classifications of the external canal, the tympanic membrane, middle ear development, and ossicular structures. Major anomalies include external auditory canal atresia involving the bony part of the ear canal, and often other anomalies such as absence of the tympanic membrane, ossicular anomalies, aberrant/dehiscent facial nerve, and microtia. Minor anomalies include a fixed/deformed ossicle, a normal or small ear canal, and possibly microtia.

External Auditory Canal Atresia (EACA)

This is a rare congenital anomaly and occurs in about 1 in 10 000 – 20 000 births. Unilateral EACA is present in about 2/3rd or more of all cases.

Ossicular Anomalies

The most common is fusion of the malleus and incus in the epitympanum, and this may occur with or without atresia. Most cases with EACA are congenital, but there are also acquired cases. Chronic infection of the external ear canal may cause stenosis of the ear canal and in advanced cases, a fibrous plug in the innermost part of the ear canal close to the tympanic membrane.

Treatment of External Auditory Canal Atresia

Surgery of EACA can be very complicated, and a grading system to predict the outcome surgical intervention of EACA has been proposed by Jahrsdoerfer et al. [21]. The system is based on CT scanning and takes into account the presence or absence of a stapes, an oval window, development of the middle ear space, anomalies of the ossicles and the facial nerve, pneumatization of the mastoid and other features. For patients with the best prognosis surgery is recommended, while others would most likely benefit from non-surgical management. Bilateral EACA usually requires surgery to restore hearing, provided that the indication for surgery is fulfilled. The selection of unilateral EACA for surgery is much stricter.

The bone-anchored hearing aid (BAHA) is the amplification system that is most suitable for EACA, as well as for patients with chronic infections and ear discharge when using conventional hearing aids. This is a percutaneous device, connected to an osseo-integrated titanium fixture. The system utilizes direct bone conduction to the inner ear and not sound transmission via the middle ear. Indications for BAHA are bilateral EACA and chronic ear infections that cannot benefit from conventional hearing aids. Indications under scrutiny at present are unilateral EACA and unilateral deafness, with the prospect to enhance directional hearing [22]. Implantable hearing aids offer also a promising possibility for the rehabilitation of EACA as well as for other types of hearing impairments.

Medical Treatment and Prevention of Sensorineural Hearing Loss

Introduction

Restoration of hearing in persons with bilateral severe deafness or profound hearing loss is often achieved by cochlear implants (CI), described in Chapter 11. Medical treatment of sensorineural hearing loss is presently based on two principles, prevention and intervention. Both are based on the prerequisite that there is no permanent severe damage affecting the inner ear prior to the treatment. Prevention is, for a long time, well established in audiological practice, and is a cornerstone in Hearing Conservation Programmes. Immunisation programmes to prevent hearing losses of infectious origins have been introduced during the last decades. Intervention include pharmacological treatment directly after an ototraumatic exposure, but before the development of permanent inner ear damage. Such treatments can preferably be applied before exposure as a preventive measure. The effect is often more pronounced compared with an intervention with the same drug. The problem is, of course, to be able to predict an ototraumatic event in advance.

Noise-Induced Hearing Loss (NIHL) Treated with Antioxidants and Other Drugs

Exposure to excessive noise is a common cause of hearing loss and tinnitus. It has been estimated that 9-16% of late-onset hearing loss in adults worldwide is due to occupational noise. The mechanisms causing noise-induced hearing loss (NIHL) have been described in detail as a result of research on animal models. Exposure to noise causes metabolic oxidative stress and the production of reactive oxygen species (ROS) resulting in cochlear injury. Free radical formation induces both necrotic and apoptotic cell death in the cochlea, affecting both types of hair cells, as well as supporting cells and the stria vascularis. This knowledge has made it possible to propose biochemical models to prevent, or even treat, NIHL. The method that is most promising for human use is to deactivate free radicals with antioxidants [23]. A number of agents with antioxidant properties have been studied in animal models. Many antioxidants are cheap to produce, and they are generally atoxic when they are administered in low or moderate dosages, as when they are used as food additives. Commonly used free radical scavengers are vitamins A, C, and E, and this combination has been shown to protects the cochlea against NIHL [24]. The antioxidant agent that has been most thoroughly investigated regarding NIHL-protection is N-acetylcysteine (NAC). If NAC is administered immediately before noise exposure it is highly effective to protect the hair cells and to reduce hearing loss [25, 26, 27, and other studies]. Antioxidants administered immediately after excessive noise exposure also reduces cochlear damage, although not as efficiently as if they are given before exposure [25, 28]. There is, however, no total agreement of the protective effect of NAC. In two animal studies NAC did not reduce the trauma produced by exposure to continuous broadband noise [29, 30]. In the first cited study the noise exposure was massive, 105 dB SPL, 8 hours a day, for 5 days. It is possible that the protective effect of NAC is limited to short noise exposures of less than maximal intensity.

The experience of NIHL- protection with antioxidants in humans is limited. Studies on people attending dicotheques have failed to demonstrate a protective effect of NAC. Quite obviously, such studies are difficult to perform, and there are other human studies of protective and intervention effects of antioxidants in progress [31]. In summary, animal research indicates that antioxidants can be used to protect the cochlea from NIHL, or even to use antioxidants for therapeutic purpose if used immediately after intense, accidental noise exposure. Moreover, antioxidants have been suggested to treat a variety of other conditions such as age-related hearing loss, Ménière's disease, and sudden hearing loss, but the level of evidence for such teatments is low.

Other drugs have been tried to treat hearing loss and tinnitus caused by accidental exposure to impulse noise. Plasma expanders have been tried more than 40 years ago with reported favourable effect [32], but the level of evidence was low. Magnesium (Mg) has been shown to have otoprotective properties. It has been observed that Mg-deficiency increases the risk of NIHL in research animals, and a diet enriched with Mg reduces the risk of both permanent and temporary threshold shift. Attias et al. [33] performed a randomised control trial (RCT) of Mg in normal hearing men. They demonstrated that oral intake of Mg reduces the noise induced temporary threshold shift, compared to placebo or no intake before noise exposure. Mg has also been used as an adjuvant to elicit the protective effect of antioxidants [24].

Sudden Sensorineural Hearing Loss

Sudden sensorineural hearing loss (SSNHL) is a diagnosis based on a symptom (sensorineural hearing loss) with a sudden onset within seconds to hours. It is usually unilateral and frequently accompanied by tinnitus and sometimes by vertigo. The aetiology of this entity is very variable. Specific diagnoses like vestibular schwannomas, neurological diseases like stroke or multiple sclerosis, must be diagnosed and treated accordingly. SSHL is idiopathic in a majority of the cases (idiopathic sudden sensorineural hearing loss, ISSNHL), Precipitating events preceding the ISSNHL such as viral illnesses, febrile states, and barotrauma, might give a hint to the cause. Several studies support the viral theory of ISSNHL. The vascular theory is another cherished approach, but with little evidence in the scientific literature. The membrane rupture theory is related to a barotrauma, like strenuous exercise or diving, or a head trauma, as a precipitating event. A perilymphatic fistula at the round the oval window has been associated to ISSNHL, and exploratory tympanotomy, with repair of an inner ear fistula is still recommended by some otosurgeons in patients with a clear history of barotrauma, or recent otological surgery. The effect of such surgery is, however, controversial.

It is difficult to validate treatment programmes for ISSNHL, since there is a considerable chance of spontaneous recovery. Roughly, $1/3^{rd}$ of the patients recover completely spontaneously, $1/3^{rd}$ recover partially, and $1/3^{rd}$ do not recover at all and have persistent hearing loss. Randomised controlled trials are necessary for treatment validations, and there are not many trials with this design. A variety of medical treatments have been based on clinical experience, most of them with low levels of evidence since they have not utilized a randomized controlled trial (RCT) design. Internationally, the most recommended treatment is administration of oral corticosteroids. Wilson et al [34] performed a RCT, and they reported a positive effect of corticosteroid treatment. The rationale for this type of treatment is an anti-inflammatory effect, a possible immunosuppressant, or improved microcirculation in the cochlea.

There are some meta-analyses of treatment outcome of ISSNHL. The Cochrane database of systematic reviews includes analyses of treatment strategies of ISSNHL [35]. Regarding treatment with steroids it was concluded that there is a benefit of treatment, but this conclusion was based one trial only. The quality of the other cited studies was low, and there was also some conflicting data. The value of steroids in the treatment of idiopathic ISSNHL therefore remains unclear [35]. Similar conclusions have been reached by the authors of three other meta-analyses of corticosteroid treatment of ISSNHL. For sudden sensorineural hearing loss it is still reasonable to recommend a course of treatment of oral corticosteroids for a short period of time, started within two weeks of onset [36]. Recently, two Swedish multi-centre studies of the effect of oral corticosteroids for treatment of ISSNHL have been reported [37, 38]. The findings of these studies is that the benefit of corticosteroids is none or negligible for the outcome of ISSNHL.

During the last decade a large number of studies in which corticosteroids have been injected in the middle ear of the affected ear have been published. Of 27 studies published between 2006 and 2011, 19 reported a positive effect of intratympanal corticosteroid treatment, and in only three no effect could be distinguished. The design of these studies was often unsophisticated, which is understandable since RCT studies are difficult to perform when an invasive procedure is applied. Intratympanic application of corticosteroids is possibly a promising treatment strategy, but with somewhat conflicting results and with a low level of evidence of so far.

Other Cochrane reviews deal with treatments of idiopathic ISSNHL with vasodilators and vasoactive substances, and hyperbaric oxygen (HBOT). The effectiveness vasodilators and vasoactive substances for ISSHL remain unproven [39]. In the acute stage of ISSHL there was some evidence that HBOT improved hearing [40]. However, this result should be interpreted cautiously because of the small number of patients and methodological shortcomings. Another treatment is inhalation of carbogen, a mixture of oxygen (95%) and CO_2 (5%), with reported variable benefit. Randomized controlled trials have not shown any benefit of antiviral treatment, e.g. with acyclovir [41].

Autoimmune Inner Ear Disease

A number of autoimmune inner ear disease (AIED) can cause of hearing loss, tinnitus, or vertigo. Two examples of autoimmune diseases than can affect the inner ear are Cogan's syndrome (hearing loss, vertigo and eye symptoms), and hearing loss in connection with rheumatoid arthritis. In spite of the multitude of diseases and syndromes AIED is rare, constituting less than 1% of cases with hearing loss and vertigo [42]. Immunological diagnosis with both tissue specific antibodies (e.g. 68-kDa bovine inner ear antigen and HSP-70) and tissue-non-specific antibodies is important (for review see Agrup and Luxon [43]).

Treatment of AIED includes corticosteroids (e.g. prednisolone). A therapeutical response should initiate a slow tapering of the steroids to a low long-term dose. The lack of a therapeutical response should initiate a rapid tapering and cessation. Patients with Cogan's syndrome are regularly treated with corticosteroids, with excellent result regarding the ocular symptoms, but often with less impressive results on the audio-vestibular symptoms.

A variety of immunosuppressive drugs have been tried to treat AIED, like cyclophosphamide, methotrexate, azathioprine, and etanercept. The effect of an aggressive immunosuppressive treatment is variable, with some evidence of stabilization and improvement, but also with serious side effects. It should be kept in mind that with the advent of CI, the administration of toxic medication to preserve hearing at all costs can be challenged.

Ototoxic Hearing Loss

There are a number of ototoxic drugs used in clinical practice. Antioxidants have a capacity to reduce ototoxic side effects regarding both hearing and vestibular function. One important group of ototoxic drugs is platinol compounds, like cisplatin and carboplatin. The ototoxicity of these drugs is related to lipidperoxidation, and they inhibit the activity of intracellular antioxidant enzymes, many of them containing glutathione. A drug that has been studied regarding platinol ototoxicity is sodium thiosulfate, a drug that stimulates the intracellular defence of reactive oxygen species. It has been shown that sodium thiosulfate reduces the decrease of intrinsic antioxidants caused by platinol compounds. Unfortunately, sodium thiosulfate also reduces the cytotoxic effect of these compounds, resulting in a decreased anticancer effect. Means to avoid this side effect have been suggested.

Intratympanal injection of sodium thiosulfate, or other agents with antioxidative properties, directly in the middle ear in a suitable vehicle, is the most promising method for targeted otoprotection without a systemic side effect [44].

Infectious and Meningitic Hearing Loss

Viral diseases like rubella, mumps and measles have been important contributors to hearing loss and total deafness in childhood. Vaccination programmes have been very successful to eradicated these causes of childhood deafness in the developed world, and more recently also in developing countries. This is important to remember in times when vaccination programmes sometimes are challenged, and there is a risk for a return of these types of hearing impairments. Bacteria like *Haemophilus influezae* type b, and *Streptococcus pneumonia* may cause severe, life-threatening diseases, meningitis and septicaemia.

Deafness belongs to the severe sequelae of these diseases. Children surviving pneumococcal meningitis have a high rate of long-term sequelae, neurological deficits in 30%, and hearing loss in 17% [45]. In recent decades vaccination programmes for these infections, as well as for Meningitis C (*Neisseria meningitidis*), have been introduced.

In bacterial meningitis and septicaemia high dose antibiotic treatment can be complemented with adjuvant treatment to reduce the risk of sequelae by reducing inflammatory response e.g. caused by arachidonic acid metabolites. The most common adjuvant treatment is to administer corticosteroids (dexamethasone). A meta-analysis of RCT-studies of treatment outcome of adult patients with bacterial meningitis demonstrated that adjuvant dexamethasone was associated with lower mortality, but only in specific subgroups, and with fewer cases of hearing impairment [46]. In a Cochrane analysis it was concluded that corticosteroids were associated with lower rates of severe hearing loss, of any hearing loss, and neurological sequelae [47]. Corticosteroids reduced severe hearing loss in *Haemophilus influenzae* meningitis. Corticosteroids reduced severe hearing loss, and any hearing loss, in high-income countries, but there was no beneficial effect of corticosteroid treatment in low-income countries.

Other drugs for adjuvant treatment have been proposed, like non-steroid anti-inflammatory drugs, antioxidants like NAC or MnTBAP, a drug that is a scavenger of both ROS and peroxide-nitrite. It has been proposed this type of treatment reduces hearing impairment and the loss of hair cells, but there are only occasional studies supporting this concept.

Future Treatment Programmes

The ultimate goal is to develop treatment programmes that can be applied in case of permanent damage to the inner ear and/or the first order neuron. In many laboratories advanced research is currently in progress. Tissue engineering is applied to increase the efficacy of Cochlear implants, e.g. by introducing nerve growth factors in the contact zone between the electrodes and the first order neuron. Future treatments are based on two principles, substitution and regeneration. Substitution can be achieved by stem cell therapy of hair cells or spiral ganglion cells. Both embryonic and adult stem cells are possible candidates for tissue implants.

The problems are monumental. It is not only necessary to design functional cells, but also to connect the biological implant to supporting structures, to the next order neuron, and to the tectorial membrane. Another line of research is gene therapy that has a potential for the treatment especially of sensorineural hearing losses of genetic origins. The method is based on the principle that a defect gene in a tissue is replaced by a functional gene by using a vector. To avoid potential dangers with a live virus vector, a Math1 protein has been suggested as a non-viral gene delivery plasmid.

Hair cell regeneration is a concept based on the biological principle that inner ear hair cells are produced throughout the entire life in fish, amphibians and birds, but not in mammals. Supporting cells appear to be transformed into hair cells in animals with the capacity for hair cell regeneration. Research is under way to revive regeneraten from progenitor cells to hair cells in mammals. The transcription factor Math1 is important for regeneration of hair cells. A realistic goal is to increase the hair cell populations in a damaged cochlea to an extent that hearing aids can be used more effectively.

All these methods are promising, but still in a stage of experimental research, clinical trials are still in the future. It must be emphasized that substitution and regeneration of inner ear hair cells and neurons are still a long way off, probably several decades.

Conclusion

Treatment of middle ear diseases causing conductive hearing loss is surgical, using middle ear surgical techniques developed about 50 years ago. These procedures have been refined during the last decades, a development that will continue. There has also been a steady evolvement of selection of patients suitable for surgery, pre-operative diagnostics, and supporting aural rehabilitation. Medical treatment of sensorineural hearing loss is still in its infancy, but a remarkable development is in progress. Medical therapy is based on prevention of hearing loss, intervention of non-reversible cochlear damage, and, in the future, on substitution and regeneration of inner ear structures.

Acknowledgments

Figures are by courtesy of Dr Piet van Hasselt (Figures 1,4,5)and the Dr Michael Hawke(Figures 2a,2b,3).

References

[1]   Merchant., S. N., Rosowski, J. J. (2008). Conductive hearing loss caused by third-window lesions of the inner ear. *Otology and Neurotology*, 29, 282-289.

[2]   Schrauwen, I., Ealy, M., Huentelman, M. J., Thys, M., Homer, M, Vanderstraeten, K., Fransen, E., Corneveaux, J. J., Craig, D. W., Claustres, M., Cremers, C. W., Dhooge, I.,

Van de Heyning, P., Vincent, R., Offeciers, E., Smith, R. J., Van Camp, G. (2009). A genome-wide analysis identifies genetic variants in the RELN gene associated with otosclerosis. *American Journal of Human Genetics, 84*, 328-338.

[3] Arnold, W., Busch, R., Arnold, A., Ritscher, B., Neiss, A., Niedermeyer, H. P. (2007). The influence of measles vaccination on the incidence of otosclerosis in Germany. *European Archives of Otorhinolaryngology, 264*, 741-748.

[4] Vessey, M., Painter, R. (2001). Oral contraception and ear disease: findings in a large cohort study. *Contraception*, 63, 61-63.

[5] Lippy, W. H., Berenholz, L. P., Schuring, A. G., Burkey, J. M. (2005). Does pregnancy affect otosclerosis? *Laryngoscope*, 115, 1833-1836.

[6] Fritsch, M. H., Naumann, I. C. (2008). Phylogeny of the stapes prosthesis. *Otology and Neurotology*, 29, 407-415.

[7] Kisilevsky, V., Bailie, N. A., Halik, J. J. (2010). Bilateral hearing results of 751 unilateral stapedectomies evaluated with the Glasgow benefit plot. *Journal of Laryngology and Otology*, 124, 482-489.

[8] Vincent, R., Sperling, N. M., Oates, J., Jindal, M. (2006). Surgical findings and long-term hearing results in 3,050 stapedotomies for primary otosclerosis: A prospective study with the otology-neurotology database. *Otology and Neurotology, Suppl.*2, 27, 25-47.

[9] Lundman, L., Mendel, L., Bagger-Sjoback, D., Rosenhall, U. (1999). Hearing in patients operated unilaterally for otosclerosis. Self-assessment of hearing and audiometric results. *Acta Otolaryngologica*, 119, 453–458.

[10] Kisilevsky, V. E., Bailie, N. A., Dutt, S. N., Halik, J. J. (2010). Functional results of 394 bilateral stapedotomies evaluated with the Glasgow Benefit Plot. *European Archives of Otorhinolaryngology*, 267, 1027–1034.

[11] Bajaj, Y., Uppal, S., Bhatti, I., Coatesworth, A. P. (2010). Otosclerosis 3. The surgical management of otosclerosis. *International Journal of Clinical Practice*, 64, 505-510.

[12] Cruise, A. S., Singh, A., Quiney, R. E. (2010). Sodium fluoride in otosclerosis treatment: a review. *Journal of Laryngology and Otology*, 124, 583-586.

[13] Swedish Council on Health Technology Assessment. (2008). Tympanostomy tube treatment of middle ear inflammation (in Swedish). *Report* 189.

[14] Information from the Swedish Medical Products Agency 5. (2010). Diagnostics, treatment and follow-up of acute otitis media AOM – A new recommendation (in Swedish).

[15] American Academy of Pediatrics. (2004). American Academy of Family Physicians, American Academy of Otolaryngology-Head and Neck Surgery and American Academy of Pediatrics Subcommittee on Otitis Media With Effusion. *Pediatrics*, 113, 1412-1429.

[16] Bluestone, C. D. (2004). Studies in Otitis Media: Children's Hospital of Pittsburgh–University of Pittsburgh Progress Report—2004. *Laryngoscope*, 114, Suppl. 105, 1–26.

[17] WHO. (2004). Chronic suppurative otitis. Burden of Illness and Management Options. Child and Adolescent Health and Development. Prevention of Blindness and Deafness. Geneva, Switzerland: World Health Organisation. Available from: http://www.who.int/pbd/deafness/activities/hearing_care/otitis_media.pdf (17 August 2011).

[18] Nadol, Jr. J. B. (2005). Chronic otitis media. In: Surgery of the ear and temporal bone (eds. J. B. Nadol Jr. and M. J. McKenna). (pp.199-218). Philadelphia, USA: Lippincott Williams and Wilkins.

[19] Battista, R. A., Shohet, J. A., Talavera, F., Roland, P. S., Slack, C. L., Meyers, A. D. (2008).Middle Ear, Ossiculoplasty. Medscape reference. Available from:http://emedicine.medscape.com/article/859889-overview (Accessed 2 March 2011).

[20] Yung, M. W. (2003). Literature review of alloplastic materials in ossiculoplasty. Editorial review. *Journal of Laryngology and Otology,* 117, 431-436.

[21] Jahrsdoerfer, R. A., Yeakley, J. W., Aguilar, E. A., Cole, R. R., Gray, L. C.(1992) Grading system for the selection of patients with congenital aural atresia. *American Journal of Otology,* 13, 6-12.

[22] Hakansson, B. (2011). The future of bone conduction hearing devices. *Advances in Otorhinolaryngology,* 71, 140-152.

[23] Henderson, D., McFadden, S. L., Liu, C. C., Hight, N., Zheng, X. Y. (1999). The role of antioxidants in protection from impulse noise. *Annals of the New York Academy of Sciences,* 884, 368-380.

[24] Le Prell, C. G., Hughes, L. F., Miller, J. M. (2007). Free radical scavengers vitamins A, C, and E plus magnesium reduce noise trauma. *Free Radical Biology and Medicine,*42, 1454-63.

[25] Kopke, R. D., Weisskopf, P. A., Boone, J. L., Jackson, R. L., Wester, D. C., Hoffer, M. E., Lambert, D. C., Charon, C. C., Ding, D. L., McBride, D. (2000). Reduction of noise-induced hearing loss using L-NAC and salicylate in the chinchilla. *Hearing Research,* 149, 138-146.

[26] Kopke, R. D., Jackson, R. L., Coleman, J. K., Liu, J., Bielefeld, E. C., Balough, B. J. (2007). NAC for noise: from the bench top to the clinic. *Hearing Research,* 226, 114-125.

[27] Coleman, J. K., Kopke, R. D., Liu, J., Ge, X., Harper, E. A., Jones, G. E., Cater, T. L., Jackson, R. L. (2007). Pharmacological rescue of noise induced hearing loss using N-acetylcysteine and acetyl-L-carnitine. *Hearing Research,* 226, 104-113.

[28] Lorito, G., Giordano, P., Petruccelli, J., Martini, A., Hatzopoulos, S. (2008). Different strategies in treating noise induced hearing loss with N-acetylcysteine. *Medical Science Monitor: International medical journal of experimental and clinical research,* 14, 159 -164.

[29] Hamernik, R. P., Qiu, W., Davis, B. (2008). The effectiveness of N-acetyl-L-cysteine (L-NAC) in the prevention of severe noise-induced hearing loss. *Hearing Research,* 239, 99-106.

[30] Davis, R. R., Custer, D. A., Krieg, E., Alagramam, K. (2010). N-Acetyl L-Cysteine does not protect mouse ears from the effects of noise. *Journal of Occupational Medicine and Toxicology,* 5 :11.

[31] Lindblad, A-C., Rosenhall, U., Olofsson, A., Hagerman, B. (2011). The efficacy of *N*-Acetylcysteine (NAC) to protect the human cochlea from subclinical hearing loss caused by impulse noise: A controlled trial. *Noise and Health,* 13:432-441.

[32] Kellerhals, B., Hippert, F., Pfaltz, C. R .(1971). Treatment of acute acoustic trauma with low molecular weight dextran. *Practica oto-rhino-laryngologica,* 33, 260 -264.

[33] Attias, J., Sapir, S., Bresloff, I., Reshef-haran, I., Ising, H. (2004). Reduction in noise-induced temporary threshold shift in humans following oral magnesium intake. *Clinical Otolaryngology*, 29, 635–641.

[34] Wilson, W. R., Byl, F. M., Laird, N. (1980). The efficacy of steroids in the treatment of idiopathic sudden hearing loss. A double-blind clinical study. *Archives of Otolaryngology*, 106, 772-776.

[35] Wei, B. P. C., Mubiru, S., O'Leary, S. (2006). Steroids for idiopathic sudden sensorineural hearing loss. Cochrane Database of Systematic Reviews 2006, Issue 1. Art. No.: CD003998. DOI: 10.1002/14651858.CD003998.pub2.

[36] Schreiber, B. E., Agrup, C., Haskard, D. O., Luxon, L. M. (2010). Sudden sensorineural hearing loss. *Lancet*, 375, 1203-1211.

[37] Nosrati-Zarenoe, R., Arlinger, S., Hultcrantz, E. (2007). Idiopathic sudden sensorineuralhearing loss: results drawn from the Swedish national database. *Acta Otolaryngologica*,127, 1168-1175.

[38] Nosrati-Zarenoe. R., Hultcrantz, E. (2011). Corticosteroid treatment of idiopathic sudden sensorineural hearing loss. Part 1: a randomized triple-blinded placebocontrolled trial. Submitted for publication.

[39] Agarwal, L., Pothier, D. D. (2009). Vasodilators and vasoactive substances for idiopathic sudden sensorineural hearing loss. Cochrane Database of Systematic Reviews 2009, Issue 4. Art. No.: CD003422. DOI: 10.1002/14651858.CD003422.pub4.

[40] Bennett, M. H., Kertesz, T., Perleth, M., Yeung, P. (2007). Hyperbaric oxygen for idiopathic sudden sensorineural hearing loss and tinnitus. Cochrane Database of Systematic Reviews 2007, Issue 1. Art. No.: CD004739. DOI: 10.1002 /14651858.CD004739.pub3.

[41] Westerlaken, B. O., Stokroos, R. J., Dhooge, I. J., Wit, H. P., Albers, F. W. (2003). Treatment of idiopathic sudden sensorineural hearing loss with antiviral therapy: a prospective, randomized, double-blind clinical trial. *Annals of Otology, Rhinology and Laryngology*, 112, 993-1000.

[42] Bovo, R., Aimoni, C., Martini, A. (2006). Immune-mediated inner ear *Acta Otolaryngologica*, 126, 1012 -1021.

[43] Agrup, C., Luxon, L. M. (2006). Immune-mediated inner-ear disorders in neuro-otology. *Current Opinions in Neurology*, 19, 26-32.

[44] Berglin, C. E., Pierre, P. V., Bramer, T., Edsman, K., Ehrsson, H., Eksborg, S., Laurell, G. (2011). Prevention of cisplatin-induced hearing loss by administration of a thiosulfate-containing gel to the middle ear in a guinea pig model. *Cancer Chemotherapy and Pharmacology*. [Epub ahead of print].

[45] Pikis, A., Kavaliotis, J., Tsikoulas, J., Andrianopoulos, P., Venzon, D., Manios, S. (1996). Long-term sequelae of pneumococcal meningitis in children. *Clinical Pediatrics*, 35, 72-78.

[46] Vardakas, K. Z., Matthaiou, D. K., Falagas, M. E. (2009). Adjunctive dexamethasone therapy for bacterial meningitis in adults: a meta-analysis of randomized controlled trials. *European Journal of Neurology*,1, 662–673.

[47] Brouwer, M. C., McIntyre, P., de Gans, J., Prasad, K., Van de Beek, D. (2010). Corticosteroids for acute bacterial meningitis (Review). *Cochrane database of systematic reviews*. 2010 Sep. 8;(9):CD004405.

In: Prevention of Hearing Loss
Editors: V. Newton, P. Alberti and A. Smith

ISBN: 978-1-61942-745-7
© 2012 Nova Science Publishers, Inc.

Chapter XI

Rehabilitation and Sensory Aids

Dianne Toe[*]

Abstract

This chapter presents an overview of the essential aspects of fitting sensory devices to adults and children. A detailed outline of the basic function, benefits and fitting outcomes for hearing aids, cochlear implants, bone- anchored hearing aids and FM Aids is provided. A programme of aural rehabilitation appears to be an important component of supporting adults in the effective use of sensory devices. Children must learn to use a sensory device in order to acquire language. This can only take place when they are appropriately supported to use audition for meaningful communication through early intervention and quality educational programmes.

Introduction

It is not always possible to prevent hearing loss. Approximately one in every 1000 children will be born with a hearing impairment, many with no family history of deafness. Other children will develop hearing loss during early childhood through susceptibility to middle ear infections or a progressive sensorineural loss. The aging populations in many developed nations are currently estimated to experience hearing loss at a rate of one person in six, many with no history of noise exposure (The Economic Impact and Cost of Hearing Loss in Australia, Access Economics, 2006). For these individuals, the fitting of a sensory device, well supported by appropriate rehabilitation, can significantly improve their opportunities to fully participate in life. Developed nations may appear to have open access to the latest technologies and techniques, while countries new to providing aural rehabilitation might begin by focusing on 'the basics'. It is, however, often the basic foundations of sensory device fitting and rehabilitative support that impact the most on the lives of individuals with hearing loss. This chapter will explore the range of sensory devices and the nature of

[*] E-mail: dianne.toe@deakin.edu.au.

rehabilitation available to children and adults. It is written in the context of a rapidly changing global technological landscape, where both medical and engineering developments often outpace reported outcomes research.

Hearing Aids

Basic Operation

Analogue and digital hearing aids operate upon similar principles but differ in the way they process the incoming sound signal. In an analogue hearing aid, a microphone converts mechanical acoustic energy into electrical current. The amplifier in the hearing aid increases the amplitude of the electrical current which corresponds to increased sound energy. The hearing aid receiver or earphone converts the amplified electrical signal into acoustic energy and delivers it to the ear via an earmould (air conduction) or a bone vibrator (bone conduction).

In a digital aid, the sound is converted to an electrical current by the microphone (an analogue procedure). An analogue/digital converter then turns the electrical signal into a series of binary numbers in the form of positive or negative electrical voltage. The central processing unit (CPU) of the digital hearing aid instructs the programming computer to manipulate this series of numbers, providing great flexibility that allows the aid to be adjusted more precisely for the hearing aid user. The computed digital output is converted back to analogue electrical impulses by a digital analogue/converter which in turn is converted by the receiver back to sound. A tiny high capacity computer chip enables the digital aid to offer a range of features and alternative programmes.

Hearing aids may be body worn, whereby the microphone and amplifier are worn on the chest and a separate receiver is worn at ear level. Ear level aids combine the microphone, amplifier and receiver and can be behind-the-ear (BTE), in-the-ear (ITE), in-the-canal (ITC) or completely in the canal (CIC). Most hearing aids require a well-fitting comfortable earmould to ensure that the aid stays in place and to prevent acoustic feedback, a high frequency phenomena created by the leakage of sound out of the ear and back into the hearing aid microphone.

Binaural Fitting

Hearing aid fittings for unilateral hearing losses are unusual and quite specialised. Nearly all hearing aid candidates have bilateral hearing losses, some asymmetrical, and consequently need a pair of hearing aids, similar to an optometrist supplying a pair of spectacles. The advantages associated with binaural hearing aid fitting include improved sound quality, improved speech discrimination in noise, reduction of the head shadow effect, loudness summation, sound localisation and spatial balance. In addition, fitting just one hearing aid to a child or adult is likely to lead to auditory deprivation over time, with the individual showing decreased speech perception scores in the unaided ear.

Earmould Selection

Children and adults with mild to moderate hearing losses may be able to use a stock or generic earmould which connects the hearing aid to the ear via a piece of tubing with a silicone ear bud, dome or plug, approximately sized to the individual's ear and sits in the ear canal. Such fittings are low cost because a custom mould is not required but will not contain acoustic feedback with more powerful hearing aids. These individuals will need a custom earmould. A well-fitting ear mould requires a good impression and the manufacture of a well-fitting custom made earmould. An audiologist must also select the most appropriate acoustic characteristics for the child or adult's earmoulds. As the earmould is the last step in the amplification system, any acoustic modifications to the earmould will affect the gain, the frequency response and the saturation response (SSPL) of the hearing aid. The three main options available to a clinician are venting, damping and fitting an acoustic horn.

Venting

Inserting a parallel vent into an earmould, allows the individual to utilise any good low frequency hearing they may have, reduces low frequency real ear gain, aerates the ear canal and may relieve a sensation of pressure. Vents are unlikely to be viable with severe and profound losses, due to the risk of acoustic feedback.

Damping

Acoustic filters or dampers of wool or sintered metal are often used to reduce the resonant peaks created by the original response of the hearing aid earphone. In theory, dampers can be placed at various points along the tubing to damp peaks at different frequencies. In practice, they are commonly placed are the tip or nub of the ear hook where they impact most on frequencies around 1000 Hz. A low resistance damper is recommended with most hearing aid fittings to reduce some of the peaks and troughs of the frequency response and thereby improve the natural quality of the sound.

Acoustic horns

An acoustic horn is a stepped piece of tubing that gradually increases in diameter from 2mm at the ear hook to 3mm or 4mm at the end of the sound bore. The Libby horn was patented in 1982. It works by matching the resistance of the ear canal more closely to the resistance of the earphone and tubing, thus enhancing the amplification of high frequency sounds.

The child or adult's ear canal must be able to accommodate at least a 3mm sound bore. Acoustic feedback and loudness discomfort can be a risk, depending upon the shape of the hearing aid frequency response and the features offered in the hearing aid. The development of digital non-linear hearing aids with an improved high frequency response has resulted in reduced reliance upon acoustic horns to match hearing aids to individual hearing aid amplification prescription targets.

Power Supply

The majority of hearing aids use one of five standard Button Cell Zinc-air batteries, operating at 1.35 volts. Battery size and type is dictated by the hearing type (BTE vs ITE etc). Hearing aid power determines battery life, with high powered aids running for 1-2 days, assuming use during all waking hours. Batteries may last up to 14 days in lower powered aids. Recently, low cost solar powered hearing aids have been developed; targeted particularly at developing countries. The cost of hearing aids and disposable batteries are prohibitive in many of the poorer nations of the world, depriving thousands of individuals of the opportunity to use their residual hearing. The World Health Organisation, in collaboration with Christoffel Blindenmission, has supported a project run by the Godisa Trust in Southern Africa to develop a low cost solar powered hearing aid [1]. In a clinical trial, these aids have been found to provide substantial benefit for individuals with moderate to severe hearing loss, although the high frequency response is limited [2]. The development and manufacture of these sustainable hearing aids at a cost of less than $100 US dollars per unit represents an enormous boon for the estimated 600 million people in developing countries with hearing loss. (Figure 11.1)

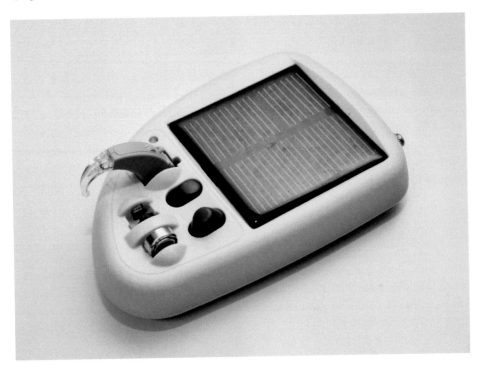

Figure 11.1 . The Solar Ear hearing aid and solar charger .

The Benefits of Hearing Aids

The aim of hearing aid fitting is to amplify speech so that it is both audible and comfortably loud. For individuals with moderate and severe hearing loss this goal is often achievable. Profound hearing losses create challenges because of the small window between just detectable sounds and those that are experienced as uncomfortably loud.

At times, audibility must be sacrificed and some individuals with profound loss may only be able to access part of the speech spectrum or a limited range of conversational speech sounds. At the other end of the continuum are individuals with a very mild hearing loss or unilateral hearing loss, some of whom experience limited hearing aid benefit due to high levels of background noise and the poor listening conditions often found in the real world [3].

Assessing hearing aid performance involves the measurement of the amount of amplification provided by a hearing aid, known as gain.

Hearing aid gain may be measured 1) in a test box with a simulated ear (the 2cc coupler); 2) in the individual's ear using a probe tube; or 3) by comparing hearing thresholds with and without hearing aids. These approaches to measurement are described in Table 11.1.

Hearing aid fitting involves a process of matching a selected hearing aid to an individual's hearing loss. In order to achieve this, an accurate pure tone audiogram must be obtained.

For young infants and individuals with severe developmental delays, electroacoustic data from Auditory Brainstem Response (ABR) testing or Steady State Evoked Potential (SSEP) testing will be used to estimate an audiogram. Based on the audiogram information, an audiologist selects a hearing aid to trial.

This selection may be based upon a "traditional" approach whereby the audiologist selects a hearing aid based on their previous experience with the degree and type of hearing loss, and fits it to their client. Following a series of assessments, involving aided thresholds or real ear measures, speech perception testing and self-report (with adults and older children) the hearing aid may be adjusted or an alternative aid trialed until a suitable fit is found.

The use of traditional approaches to hearing aid fitting has declined [4] and many audiologists now adopt a prescriptive approach to aid fitting. This involves the use of a hearing aid "prescription", based upon a theory or model that attempts to maximize audibility of speech for the degree and configuration of the audiogram. Some familiar examples of these are NAL (NAL-RP, NL1 and NL2) [5, 6] and DSL [7, 8].

Algorithms for these prescription procedures are built in to the software in hearing aid analyzing equipment, making it simple to generate a set of targets and adjust the individual's hearing aid to those targets. In addition, many hearing aid manufacturers have developed their own aid fitting algorithms that are incorporated into hearing aid software and compatible with aid fitting equipment. These generate targets for coupler measures and/ or real ear measures and guide the audiologist through each step of the hearing aid fitting process. Some form of real ear validation of the aid fitting is a critical component of the aid fitting process. Aid fittings based only on 2cc coupler measures will not take the individual characteristics of the listener into account and can be quite inaccurate in young children [4].

Table 11.1. Methods of measuring hearing aid performance

Method	Description	Equipment	Applications	Issues
Coupler Measures	The hearing aid is placed inside the sound proof chamber of a hearing aid test box and attached to a 2cc coupler. A 2cc coupler is a small metal chamber that simulates the volume of an adult ear canal (2 cc). At the base of the 2cc coupler is a microphone. The hearing aid and coupler are placed inside the soundproof test chamber and a tone or speech weighted noise at a specific input level (50 or 60 dB) is generated in the test box at the hearing aid microphone. The output of the aid is measured in the microphone in the base of the coupler. The gain of the hearing aid is measured by the test box by subtracting the input level from the measured output across the frequency range of the hearing aid. The maximum power output (MPO) can also be measured in the test box by using a higher input level of 90 dB.	A hearing aid and test box with 2cc coupler	Checking aid against manufacturers specifications Pre-selection of hearing aids for fitting Checking hearing aid performance against an the gain, frequency response and MPO established at initial fitting.	The 2cc coupler simulates an average ear. There may be significant variation in individuals, particularly infants with much smaller ear canals.
Real ear probe tube measures	Real ear gain is measured using a thin rubber probe that is initially placed in an unaided ear canal with the person seated in front of a loudspeaker. The loud speaker generates a test signal (warble tone, NB noise or speech weighted noise) and the output is measured in the ear canal. The hearing aid is turned on and placed in the ear canal, keeping the probe tube in place.. The signal from the loudspeaker is repeated and the gain of the aid can be calculated by the real ear analyzer by subtracting the SPL in the unaided ear canal from the SPL in the aided ear canal.	Real ear gain analyzer	Validation of hearing aid fitting against a set of theoretical targets generated by prescriptive model of hearing aid fitting	Probe tube measures are quick, reliable and accurate. The probe tube may be rejected by active young children. Probe tube measures can be used to verify aid fittings with a range of inputs and are therefore well suited to nonlinear digital aid fittings. Real ear equipment that offers a speech signal is required for non linear digital aid fittings
Soundfield thresholds and functional gain	Hearing thresholds are measured in the unaided condition, either under headphones (dB HL) or in the soundfield. The hearing aid is worn on user volume and aided hearing thresholds are tested in the soundfield. Functional gain is calculated by subtracting the aided thresholds from the unaided thresholds.	Audiometer with loudspeaker.	Verification of hearing aid fitting against a set of frequency targets generated by the prescriptive model of aid fitting	Soundfield thresholds obtained with non-linear hearing aids can be misleading because higher gain is provided for soft inputs. Test-retest reliability of aided thresholds can vary by up to 15 dB.

The rapid development of hearing aid technology can be overwhelming. The move from analogue signal processing to digital processing has ushered in a range of new features and opportunities. Analogue hearing aids often provide linear amplification, whereby they increase the output for all input levels by a fixed amount of gain up to the point when the Maximum Power Output (MPO) is reached. These aids may employ a simple form of peak clipping to limit the output and protect the listeners hearing and loudness discomfort. This is where the peaks of the amplified sound signal are clipped when MPO is reached. Alternatively, compression limiting is used whereby automatic gain control is used to reduce gain when the MPO is reached. Analogue aids can be easier to fit because they offer a limited range of options. They may employ either a basic screwdriver adjustment or use a computer interface for more precise matching of gain to audiogram. Their advantages revolve around reduced costs, in terms of initial outlay, equipment requirements for basic fitting and also repair costs. For many individuals with hearing loss the differences between a well fitted analogue hearing aid and highly sophisticated digital hearing aid are small [9] and the cost-benefit equation should be kept in firm focus.

The march towards a fully digital world is on, however, and in step with photography, home entertainment and telephony, hearing aids will soon be exclusively digital. In developed countries such as the USA, recent estimates suggest that 97% of all aids manufactured were digital [10]. Digital hearing aids offer individuals with hearing impairment a range of useful features. They use non- linear compression circuits to increase listeners comfort and the audibility of speech by providing higher gain for soft inputs and less gain for loud inputs. Thus, soft phonemes may become audible and loud sounds potentially less jarring. Multiple channels are a common feature of digital aids. They aim to improve the signal to noise ratio in the low frequencies and reduce the impact of recruitment (abnormal growth of loud sounds) in the high frequencies, Although some hearing aids offer more than 20 individual channels, more is not always better. For some listeners, increased compression channels may reduce vowel identification by smoothing out spectral contrasts [11]. Other special features include automatic feedback control, multiple programmes to be used in different noise environments, directional microphones, wireless links between binaural aids, noise reduction, and speech enhancement. A recent and exciting development involves trainable hearing aids that can adapt to the users preferred volume in different listening environments. These aids can measure sound levels and spectral shape of the listening environments experienced in real life and adjusts the aid gain and frequency response according to individual preferences. After a short period of training by the user the aid can be truly customized to self-adjust for each listening situation. Such devices will reduce aid fitting time and have considerable potential to increase client satisfaction [12].

The benefits of digital hearing aids have proved difficult to clearly establish. At a superficial level they should be analogous to the move from VHS to DVD home movies and therefore sound clearer, provide better access to more sound input across a range of listening environments and offer more features. In practice, several studies comparing analogue and digital aid fittings have failed to show any significant differences [13, 14], however, other blinded studies have demonstrated clear benefits for digital signal processing hearing aids in terms of speech perception scores, rating scales and overall preference [14,15]. It seems likely that study design and the sensitivity of the measures used need further refinement if the benefits of the latest digital aids are to be effectively assessed.

Measuring Hearing Aid Benefit Outside of the Audiology Clinic

Validation of hearing aid fitting may occur inside the audiology clinic but it is out in the real world that hearing aids must prove their value to the user. In the adult population, a very simple measure of value is how frequently the aid is used. More sophisticated self report outcome measures have been developed in an effort to quantify the impact of hearing aid use on quality of life. These instruments might be used to justify budgets or demonstrate the efficacy of treatment to consumers [16]. Often referred to only by their acronym, examples include the Abbreviated Profile of Hearing Aid Benefit (APHAB) [17], the Client Oriented Scale of Improvement (COSI) [18] and the Satisfaction with Amplification in Daily Life (SADL) [19] and a recently developed brief instrument, the International Outcome Inventory for Hearing Aids (IOI-HA) which has been translated into at least 21 languages [20]. Such measures, based on self- report, appear to be straightforward tools that could provide a useful and valid measure of hearing aid benefit. Saunders, Chisolm and Abrams [16], however, suggest that measuring hearing aid outcomes is, in fact, highly complex. It is influenced heavily by client expectations, attitudes, personality and even the high technology label ascribed to an aid [21]. Moreover, there is a widely reported disconnect between measures of benefit for speech perception and functional outcomes [22, 23] begging the question of what it is that is actually being measured by these self- report instruments.

Measuring the benefits of hearing aid fitting beyond the audiology clinic is even more problematic for children. Infants and toddlers are fitted with aids for the critical task of acquiring spoken language. In order for them to have the language to provide a self- report on aid efficacy, the aid fitting must have done its job well. In the interim, parents and teachers must take on the role of observing a child's listening behaviour and giving feedback to the audiologist. There have been a number of rating scales and questionnaires developed for this purpose including the Parent Evaluation of Aural/Oral Performance of Children (PEACH) [24] and the Meaningful Auditory Integration Scale (MAIS) [25]. These scales have been used to compare different hearing aids and to monitor cochlear implant fitting, but they cannot replace careful monitoring of listening, speech and language development and milestones throughout a programme of aural habilitation.

Special Issues for Children

Very young children have small ear canals. Unless taken into account, the difference between the 2cc Coupler and the real ear in young infants could lead to over amplification. This highlights the importance of real ear verification of aid fitting targets with very young children. In addition, it has been suggested that young children require a better signal-to noise ratio than adults. Nozza, Rossman, Bond and Miller found that infants required a signal/noise ratio that was 6-12 dB higher than adults for a similar speech discrimination task [26]. Based on this finding, it seems possible that young children may require more gain than adults to ensure they have optimum access to the speech signal. Moreover, unlike adults with acquired hearing loss, young children are not using a hearing aid to relearn how to listen to speech in a well- established language base. Infants must use the sensory input from their aids to acquire language, speech and their understanding of the world.

In this context, there is little room for error, the young child's potential for learning spoken language is dependent upon optimizing their sensory input.

Special Issues for Adults

Hearing aid fitting in adults has its own challenges. Motivation has been shown to be a key predictor of successful outcomes. Adults who see themselves as a person with hearing difficulties and are motivated to hear better are much more likely to keep wearing their aids and see them as valuable than adults who do not view themselves as needing hearing help [27]. It is very important, then, that hearing aids are fitted to the right people (i.e., those that actually want them), rather than using some apparently relevant criteria such as degree of hearing loss that might be imposed by policy makers. Another task for adults with acquired loss relates to the overblown expectations that can be created by creative advertisers trying to persuade individuals that new technology can overcome all of their hearing difficulties. With something as truly complex as communication, technology can only ever be part of the solution.

Best Practice and Future Developments

It is easy to become overly focused upon the new advances in hearing aid technology but it is the total package of hearing aid fitting that will ultimately make the difference to the lives of adults and children with hearing loss. The accurate assessment of hearing, education prior to fitting to ensure realistic expectations, the pre-selection of the aid and its validation post-fitting using a well- researched fitting algorithm, and finally the ongoing follow up to ensure the aid is improving listening opportunities at school, work or play. Countries that are new to the task of addressing the needs of their population with hearing loss need to focus on the effective implementation of this package. It will require excellent training, a realistic budget and time allocation and long term support and evaluation. Similarly, countries with long established hearing aid fitting programmes need to resist the temptation to cut costs in these areas in order to focus funding exclusively on paying for the latest technological development.

The exciting future of hearing aid fitting includes increased connectivity to all things electronic, wireless aids that enhance hearing for individuals with normal hearing and aids that not only train themselves but have their own fitting software and hardware. Such developments will help to empower children and adults with hearing impairment in the process of aid selection and use and this in turn should lead to better hearing aid outcomes.

Implantable Devices for Individuals with Conductive Hearing Loss

Adults and children with conductive losses may be able to benefit from a bone anchored hearing aid. Children born with bilateral atresia or chronic suppurative otitis media cannot wear conventional hearing aids. Historically, these children have been fitted with a bone conduction hearing aid comprising a bone conduction transducer, powered by a BTE or body worn hearing aid and held in place by a steel spring band, worn over the head. Pressure created by the steel headband makes these aids uncomfortable to wear. An alternative device for children over the age of the age of three is the bone anchored hearing aid (BAHA). These surgically implanted devices have been in use for over 30 years. A titanium screw is implanted into the mastoid process. Following osseo-integration of the screw (three months for adults and six months for children) a pedestal and vibrating hearing aid are attached. The vibrating hearing aid allows sound to be transmitted directly to the cochlea (Figure 11.2), effectively bypassing the middle ear. The BAHA can be fitted monaurally or binaurally with binaural fittings showing significant benefits for individuals with bilateral hearing loss [28].

More than 15000 people have received a BAHA [29] and they are now considered viable for a wide range of hearing losses including bilateral conductive hearing loss, mixed loss, and unilateral severe-profound sensorineural loss [29]. In a recent study of long term outcomes with these aids, Badran, Arya, Bunstone and McKinnon [30] found that 91% of 165 patients had continued to use their BAHA, despite one third of them requiring some kind of revision surgery during the life of the implant. Reasons for revision surgery include skin reactions, thickening or overgrowth of the skin and failure of osseo-integration. This finding is consistent with a study of 15 children with Down's syndrome who were fitted with BAHA. Despite a tissue rejection rate of 20%, all 15 children wore their BAHA for more than eight hours per day and reported improved quality of life [31].

A very interesting group, who have recently been shown to benefit from BAHA, are individuals with severe to profound unilateral sensorineural hearing loss (UHL). The BAHA device is placed on the side of the deaf ear. It transmits sound through bone conduction, and stimulates the cochlea of the normally hearing ear. A case study with three teenagers showed a 43% improvement in speech discrimination in noise by BAHA users with significant UHL as well increased satisfaction in difficult listening situations [29].

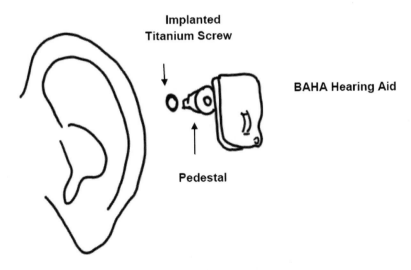

Figure 11.2. Diagram of bone anchored hearing aid (BAHA).

The minimum age for implantation of this device in the cranium is three years. Children born with congenital bilateral atresia can use a BAHA softband whereby the vibrating transducer is worn on a soft headband and no invasive surgery is required. This device may also prove useful for individuals wishing to trial a BAHA prior to surgery. Positive results have been founds with 12 children using the BAHA softband indicating improved language development and aided thresholds, along with extensive daily usage [32].

Middle Ear Implants

Many years after 1935, when Wilska experimented with iron particles on the tympanic membrane stimulated via a magnetic field, wearable middle ear implants have become a practical option for some individuals with hearing loss. These devices may take the form of a fully implanted device or partially implanted electromagnetic system.

A much more recent development is the fully implantable middle ear implant. An example of this device is the ESTEEM. It uses the tympanic membrane as a microphone. A sensor is placed at the body of the incus and it sends an electrical signal to a fully implanted sound processor. The signal is amplified and filtered, converted to a mechanical signal and directed to the stapes. This system utilises the natural ear canal resonance and has a battery life of up to 8 years. It received FDA approval in March 2010 but will continue with clinical trials in order to further evaluate post-implantation complications and device effectiveness. This device is designed for individuals with moderate to severe hearing loss with an estimated cost of $30,000 US dollars for surgery, device and habilitation. [33]

Cochlear Implants

A Brief History

The first cochlear implant operation took place in France in 1957, reported by Djourno and Eyries [34]. They placed an electrode on the auditory nerve and provided the patient with some basic pitch discrimination. In 1964, at Stanford University, Blair Simmons implanted some recipients with a six-channel device. It used a percutaneous plug so that the electrodes could be individually stimulated. Although, recipients could not understand speech through the device, Blair Simmons [35] was able to observe that stimulation in different areas of the cochlea produced different pitch percepts. House began experimenting with single channel devices in Los Angeles in the early 1960s. Between 1972 and the early 1980s more than 1000 people, including several hundred children, had received the House commercial single channel implant [36]. These devices were a useful aid to lip- reading but provided no spectral cues.

Meanwhile, three different groups in Europe and Australia were working on a multichannel implant. In 1978, the first multiple channel cochlear implant (10 channels) was implanted in an adult at the University of Melbourne. Results were very promising and collaboration with Nucleus Limited led to the implantation of six adults with a commercial 22 channel device in 1982. Recipients were able to understand running speech without the aid of lip reading. By 1985, the Nucleus device had been approved by the USA Food and Drug Administration. The first child was implanted in Australia in 1985 at the age of ten. Since then the multiple channel cochlear implant has been refined in terms of assessment, hardware, speech processing strategy and safety considerations. There has been a steady drop in the age of first implantation with the youngest Australian cochlear implant recipient being four months at the time of writing this chapter. Three manufacturers currently produce cochlear implants; Cochlear, Med-EL and Clarion. According to the Food and Drug Administration (FDA) of the USA, as of April 2009, approximately 188,000 people have received implants worldwide.

Basic Function

A cochlear implant comprises external as well as surgically implanted, internal components. The external components of the cochlear implant consist of a microphone to pick up sound, a speech processor (ear level or body worn) to extract critical components of the speech signal and a transmitter. The transmitter is a coil held in place by a magnet on the skull, just behind the ear. The transmitter coil sends a signal to the internal receiver using radio waves. The internal components involve the surgical implantation of a receiver stimulator that is placed into a drilled out section of the mastoid bone. This is attached to the electrode array which passes through the middle ear and is wound around the first one and a half turns of the cochlea. The receiver passes the sound signal to the electrode array. Depending on the speech sound heard, stimulation occurs at a tonotopically organized position along the cochlea that approximately corresponds to the place that frequency is coded in a normally functioning cochlea.

Much of the development of cochlear implants over the last 25 years has focused upon speech processing strategies. The early Nucleus device extracted out the fundamental frequency and second formant from the speech signal. The first formant was then added (F0F1F2 strategy) followed by the Mulitpeak strategy with three high frequency bands. Then came SPEAK, a digital speech processing strategy that extracted the six maxima spectral peaks from the running speech input [34] More recently, different devices have offered implant recipients a choice of speech processing strategies including (Continuous Interleaved Sample) CIS, which selects 6-8 electrodes and fires them in sequence at a high stimulation rate (20,000 pulses per second) to deliver sound to the cochlea in a way that reflects the original sound signal. Another processing strategy, Advanced Combination Encoders (ACE) combines the higher stimulation rate of CIS with the way SPEAK highlights spectral frequency peaks.

Candidacy

Initially, only profoundly deaf individuals were considered to be cochlear implant candidates but criteria have been adjusted as implants have developed. These adjustments are based on outcomes for both children and adults who use hearing aids compared to outcomes for those with cochlear implants. Children and adults with moderate hearing loss are not currently considered to be implant candidates because they obtain better speech perception test results with hearing aids than would be likely with a cochlear implant. This may change in the future, if outcomes with cochlear implants continue to improve.

Although some variation occurs from clinic to clinic and across countries the following basic candidacy criteria are reasonably standard at the time of writing.

Adults

- Bilateral severe to profound sensorineural hearing loss (thresholds of 70 dB HL or greater)
- Receives limited benefit with appropriately fit hearing aids
- No physical contraindications for placement of the implant (based on CT scan results)
- No medical contraindications for surgery
- Realistic expectations

Children

- Bilateral severe to profound sensorineural hearing loss (thresholds of 70 dB HL or greater)
- Hearing aids provide little or no benefit despite consistent use and appropriate intervention
- No medical contraindications for surgery

The Benefits of Cochlear Implants

Adults

Cochlear implantation has become a well-established method of restoring hearing sensation to postlingually deafened adults with a severe to profound sensorineural hearing loss. Nearly all adults with cochlear implants achieve sound awareness, and improved closed set speech perception [37, 38] while many experience open set speech discrimination via audition alone and some telephone use. For example, Bassim et al. showed that 64 people who received a unilateral Med-El cochlear implant improved their speech perception scores from a pre-implant mean score of 1% (Consonant- Nucleus-Consonant (CNC) words) and 12% (Sentence recognition in quiet (CUNY)) to a one year post implant mean score of 54% (CNC) and 96% (CUNY) [39].There are, however, also a significant number of individuals for whom the implant provides limited assistance with speech perception. A number of studies have endeavored to establish predictive factors for post- operative performance. Age at implant, aetiology of deafness, pre-implant speech perception scores and amount of pre-implant residual hearing have not been consistently found to predict post- implant speech perception scores [38]. Duration of deafness prior to receiving an implant is a predictive factor with individuals with a shorter duration of deafness experiencing better outcomes. The rapid development of cochlear implant technology, including surgical procedures, speech processing strategies, hardware and candidacy criteria makes it difficult to compare studies or to be sure that the impact of the latest best practice in cochlear implant provision has really been rigorously studied and reported. Individuals with more residual hearing are benefitting from cochlear implants, despite having some open set sentence perception pre-implant and all three manufacturers consider individuals with severe hearing loss or moderate-profound hearing loss to be implant candidates [37].

Children

As noted above, children with significant hearing loss must learn how to listen with a sensory device in order to acquire language. The benefits of cochlear implants for children with severe and profound hearing loss are substantial. Prior to the development of the cochlear implant, children with profound hearing loss typically acquired language at half the rate of their hearing peers. Now, after receiving an implant at a young age, more than half of these children exhibit spoken language that is similar to their hearing age-mates [40]. Like adults, however, there is a wide range of speech perception performance and language outcomes for children with cochlear implants. Children implanted at a younger age (at least below four years) typically achieve better outcomes in speech perception [41], speech production [42] and in expressive and productive language [43]. Implantation before two years has been shown to be a strong predictor of spoken language skills at age 3 [44]. Profoundly deaf children who receive cochlear implants in the first 2 years of life produce highly intelligible speech before the age of 6 [45]. A recent study by Schauwer, Gillis and Govaerts has shown that the qualitative babbling characteristics of early implanted children are very similar to those of hearing children [46]. Children who receive cochlear implants in the first year of life, before 12 months, have also demonstrated highly intelligible speech and receptive language skills on par with their hearing peers, particularly in the area of syntax [47]. In Australia, and increasingly in other developing countries many young children now receive simultaneous bilateral cochlear implants, providing them, with them with improved localisation and speech perception in background noise. These additional advantages will further enhance opportunities to develop language skills more similar to their hearing peers.

The search for predictors of language development outcomes has indicated that a range of predictive factors are at play, including family factors such as socioeconomic status and family composition, and also IQ, gender and communication mode [44]. More recent investigations have undertaken detailed comparisons of language skills between school- aged children with cochlear implants and their age- matched hearing peers [48]. Efrat, Schorr, Roth and Fox [48] found that, while these two groups showed no mean differences in terms of speech intelligibility or on some general language measures, significant delays were observed in the children with cochlear implants in the areas of syntax, morphology and more sophisticated metalinguistic skills such as knowledge of idioms.

These issues are explored in more detail by Pisoni and colleagues [49]. They contend that the assessment of the benefits of cochlear implants in children must now move to a new 'higher' level, whereby the impact of much improved speech perception on central cognitive processes such as attention, memory, learning and categorization in young deaf children is explored in considerable depth [49]. Working memory seems to be influenced by early auditory and spoken language experience suggesting that specific experience with spoken language and exposure to spoken words affects working memory and more specifically the sub-skill of speed of rehearsal [49].

This suggests that very early implantation and consistent exposure to quality spoken language input may further improve outcomes for children with severe to profound hearing loss, however, merely receiving an implant is insufficient to maximize its benefits. Intensive intervention in terms of language acquisition and family-centered support continues to be critical.

Bilateral cochlear implants may be the preferred sensory device for children and adults with severe to profound hearing loss in many countries but the cost of safe, expert cochlear implantation and appropriate follow up and support is often prohibitive in some developing countries [50].

Alternatives such as the use of cheaper, older technology such as single channel implants or locally developed inferior products have been shown to be risky and unacceptable [51]. This raises a much bigger moral, global issue of how to provide access to life changing technology to meet the needs of all people with hearing loss, regardless of where they live.

FM Hearing Aids and Other Assistive Listening Devices

Many individuals with hearing aids and cochlear implants find listening in the real world challenging. Despite the development of noise cancelling microphones and directional microphones in modern sensory devices, the presence of background noise (particularly unwanted speech), poor acoustic conditions and the effort of listening at a distance reduces the effectiveness of the hearing instrument. The classroom is one environment that is often characterized by difficult listening conditions. Over the last 40 years or more, a range of classroom amplification devices have been used including bulky hardwired headphone systems, loop systems that used electromagnetic conduction and more recently and most successfully, personal FM systems. Personal FM systems, also known as radio aids, are two part systems that use a microphone/transmitter worn by the speaker and a receiver worn by the individual with a hearing loss. Sound is picked up via the microphone (headworn or lapel), worn close to the lips, and converted into Frequency Modulated (FM) radio waves that are transmitted on a specific frequency to a receiver. The signal is then transformed back to a speech signal and delivered to the listener's hearing aids/cochlear implants.

FM systems have been shown to be beneficial for children in classrooms provided they are appropriately calibrated with the child's hearing aids or cochlear implants [52, 53]. Lewis recommends that the output of the FM system should be measured with an input level of 85-90 dB (to simulate the proximity of the microphone to the mouth) while the output of the hearing aid is measured with a 70 dB input level. The output of the FM aid is set to provide an FM advantage of 10-15 dB so that when both the hearing aid microphone and FM microphones are activated, there is always an FM aid advantage [54]. FM systems have great potential to benefit students with hearing impairment. Bringing the microphone close to the speaker is a highly effective way of providing a clear auditory input; however, they require careful management. Whoever wields the FM aid transmitter has control of the hearing aid user's ear. Unless the HA/CI user turns off the FM receiver they must listen to what is said into the FM transmitter. This places significant responsibility on the teacher, particularly with very young children, to ensure that the FM transmitter is worn and used by someone who is speaking to the child with the FM receiver It is all too easy to forget to switch off the transmitter and provide the young child with hearing impairment with unnecessary side conversations and irrelevant input.

More recently interest has grown in the potential for adults who use hearing aids and cochlear implants to benefit from an FM system. FM aids have been miniaturized so that they can be attached to a BTE aid via a small shoe or built into the hearing aid itself. A small microphone/transmitter is worn by the speaker. For adults, this may be a work colleague, partner or relative. Adults often report difficulty with hearing in noise and in a variety of challenging environments, including restaurants, meetings, places of worship, in the car and a range of group of social settings. Boothroyd [55] assessed the benefits of FM use for a group of 12 adults with mild to severe hearing loss for speech perception in the clinic and benefits in daily life through questionnaire. Although all participants benefitted from using the FM aid and many found it very helpful for distance listening and in noisy settings, none indicated that they had any intentions of buying the FM system. This may be partially due to noise problems that were experienced with the particular device being trialed but also related to practical issues such as the difficulties associated with handing the transmitter around at meetings, or at dinner and its limitations for picking up only one speaker when what was desired was the capacity to hear several speakers, often in rapid succession. A more recent study by Chisholm, Noe, McArdle and Abrams [56] with 36 participants demonstrated that highly positive outcomes could be achieved by adults with FM aids. FM systems were fitted at no cost to older adults (veterans) with hearing aid experience. Several focused support sessions were provided in order to effectively train the recipients to use the device well. Under these conditions, the FM aids were used consistently for a wide variety of activities, including restaurants, the car, small groups and outdoors, and provided substantial reported benefit as compared to hearing aids alone. This finding underlines a basic principal of sensory device use; adults and children can only optimize the benefit of a sensory device when they are well supported during fitting, evaluation and long term follow up.

Rehabilitation for Adults

Ross [57] defines aural rehabilitation as " any device, procedure, information, interaction or therapy which lessens the communicative and psychosocial consequences of a hearing loss". Traditionally, aural rehabilitation for adults with acquired hearing loss included several clearly defined components including speech reading and auditory training, information on assistive devices, counselling, and detailed instruction to ensure effective use of the sensory device. This approach was taught routinely and implemented in clinics on a one-to-one basis or in small groups. In Australia, not-for-profit organizations also ran aural rehabilitation classes and these had the added benefits of empowering adults through the process of interacting with others with mutual interests. In 1988, Erber published *Communication Therapy for Hearing-Impaired Adults* [58]. This ground-breaking book focused upon conversational skills and improving pragmatic skills in adults with hearing loss in order to increase their communicative satisfaction and decrease social isolation. This more holistic approach to rehabilitation acknowledges that adults with hearing loss need more than just a sensory device.

Unfortunately, the provision of holistic aural rehabilitation seems to have lost popularity in recent years. The four components of AR, described by Boothroyd [59], sensory management, instruction, perceptual training and counselling are often distilled down to the fitting of a sensory device with one appointment for follow up or possibly just a brief follow up telephone call. Surveys cited by Bally and Bakke [60] suggest that formal AR is infrequently provided by contemporary audiologists. According to Ross, as hearing aid fitting has become more and more the domain of audiologists, streamlining of services and profit maximization have also become a focus [61]. Organizations strive to find ways of fitting hearing aids with the smallest number of appointments. Contrast this to the support frequently provided to adult recipients of cochlear implants, where auditory training, ongoing counselling and substantial device follow up appear to be standard practice [61]. Of course, cost is also an important component of this equation. Many cochlear implant programmes have been research driven with a strong focus on outcomes. The cost of providing communication training may be picked up by a third party or built in to the cost of the implant. In addition, a client who has undergone surgery to receive an implant is likely to be highly motivated to learn to hear well with their new sensory device and is therefore prepared to invest hours in attending aural habilitation sessions. Post- hearing aid fitting, both clients and providers often view this kind of follow up as optional, yet there is no real reason that rehabilitation support post- implant and post- hearing aid should differ. The fact that many expensive hearing aids end up in drawers rather than worn by recipients suggests that aural habilitation should never be optional. If both private payment and funding bodies pegged their funding/ final payment to medium and long term outcomes rather than paying for the hearing aid fitting process itself, hearing aid providers might suddenly develop a renewed enthusiasm for the provision of aural rehabilitation. Rigorous research studies that assess the efficacy of different types of rehabilitation for adults are urgently required [59].

Cost restraints, and poor motivation by both hearing aid providers and clients has led to the development of a number of innovative approaches. There are some home-based computer-controlled communication training programmes [61] but these seem unlikely to simulate the complexities of communicating with real people. Another exciting approach at Gallaudet University, involves the training of peer mentors who work with hearing-health professionals to provide extensive aural habilitation/rehabilitation to adults [60]. The two year programme prepares individuals with hearing impairments to provide comprehensive aural habilitation/rehabilitation including family support and counselling, extensive advice on assistive listening devices, communication strategy training and one to one counselling. This exemplary programme might not be so easily transferred to other settings but the underlying concept of peer supported aural rehabilitation programmes could be easily adapted in other settings.

Habilitation of Children

Unlike adults, who already have a well- developed language prior to the loss of hearing, young children with a prelingual hearing impairment use their sensory aid to learn language and to acquire world knowledge. Habilitation of children is synonymous with language acquisition. Learning to listen with hearing aids or cochlear implants is only purposeful when it is linked to meaningful communication. Consequently, any discussion of approaches to habilitation must include methods of communication and orientation in the provision of early intervention and education services to children with hearing loss. These have been an ongoing source of controversy at least as far back as the 1800s when Alexander Graham Bell and Thomas Gallaudet held diametrically opposed views on the comparative value of oral/aural education compared to communication via sign language.

Despite acknowledging the enormous heterogeneity of deaf children, there remains a range of strong beliefs about the most effective way to support young children to use a sensory device to develop spoken language skills. A brief description is contained in Table 11.2. Only approaches that utilise audition and a sensory device are included in this list, as the focus of this chapter is on auditory habilitation in children.

Due to the complexity of the issue, few studies have attempted to determine the most effective approach for developing a child's use of their sensory device and their language skills. Moreover, outcome studies are fraught with traps for the uninitiated researcher.

Lynas [62], when undertaking a longitudinal study of eight profoundly deaf children to explore the impact of educational practice on outcomes, commented on the difficulties associated with establishing a relationship between communication approach, teaching practice and other background factors and educational outcomes. A range of factors are implicated in these outcomes including the amount of family support and involvement, the age of diagnosis and commencement of early intervention, the quality of teaching, the child's IQ, the sensory device used (i.e., hearing aid or cochlear implant) and the approach to communication that is adopted. In order to develop the auditory pathway for spoken language, early intervention needs to begin early, before six months of age if possible [63].

Table 11.2. Methods of communication/auditory habilitation for children who are deaf or hearing impaired

Approach	Description
Auditory/Verbal	This approach aims to develop spoken language through the primary channel of listening. Parents are supported to learn the techniques of focusing their child on auditory input and highlighting and enhancing what is heard. Parents are seen as the primary interventionist with the teacher or therapist as a guide and support. This approach uses techniques that limit some visual cues by directing the child to auditory stimuli. Children begin with activities that promote sound awareness and quickly move on to meaningful interactions using joint attention to limit visual cues.
Auditory oral	The auditory-oral approach is a method in which children learn to use whatever hearing they have, in combination with speech reading and contextual cues to learn spoken language. As with an Auditory/Verbal approach, the goal is for a child with hearing impairment to develop spoken language skills that ensure they will function independently in the hearing world.
Simultaneous communication	Simultaneous Communication is an approach where both a spoken language and a manual variant of that language (such as Manually Coded English or Sign in English word order) are used simultaneously. It can be challenging to produce both languages perfectly. The native language of the user may be stronger. In hearing parents this will be spoken language. With this approach, children with limited access to spoken language are ensured a visual language input while still developing spoken language skills through a sensory aid.
Cued Speech	Cued speech is a visual communication system designed to enhance speech reading ability. It combines the natural mouth movements of speech with eight hand shapes or cues that represent different sounds of speech. For example, the hand shapes help the child distinguish sounds that look the same on the lips- such as "t" and "d". Vowel sounds are represented by four positions around the mouth. Cued Speech may be used in conjunction with sensory devices to support the development of spoken language.

When children are identified early, participate in high quality early intervention and, for severe-profoundly deaf children, receive early cochlear implantation, language outcomes are optimized [64]. All families of children who are deaf or hearing impaired need to be well supported with a family-centered approach that adapts the support to the family rather than trying to mould the family to the habilitation programme [65, 66].

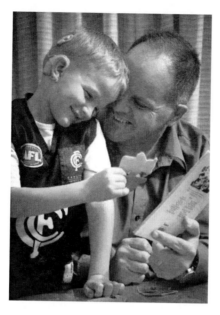

Figure 11.3. A father and son share a special moment at Taralye – the oral language centre for deaf children, Victoria, Australia.

Conclusion

Supporting individuals with hearing impairment to optimize their use of a sensory device is a lifelong process. Children develop and grow, moving through school to adulthood and their need for support in habilitation and their use of sensory devices will ebb and flow. Similarly, adult needs will change depending on their current life circumstances. Matching the sensory device and the nature of the intervention or rehabilitation to the individual is the key. Hearing loss cannot always be prevented, but its impact on people's lives can be reduced through carefully selected sensory devices and a client or family centered approach to support.

References

[1]   McPherson, B., and Brouillette, R. (2004). A fair hearing for all: providing appropriate amplification in developing countries. *Communication Disorders Quarterly*, 25: 219-223.

[2]   Parving, A., and Christensen, B. (2004). Clinical trial of a low-cost solar powered hearing aid. *Acta Oto-laryngologica, 124*, 416–420.

[3]   McKay, S., Gravel, JS., Tharpe, A.M. (2008). Amplification considerations for children with minimal or mild bilateral hearing loss and unilateral hearing loss. *Trends in amplification, 12*, 43-54.

[4] Seewald, R.C.(1998). Infants are not average adults: Clinical procedures for individualizing the fitting of amplification in infants and toddlers. Presented at the international conference *A Sound Foundation through Early Amplification*, 1998, October, Chicago

[5] Byrne, D., Parkinson, A., Newall, P. (1990). Hearing aid gain and frequency response requirements of the severely/profoundly hearing-impaired. *Ear and Hearing*, *11*, 40-49.

[6] Byrne, D., Dillon, H., Katsch, R., Ching, T., Keidser, G. (2001). The NAL-NL1 procedure for fitting non-linear hearing aids; Characteristic and comparisons with other procedures. *Journal of the American Academy of Audiology, 2,* 37-51.

[7] Cornelise, L.E.,Seewald, R.C.,Jamieson, D.G. (1995).The input/output formula: A theoretical approach to the fitting of personal amplification devices. *Journal of the Acoustical Society of America, 97,* 1854-1864.

[8] Scollie, S., Seewald, R., Cornelisse, L., Moodie, S., Bagatto, M., Laurnagaray, D., Beaulac, S., Pumford, J. (2005).The Desired Sensation Level Multistage Input/Output Algorithm, *Trends in Amplification, 9,* 159-197.

[9] Humes, LE., Christenson, L., Thomas, T., Bess, F., Hedley-Williams, A., Bentler, R. (1999). A comparison of the aided performance and benefit provided by a linear and a two channel wide dynamic range compression hearing aid. *Journal of Speech, Language, and Hearing Research, 42,* 65-79.

[10] Smaka, C. (2009). Digital hearing aids. Healthy hearing computer guides. Available from http://www.healthyhearing.com/questions/40715-digital-hearing-aids (Accessed 21 July 2011).

[11] Bor, S., Souza, P., Wright, R. (2008). Multichannel compression: effects of reduced spectral contrast on vowel identification. *Journal of Speech, Language, and Hearing Research,* 2008, *51,* 1315-1327.

[12] Dillon, H., Zakis, J.A., McDermott, H., Keidser, G., Dreschler, W., Covery, E. (2006). The trainable hearing aid: What will it do for clients and clinicians? *The Hearing Journal, 56,* 30-36.

[13] Marriage, J.E., Moore, C.J., Stone, M.A., Baer, T. (2005). Effects of three amplification strategies on speech perception by children with severe and profound hearing loss. *Ear and Hearing, 26,* 35-47.

[14] Schum, D.J., and Pogash, R.R. (2003). Blinded comparison of three levels of hearing aid technology. *Hearing Review*, *10,* 40-43, 64, 65.

[15] Wood, S., and Lutman, M. (2004). Relative benefits of linear analogue and advanced digital hearing aids. *International Journal of Audiology*, *43,*144-155.

[16] Saunders, G., Chisolm, T., Abrams, H. (2005). Measuring hearing aid outcome — not as easy as it seems. *Journal of Rehabilitation Research and Development, 42,*157-168.

[17] Cox, R.M., and Alexander, G.C. (1995).The Abbreviated Profile of Hearing Aid Benefit (APHAB). *Ear and Hearing, 16,* 176-186.

[18] Dillon, H., James, A., Ginis, J.A. (1997). The client-oriented scale of improvement (COSI) and its relationship to several other measures of benefit and satisfaction provided by hearing aids. *Journal of American Academy of Audiology, 8,* 27-43.

[19] Cox, R.M., and Alexander, G.C. (1999). Measuring satisfaction with amplification in daily life: The SADL Scale. *Ear and Hearing, 20,* 306-320.

[20] *Cox,* R.M., Stephens, D., *Kramer,* S.E. (2002).Translations of the international outcome inventory for hearing aids *(IOI-HA)*. *International Journal of Audiology, 41,* 3–26.

[21] Bentler, R.A., Niebuhr, D.P., Johnson, T.A., Flamme, G.A.(2003). Impact of digital labelling on outcome measures. *Ear and Hearing, 24*, 215-224.

[22] Cox, R.M., and Alexander, G.C.(1992). Maturation of hearing aid benefit. *Ear and Hearing, 13*, 131-141.

[23] McClymont, L.G., Browning, G.C., Gatehouse, S. (1991).Reliability of patient choice between hearing aid systems. *British Journal of Audiology, 25*, 35-39.

[24] Ching, T. (2003). Selecting, verifying and evaluating hearing aids for children. *Audiological Medicine, 1*, 191-198.

[25] Robbins, A.M., Renshaw, J.J., Berry, S.W. (1991). Evaluating meaningful auditory integration in profoundly hearing-impaired children. *American Journal of Otology, 12* (Suppl), 144-150.

[26] Nozza, R.J., Rossman, R.N.F., Bond, L.C., Miller, S.L. (1990). Infant speech-sound discrimination in noise. *Journal of the Acoustical Society of America, 87*, 339-350.

[27] Dillon, H. (2008). Outcomes for wearers of hearing aids and improving hearing aid technology: Denis Byrne memorial Oration. Paper presented at the 18th Audiological Society of Australia National Conference, Canberra, 2008, May. Available from http://www.nal.gov.au/Publications/conference_presentations.htm

[28] Priwin, C., Stenfelt, S., Edensvard, A., Granström, G., Tjellström, A.H., Kansson, B. (2005). Unilateral versus bilateral bone-anchored hearing aids (BAHAs).*Cochlear Implants International, 6* Suppl, 79-81.

[29] Christensen, L.V., and Dornhoffer, J.D. (2008). Bone-anchored hearing aids for unilateral hearing loss in teenagers. *Otology and Neurotology, 29*, 1120–1122.

[30] Badran, K., Arya, A.K., Bunstone, D., Mackinnon, N. (2009). Long-term complications of bone-anchored hearing aids: a 14-year experience. *The Journal of Laryngology and Otology, 123*, 170-176.

[31] McDermott, A., Williams, J., Kuo, M., Reid, A., Proops, D. (2008). The role of bone anchored hearing aids in children with Down syndrome. *International Journal of Pediatric Otorhinolaryngology, 72*, 751-757.

[32] Verhagen, C.V., Hol, M.K., Coppens-Schellekens, W., Snik, A.F., Cremers, C.W. (2008).The Baha Softband. A new treatment for young children with bilateral congenital aural atresia. *International Journal of Pediatric Otorhinolaryngology, 72*, 1455-1459.

[33] Esteem: the hearing implant, 2010. Available from http://www.envoymedical.com/

[34] Clark, G.M.(1995). Cochlear implants: historical perspectives. In: G Plant, and K Spens, (Eds.). *Profound deafness and communication.* (pp.165-218). London: Whurr.

[35] Blair Simmons, F. (1966). Electrical Stimulation of the Auditory Nerve in Man. *Archives of Otolaryngology, 84*, 2–54.

[36] Niparko, J.K., and Wilson, B.S. (2001).History of Cochlear Implants. In: J. Niparko , K. Kirk, N. Mellon, A. Robbins, D. Tucci, B. Wilson. (Eds.). *Cochlear Implants: Principles and Practices.* (pp.**103-107).** Philadelphia, Lippincott, Williams and Wilkins.

[37] Cullen, R.D., Higgins, C., Buss, E., Clark, M., Pillsbury, H.C., Buchman, C.A. (2004).Cochlear implantation in patients with substantial residual hearing. *Laryngoscope, 114*, 2218-2223.

[38] Green, K.M.J., Bhatt, Y.M., Mawman, D.J., O'Driscoll, M.P., Saeed, S.R., Ramsden, R.T., Green, M.W. (2007). Predictors of audiological outcomes following cochlear implantation in adults. *Cochlear Implants International, 8,* 1-11.

[39] Bassim, M., Buss, E., Clark, M.S., Kölln, K.A., Pillsbury, C.H., Pillsbury, H.C., Buchman, C.A. (2005).MED-EL Combi40+ Cochlear implantation in adults. *Laryngoscope, 115,* 1568-1573.

[40] Geers, A.E., Moog, J.S., Biedenstein, J., Brenner, C., Hayes, H. (2009). Spoken language scores of children using cochlear implants compared to hearing age-mates at school entry. *Journal of Deaf Studies and Deaf Education, 14,* 371-385.

[41] Waltzman, S.B., Cohen, N.L., Green, J., Roland, J.T. (2002). Long-term effects of cochlear implants in children. *Journal of American Academy of Otolaryngology-Head and Neck Surgery, 126,* 505-511.

[42] Tye-Murray, N., Spencer, L., Woodworth, G. (1995). Acquisition of speech by children who have prolonged cochlear implant experience. *Journal of Speech, Language and Hearing Research, 38,* 327-337.

[43] Svirsky, MA., Teoh, S., Neuburger, H. (2004). Development of language and speech perception in congenitally, profoundly deaf children as a function of age at cochlear implantation. *Audiology and Neurotology, 9,* 224-233.

[44] Nicholas, J., and Geers, A. (2006). Effects of early auditory experience on the spoken language of deaf children at 3 years of age. *Ear and Hearing,* 27, 286-398.

[45] Habib, M.G., Walzman, S.B., Tajudeen, B., Svirsky, M.A. (2010). Speech production intelligibility of early implanted pediatric cochlear implant users. International *Journal of Pediatric Otorhinolaryngology,74,* 855-859.

[46] Schauwers, K., Gillis, S., Govaerts, P.J.(2008). The characteristics of prelexical babbling after cochlear implantation between 5 and 20 months of age. *Ear and Hearing,* 29, 627-637.

[47] Colletti, L. (2009). Long-term follow-up of infants (4-11 months) fitted with cochlear implants. *Acta OtoLaryngologica, 129,* 361-366.

[48] Efrat, A., Schorr, F.P., Roth, N.A., Fox, A. (2008). Comparison of Speech and Language Skills of Children with Cochlear Implants and Children with Normal Hearing. *Communication Disorders Quarterly, 29, 195-210.*

[49] Pisoni, D., Cleary, M., Geers, A., Tobey, E. (2000). Individual differences in effectiveness of cochlear implants in children who are prelingually deaf: New process measures of performance. *The Volta Review, 101,* 111–164.

[50] Tarabichi, MB., Todd, C., Khan, Z., Yang, X., Shehzad, B., Tarabichi, M.M. (2008). Deafness in the developing world: the place of cochlear implantation. *The Journal of Laryngology and Otology, 122,* 77-80.

[51] Zeng, FG. (1995). Cochlear implants in China. *Audiology, 34,* 61-75.

[52] Toe, D. (1999). Impact of FM aid use on the classroom behaviour of profoundly deaf secondary students. *Seminars in Hearing, 20,* 223-235.

[53] Boothroyd, A., and Iglehart, F.(1998). Experiments with classroom amplification. *Ear and Hearing, 19,* 202-217.

[54] Lewis, D. (1997).Selection and assessment of classroom amplification. In: W. McCracken, S. Laoide-Kemp (Eds). *Audiology in Education.* (pp 323-347). London: Whurr Publishers Ltd.

[55] Boothroyd, A. (2004). Hearing aid accessories for adults: the remote FM microphone. *Ear and Hearing, 25,* 22-33.

[56] Chisholm, T.H., Noe, C.M., McArdle, R., Abrams, H. (2007).Evidence for the use of hearing assistive technology: The role of the FM system. *Trends in Amplification, 11,* 73-89.

[57] Ross, M. (1997). A retrospective look at the future of aural rehabilitation. *Journal of the Academy of Rehabilitative Audiology, 30,* 11-28.

[58] Erber, NP. (1988). *Communication Therapy for Hearing-Impaired Adults.* Abbotsford, Australia, Clavis Publishing.

[59] Boothroyd, A. (2007). Adult aural rehabilitation: what is it and does it work? *Trends in Amplification, 11,* 63-71.

[60] Bally, S.J., Bakke, M.H. (2007). A peer mentor training program for aural habilitation. *Trends in Amplification, 11,* 125-131.

[61] Ross, M. (2007). A look at AR in the last decade. *The ASHA Leader, 12,* 5, 30.

[62] Lynas W. (1999). Supporting the deaf child in the mainstream school: Is there a best way? *Support for Learning, 14,* Supp, 113-121.

[63] Yoshinaga-Itano, C., Sedley, A.L., Coutler, D.A., Mehl, A.L. (1998). Language of early and later-identified children with hearing loss. *Pediatrics, 102,* 1168-1171.

[64] Nicholas, J., and Geers, A.E. (2006). Effects of early auditory experience on the spoken language of deaf children at 3 years of age. *Ear and Hearing, 27,* 286-298.

[65] Calderon, R. (2000). Parent involvement in deaf children's education programs as a predictor of child's language, early reading, and social-emotional development. *Journal of Deaf Studies and Deaf Education, 5,* 140–155.

[66] Moeller, M.P. (2000). Early intervention and language development in children who are deaf and hard of hearing. *Pediatrics,106,* E43.

In: Prevention of Hearing Loss
Editors: V. Newton, P. Alberti and A. Smith

ISBN: 978-1-61942-745-7
© 2012 Nova Science Publishers, Inc.

Chapter XII

Industrial Hearing Conservation

Peter W. Alberti[*]

Abstract

This chapter deals with the prevention of hearing loss (HL) of occupational origin, the result of exposure to excessive levels of sound alone, or chemicals: volatile hydrocarbons, asphyxiants and organic pesticides, or a combination of noise exposure and chemicals acting synergistically. Occupational hearing loss (OHL) is extremely common in all parts of the world and should be entirely preventable. The chapter reviews the establishment of safe exposure levels, types of noise and means of controlling it. It identifies the components of a successful hearing conservation programme (HCP), of which the most important is to engineer out or separate the worker from the noise. The use of personal hearing protectors (PHP) is described as are the various types including those used in intermittent levels of noise or where communication capability is required. Measurement of sound and engineering controls is described; so are particular issues with personal hearing protectors (PHP). Some comment is made about hearing conservation in the developing world and the results of hearing conservation programmes are reviewed.

Introduction

Intense external physical stimulation may damage the body acutely or chronically,whether it be ultraviolet radiation from sunshine, infrared radiation from steel smelting or sound. To a greater or lesser extent all of these stimuli are part of everyday life and all have the potential to cause harm. Sunshine may cause sunburn and lead to the development of cancer later: whether the exposure is experienced working on a farm or on a golf course is irrelevant; the sunshine may be harmful. The same is true for sound which will be examined in detail in this and other chapters. Very intense sound can produce temporary threshold shift (TTS) or permanent threshold shift (PTS), immediate and chronic hearing loss,

---
[*] Corresponding author: peter.alberti@rogers.com.

tinnitus and in the long run hearing that worsens more rapidly than would be expected from aging alone. These are all under the rubric'noise induced hearing loss (NIHL)'. The sound exposure may occur at work, military service or during leisure pursuits. If avoidance is impossible, a hearing protective device HPD may be required.

Excessive noise, even if not severe enough to affect hearing, may interfere with communication, concentration, the ability to relax and to sleep; this is dealt with in chapter 13.

Hundreds of millions of people suffer from hearing loss produced by noise trauma, which when added to normal ageing, unnecessarily disables a large cohort of the middle aged and elderly population. It is totally preventable, yet it is globally the most common cause of acquired adult onset HL. In the United States alone it is estimated that over 20 million people are exposed to hazardous levels of industrial noise – this excludes agriculture, the construction industry, oil and gas drilling and the military. In Europe about 40 million people are exposed to hazardous sound [1]. Numbers in the developing nations are unknown but are likely to be higher. Added to this is the overwhelming noise exposure experienced by those serving in the armed forces, plus recreational noise from such diverse hobbies as hunting, woodworking and recreational music; this is a globally pervasive public health problem.

There are sufficient publications from all over the globe to indicate that NIHL is taken seriously by some in virtually all countries, but in reality, active prevention has taken place only in a few, and then usually only in large industries. The textile industry is widespread especially in the developing world and cotton mills are amongst the loudest workplaces. Diesel engines and pneumatic equipment are globally ubiquitous. As newly emerging countries industrialize, their workers are exposed to an increasingly cacophonous life. Many workers are unaware noise exposure produces hearing loss and in large portions of the world, society does not care. There are other ototraumatic agents, particularly certain inhaled chemicals which are individually ototoxic and also act synergistically with sound to produce problems in hearing.

Avoidance of toxic exposure, noise and chemicals, is by far the best and probably the most economical way of retaining a workforce in good hearing health. If all industrial safety was left to personal protection the worker would be fitted with heavy boots, probably a fireproof apron, hardhat, safety glasses, hearing protectors and respirator and lack mobility in the workplace. Ideally what is required is attention to total safety and health and not piecemeal efforts to remediate each individual hazard.

Establishing Safe Exposure Levels

In Britain and the European Union (EU) it was concluded that, between reasonable limits, the amount of NIHL was directly related to the total daily sound exposure; this became known as the equal energy concept (L_{ea}). Three dB added to a sound, any sound, doubles its intensity, three dB removed from a sound halves its intensity (remember that the decibel scale is logarithmic), so it was concluded that an exposure of 90 dBA for eight hours was equally safe (or hazardous) as a four hour exposure at 93 dBA, a two hour exposure at 96 dBA or a 16 hours exposure at 87 dBA. In the United States multiple approaches were taken [2].

Table 12.1. Safe exposure levels, Leq and Losha

Safe exposure (hours)		
Sound level dBA	Leq	Losha
85	8	16
87	5	13
90	4	8
92	1.5	6
95	47 min	4
97	30 min	3
100	15 min	2
102	9 min	1.5
105	4.75 min	1

A five dB trading relationship was adopted by OSHA (Losha) because it was argued that noise at work is usually intermittent through the day with small periods of recovery occurring, enabling the ear better to withstand somewhat higher noise levels than predicted by the equal energy hypothesis. These decisions were and are made in the political and economic arena as well as in the laboratory.

The differences in the regulations pertaining to the EU and the United States of America (USA) are great. For example a worker in Europe exposed to 91 dB in the workplace would only be allowed to work there without hearing protection for two hours, whereas his confrères in the United States, undertaking the same job under the same conditions would be allowed to work for seven hours unprotected (Table 12.1).

Tables like this are frequently published but in some ways are specious – if the sound levels are above 85 dBA, a hearing conservation programme should be initiated and if above 87 dBA, HPDs should be worn. By far the best solution is not to expose workers to sound which is so intense that it is damaging. The vagaries of the US regulations are well reviewed by Suter [2].

Chemical Ototoxins

There is increasing evidence that exposure to other workplace chemicals, volatile hydrocarbons, asphyxiants and organo-pesticides is producing hearing loss [3 -5]; in some instances they also produce central sensory disturbances, especially neuronal toxic vertigo and nephrotoxicity (which are beyond the scope of this book).Their mechanism of action appears to be the generation of reactive oxygen species (free radicals) similar to the damage caused by noise trauma.

It is not surprising that noise and chemicals may act synergistically i.e. exposure to both simultaneously (all within a relatively few hours of each other) produces more damage than would be expected from either one on their own. There is an excellent overview published by the EU [5]. The mechanisms involved are described in Chapter 3.

Ototoxic chemicals are widely used and include solvents, such as toluene (used in printing), styrene and xylene (used in chemical manufacture), benzene, whites spirit, carbon disulphide (used in textile manufacturing) [6] and fuels, especially jet fuels [7]; asphyxiants such as carbon monoxide, a by-product of steel making and hydrogen cyanide used in ore extraction [8]; metals such as cadmium, lead and mercury [9] and finally pesticides especially organophosphates and paraquat [10, 11].

Anecdotal accounts of hearing loss in these industries and epidemiological studies in industrial plants and experimental animals reveal that these agents may produce or exacerbate occupational hearing loss [12]. These include studies of petrochemical workers [13]; a printing plant where it was demonstrated that hearing loss rate was double in people exposed to toluene and noise together as it was to each on their own [14], a number of paint manufacturers in Poland [15] and an auto manufacturing facility in Iran [16]. Not all studies have shown damage [17]; in some industries, at least, appropriate ventilation and work practices are effective.

In certain industries a great deal of work has been undertaken to make safer products, which also reduces the risk to hearing. The paint industry has had massive product development with the introduction of water-based paints and the substitution of compounds with fewer volatile hydrocarbon solvents [18] and heavy metals, especially lead. This protects workers in occupations as divergent as automobile manufacturing and home improvement. There have been changes in ink diminishing the use of toluene, making printing safer.

It is possible that the tables of risk for hearing damage from noise exposure have been contaminated by including workers who have also been exposed to ototoxic chemicals; the type of noise is important, impact noise embedded in steady state sound produces more damage than either steady state or impact sound of equal energy on their own. These matters are reviewed by Henderson et al [19]. With the knowledge of the additional deleterious effect of chemicals and noise combinations it should be possible to produce modified tables to provide a better assessment of risk in the workplace.

Types of Noise

1. Steady-State High Level Sound

Broad-spectrum atonal noise is the best understood and most studied cause of noise trauma. Not many workers spend all their workweek in steady-state/steady level sound, often sound levels vary during a production cycle and it may be intermittent. However in terms of hearing conservation it is assumed that a more or less constant noise is steady-state noise.

a   pure tone – rare in industry
b   complex (a mix of pure tones) – also rare in industry
c   broadband (a potpourri of sounds) – common industrial background sound

2. Impact Noise

Some industrial noise is produced by an impact, hammering, riveting drop forging or in the military, a gun fire. The sounds are frequently of high intensity and by definition of short duration although the decay time may vary significantly. The intensity of impact noise is more difficult to measure than steady-state sound. The risk to hearing depends on the absolute intensity and the decay time.

3. Combined Steady State and Impact Sound

The amount of damage caused by impact noise is greater for a given noise level if it is embedded within steady-state noise than if the same total sound was delivered only by the impact noise; examples include drop forging against a background of high level steady state sound, or firing a gun from a moving tank [20].Technical definitions of various sound types can be found in more detailed texts [21].

There are other complicating factors. Work shifts vary in length; for example some people are exposed to 12 hours of continuous noise interspersed with a 12 hour rest period, others work overtime, often for long stretches. If the noise levels are fairly high, does 12 hours allow time for adequate recovery before the next workday? It would appear that most, if not all TTS from occupational noise exposure has disappeared after 12 hours so it is suggested that a minimum of 12 hours of rest from all noise exposure is required between work shifts.

In some occupations workers do not escape from noise for days on end as, for example, crew on some tugboats and workers on offshore drilling rigs. The writer knows of no published trading relationship for workweeks organized differently than an eight hour workday.

Engineering Controls

These are feasible: in some instances technologies have changed sound from intense to quieter, as for example replacement of riveting by welding in the shipbuilding industry and pneumatic drills in hard rock mines by quieter electric hydraulic ones. In both there is economic benefit from the change. Unless new technology is as cost effective as the one it replaces, it will not be voluntarily adopted. Pneumatic drills used in road repairs can be muffled as can compressors but they rarely are; they cost more and are marginally less efficient.

However, they seem to be superseded by more powerful jack hammers attached to backhoes and bulldozers, picking up large slabs and producing much less total sound for a given unit of work than the incessant noise of multiple small drills. Often excessive sound affects uninvolved workers with quieter jobs sited in a noisy environment. That is the realm of Hearing Conservation (HC). This chapter deals with occupational HC, mainly civil but also some military; the problems of and solutions to social and recreational noise are dealt within chapter 13.

Hearing Conservation Programme

Industrial and military HCPs are designed to protect hearing and maintain the ability to receive wanted or necessary sound. They require time and effort to establish and to maintain

They consist of:

1   Identifying and quantifying a hazard
2   Removing, or at least reducing the hazard to a safe level
3   Discussion with and education of the workforce about the problem and solutions
4   Hearing screening
      pre-employment
      regularly during employment
      on retirement
5   Provision of personal hearing protectors (HPD)
      instruction in their use
      ensuring HPDs are properly maintained and used
6   Monitoring:
      a. workplace sound
      b. hearing tests of workforce
      c. other hazards to hearing e.g. volatile hydrocarbons
7   Keeping accurate records
8   Engineering out the hazards
9   Monitoring the effectiveness of the programme by repeated hearing testing and repeated sound level measurement

1. Recognize the Potential Hazard

Sound levels are measured by sound level meters. These are electronic devices that measure the overall sound level and also the intensity at various frequencies. They must be calibrated and sheltered from wind. Several types exist and the more elaborate ones can also integrate sound over a period of time to give the L_{osha8} or L_{eq8} measurements. Such sound measurements may be made inside the factory as a whole and close to specific work sites. It is good practice to make sound contours of the plant where a hearing conservation programme is being implemented; this allows easy identification of sound hotspots and when repeated year-over-year enables the monitoring of the soundscape within the plant. This will help identify areas where workers are at risk from excessive noise. Where the sound level is above 85 dBA a hazardous sound warning should be posted so that anyone entering the area wears hearing protection.

It is important to distinguish between the overall sound level and the sound exposure of the worker. It is necessary know the total noise dosage received during a shift:because the sound can vary: the worker may move around to quieter or louder areas. An individual's sound exposure is measured using an individual noise dosimeter These small devices worn during a work shift, take and store repeated spot recordings of the sound intensity for later downloading and analysis. They indicate the 8 hour $L_{eq)}$ (or L_{osha}) exposure and the intensity distribution throughout the time they are worn. They are too expensive to be worn by every worker. Most have an integral microphone; the device is body worn and thus the microphone is not at ear level. The worker with his face close to a noisy machine may receive a higher level of sound than is recorded. Recently ear plugs have been produced with built in microphones deep in the ear canal able to measure directly both the attenuation of protectors and the sound level within the ear canal. Such devices have been used to the present to help fit plugs rather than to characterize work place noise; those reports no doubt will follow.

Plants using hazardous chemicals should monitor the levels. Further discussion is outside the scope of this book. Attention should also be paid in the agricultural industry where organo -phosphates are used as pesticides and where there are also high levels of sound. All can be a potent synergist to noise and produce significant hearing losses.

2. Reduce the Toxic Sound Level

By far the best way of reducing OHL is to remove or separate the worker from the excessive noise. This is best undertaken when starting new or restructuring older plants. Management has to acknowledge the need, and have the will to implement such changes. Those who design machinery should be aware of the hazards of excessive sound and those who purchase machinery should write sound specifications into the contract. Unfortunately the impetus is more frequently the stick rather than the carrot, tough regulations and regular inspection are frequently necessary. The means of doing this are listed:

a   use quieter machinery
b   sound dampen existing machinery
c   enclose the machinery
d   automate the process
e   separate the worker by using
     sound treated control rooms
     sound enclosures around machine
f   change the process

Use Quieter Machinery

Over the last 50 years machinery became more efficient, larger and louder. No attention was paid to sound pollution until it became a safety and health issue. Gradually, in some jurisdictions, maximum sound specifications were included in contracts for new machinery and in many instances have resulted in a quieter workplace. Regulations about machinery sound levels are described in Chapter 12. It is also helpful to pay attention to machinery mounts, which may insulate them from transmitting sound and vibration. It may be possible to retrofit sound baffles. Economics can be a powerful force in quietening (or not) the workplace.

Automating processes within sound baffled areas also protects hearing. Much of the noisy work on car assembly plants, done by hand two decades ago, is now undertaken with the help of robots, so far fewer workers are exposed to noise.

An enlightened management and a persistent, informed workforce may frequently initiate local changes, such as the inclusion of sound damping material around a particularly loud machine or the movement of workers away from its proximity, especially if their own task could be undertaken in quieter surroundings [22].

Now, in many semi-automated processes the equipment operators work within sound-proofed cubicles or control rooms and only occasionally must go in to the hazardous sound area. Two examples are paper mill and oil refinery operators who now work in sound isolated control rooms, rather than on the plant floor. Frequently workers are vicariously exposed to excessive sound not related to their own job which may not be sound intense, if their work station is placed beside loud machinery only because space is available, they should be moved. Baffles inside large spaces to prevent the reflection of sound from noisy machinery to quieter areas are also helpful.

The most successful hearing conservation programmes are those with a 'win win' situation, in which the noise is reduced below hazardous levels and productivity increases. This has occurred in a wide range of industry;e.g. in shipbuilding welding replaced riveting,and computer controlled metal forming equipment reduced the number of workers on the shop floor. In the aerospace industry panels are now glued and workers are no longer deafened lying inside wings while panels are being riveted. Better metal forming in the auto industry means that panels can be attached to each other without having to be hammered into place as was the custom as recently as 15 years ago. In information technology (IT) during the second half of the last century computer rooms were ubiquitous and had ear damaging sound levels produced by fans and impact printers. Both sound sources disappeared as more powerful, smaller, more efficient computers were introduced with lower ventilation requirements and different printing techniques.

3. Instruct Personnel about Risk

Any programme is more effective, whether it be sorting domestic garbage, routinely wearing safety helmets cycling, using seat belts or wearing safety boots at work, if the participants accept the need and have 'bought into' it. The same is true for hearing conservation. Still too many workers are uninformed about the potential harmful effects of noise exposure and that it is possible to prevent it. NIHL is insidious in onset and like virtually all hearing loss, in the early stages is easily ignored. Hearing loss in industry suffers from the same problems that bedevil most adult onset hearing loss: it is recognized, but shrugged off, "it doesn't matter, one can't do anything about it any way'. This is wrong on both counts. The pioneering work of people like Hetu[23] and his colleagues have clearly shown that a great deal of individual and family misery is created by preventable industrial hearing loss. There are many examples of good educational programmes for workers and some of long term effective hearing conservation systems. It is not the function of this text to promote commercial programmes; they can be found on the web. Some examples include the peer reviewed journal Noise and Health, the National Hearing Conservation Association, NIOSH and EU web sites. There is disappointingly little information about the effectiveness of instructional programmes for hearing protector use [24], although there are many descriptions in the literature.

One of the most important steps is to educate, empower and enlist the workforce into caring for its own safety. Management instruction is much more effective with assistance from the workers own safety committees which includes members working on the shop floor. For example, the Province of Ontario (Canada),mandated worker safety and health committees headed by a worker in every larger workplace, with enormous benefit to all concerned. People realize that what is being attempted was beneficent, not just another top down directive and responded positively. As a result, certainly in the field of hearing conservation, the proper use of hearing protectors increased significantly. Well unionised large industries have more effective programmes than smaller less organised ones [25].

4. Hearing Testing

Industrial hearing screening is designed to:

- screen hearing thresholds
- detect abnormal thresholds
- detect changes in threshold over time in individuals
- monitor programme effectiveness

There are issues related to industrial hearing testing. The equipment must be regularly calibrated and the tests conducted in a quiet area, preferably meeting national standards for such testing. Domed headphones are sometimes used to help mask out unwanted sound; insert earphones are also very effective but may not be valid in some jurisdictions. These are screening tests and only quantify the air conduction threshold. Large plants have their own test resources and testers, smaller ones are frequently serviced by mobile hearing testing facilities.

Ideally the tests should be undertaken after 12 hours away from noise to avoid the result being contaminated by TTS. This is difficult to implement. It is the writer's view that annual tests can be undertaken during the work shift as long as hearing protection has been used – those whose hearing has worsened can be recalled for further testing after a minimum of 12 hours in quiet. After all, if the programme is effective, it should not matter when the test is undertaken. The pre-employment test should be taken with the risk of TTS removed, ideally within three months of hiring although if testing is contracted out, it may have to wait for the annual visit of the mobile facility.All tests are opportunities to reinforce proper wearing practices and to discuss individual problems

5. The Provision of Personal Hearing Protection

The function of HPDs is to protect the ears from unwanted and potentially damaging sound. They consist of sound deadening material either in the form of plugs which fit into the ear canal or domed cups lined by foam which cover the ear to prevent sound reaching to the tympanic membrane. Depending upon the type and material of which they are made, the usual protection in practice is between 10 and somewhat over 30 dBA. As much industrial sound is in the low to mid 90 dBA range, they can be quite effective. Problems arise with impact sound, heavy industry and the military where sound levels may be much higher. If the sound is intense enough it may even be transmitted by bone conduction to the ear.

HPDs can mitigate the effect of high sound levels but only if they are worn!The devices are inherently uncomfortable and only protect the individual user, but leave bystanders at risk. The ideal protector must be comfortable, appropriate for the particular sound level, should not interfere with worker safety and allow necessary communication. It should be compatible with other safety equipment, for example hardhat and safety glasses. In practice there are problems including fit, hostile working conditions and the ability to communicate. Thus HPDs may not be particularly effective on a workforce wide basis. However, with perseverance, programmes based upon their use can be successful.

The various types of HPD will be described, following which special needs and problems will be dealt with.

Types of HPDs

1   Simple hearing protectors
      Plugs
      Muffs
2   Special purpose protectors
      Level dependant (passive and active)
        Plugs
        Muffs
      Musician's plugs
      Active noise reduction (frequently combined with a communication function)
      Protectors with active communication ability
      Multifunction protectors

Simple HPDs

There are three basic types, a sound excluding earplug: a sound excluding earmuff covering the ear and a semi-inserted small plug on a spring, similar to a plug which will not be discussed further. There are many manufacturers of HPDs, more than 400 different types are available in the EU alone [26], a testament both to the widespread need and that no one type is effective for all.

Earplugs

Pre-formed flanged earplugs were introduced during World War II. The modern version of these plugs, now made of a soft silicone rubber, with usually four or more flanges known as ear or skull screws (!), are one size fits all and quite effective. They are washable and reusable. They frequently have a cord attached for safe keeping.

Individually moulded plugs were popular and used widely in the 1960s and 70s, They were accepted by the workers, in part because management cared enough to provide something on an individual basis, and by management, because once fitted, they should have lasted for a long time. They consisted of a personally moulded silicone rubber plug, rather like a solid ear mould for a hearing aid, coated with a soft silicone dip to create the absolute acoustic seal required for sound occlusion. They were abandoned in favour of simpler foam cylinders or multi-flanged plugs because they hardened and lost their seal. Now personally moulded plugs are making a return appearance with a new preparation technique and material, produced by the largest manufacturer of the foam plugs. Foam insert plugs are ubiquitous and can be extremely effective.

They consist of a cylindrical piece of plastic foam which is rolled up, inserted into the ear canal and expands to fill the crevices thereby acting as an excellent sound seal. They can be washed and reused and are relatively comfortable to wear; they may come with cords attached for reuse but on hygienic grounds, are frequently only used once. As sold to industry in bulk, they cost only pennies, but the cumulative cost over months and years is quite high.

Ear Muffs

Ear muffs consist of a domed enclosure lined with sound absorbing material with soft, replaceable seals that fit comfortably and tightly to the irregular outline of the skull and jaw to prevent sound entering the ear canal; they require force to hold them against the skull, usually provided by a spring band which may be worn over the top of the head or at the back of the skull, in which case a strap over the top of the head attached to the upper edge of the muffs supports the cups while the spring presses them firmly to the head to allow other head coverings to be worn. Muffs may also be attached by a spring to a hard hat to combine head and ear protection.

In intermittent noise the muff can be swung over the hardhat; this combination has the disadvantage that moving the hat inevitably moves the muff and frequently breaks the sound seal. Ear muffs are effective as long as the dome is of sufficient size (which leads to trouble with earmuffs designed to fit under combat helmets) and contains sound absorbent foam. The disadvantages include forming a proper seal between the irregular shape of the head and the muff, hardening of the soft plastic used for the seal over time so that the seal is no longer properly formed, and leakage past some safety glass temple bars.

The amount of protection provided will be discussed below, but under ideal conditions, muffs are more effective than plugs and both types provide more attenuation in the higher than in the lower frequencies.

In most industrial noise backgrounds almost all protectors are effective and care should be taken not to protect too much for this isolates unnecessarily. In the highest levels of industrial noise as may occur in drop forges or bottling plants, double protection may be necessary, plug and muff together which should provide about 30dBA of attenuation in the field. There is however a limit to the amount of protection which HPDs can give; if sound is intense enough it is transmitted by bone conduction to the ear with sufficient energy to be damaging.

Simple HPDs do not meet the requirements of all users; high sound levels may be intermittent, it may be important to hear voices or to communicate electronically and it maybe helpful to remove the distortion of sound produced by the uneven frequency response of the protective device.

A variety of specialized protectors have been developed to cope with these circumstances.

Special Purpose Protectors

Level Dependant Protectors, Passive and Active

It may benecessary to protect the ear from intense intermittent sound but retain normal hearing for environmental sounds and speech between impulses. Good examples are hunters, landscape gardeners, firefighters, some construction workers and infantrymen.

There are two types of passive plug designed for this purpose. The first is an old design, a plug with a central metal diaphragm with a fine hole pierced in it (Sonex is a well-known example); normal sound passes through without turbulence; an explosive sound produces turbulent sound waves and is blocked. Major efforts have been made by the military to produce passive earplugs which can be a turned on and off. Flanged earplugs similar to conventional ones have been provided with a central filter switch that opens or closes at finger touch. The combatant can reduce sound when near a helicopter or firing guns and leave it open at other times. There seems to be a fairly constant redesign of these devices based on experience in the field (the latest models described in a variety of webpages [27]). In normal hearing listeners speech can be understood well using either device in normal background sound [28].

There are also earmuffs which transmit external sounds to the ear except when the external sounds exceed a hazardous level. They are good earmuffs with an external microphone wired to a small amplifier within the earmuff. The amplifier has an electronic peak limiter which switches it off momentarily when sounds exceed the safe level. They allow the wearer to hear environmental sounds, but have a serious drawback, directional hearing is not as good as normal while using them. They are also used in industry like quarrying where there is intermittent blasting and rock drilling but where it is also necessary to hear the appropriate warning signals. A similar but 'reverse' device is available: a good muff with a microphone and amplifier built in which is manually activated when the wearer wishes to hear something and which switches itself off after about 30 seconds.

Musician's Plugs

Standard earplugs and muffs are more effective at protecting the ear from high frequency than from low-frequency sound. Sound that passes through them is perceived as muffled, masking a disproportionate amount of high-frequency sounds such as the sibilants in speech and higher pitched tones; music perception is distorted. There are certain occupations in which environmental sound levels are very high but it is still necessary to hear (albeit more quietly) the sound and the environment. Pop musicians are good examples; if playing on a regular basis they expose their ears to damaging levels of sound but if they wear ordinary muffs or plugs, the sounds they hear are sufficiently distorted that it impacts their music making. To overcome this, HPDs have been devised (by a musician acoustician) with filters which allow some high-frequency sound to the ear, flattening the response. In visual terms it is akin to trading tinted dark sunglasses for slightly less tinted neutral gray ones. They have been given the name "musician's plugs" [29], are reusable and fairly expensive. They have been more widely adopted by 'pop' musicians than classical ones for the amplified sound levels are higher and the exposure longer amongst the former. The most popular type is available with three levels of attenuation, depending upon need. They require a deep impression in the ear canal to prevent an 'occlusion effect' (a sometimes annoying echo like sound generated in the air trapped deep to the plug).

Active Noise Reduction (ANR)

The basic design is of good earmuffs with the microphone inside the muff and another outside. A small microphone inside the muff monitors the sound that is passed through the dome; it is phase inverted and the inverted signal is played into the muff through a small speaker. This sound will have the opposite phase to the sound inside the muff so it cancels out that sound, reducing the sound level significantly. This is technically difficult and works best at low frequencies, important in many military applications such as armoured vehicles and jet aircraft cockpits. The ear muffs themselves protect more against high-frequency sound so the combination provides protection across the frequency spectrum. Speech signals transmitted into the dome are not affected because there is no external speech signal to cancel out. The devices are expensive and only used with special needs: helicopter pilots, crew of armoured vehicles, jet fighter pilots and the pilots of light aircraft where cockpit noise from the propeller and engine during the take-off creates communication difficulty with the control tower. There is an excellent review of these devices published as a symposium - RTO HFM (Research and Technology Organisation/ Human Factors Medicine) lecture series [30].

It should be emphasized that military noise is much greater than that found in industry and so is the need for communication in a noisy environment. Berger [31] evaluated ANR hearing protection against 300 representative industrial soundscapes and concluded that they added very little to well-fitting conventional ear muffs in terms of protection and their initial and operating costs were much higher.

HPDs with Communication Ability

Even in high sound levels it may be necessary to converse and to hear instructions, as for example pilots, infantry men and construction equipment operators. HPDs with communication capability are available as muffs and plugs. One of the simpler versions is an earmuff with the transmitting headset inside. If two-way communication is required some form of noise cancelling boom microphone is frequently used. This sort of device has been used for pilots of small planes and has wide military application. Frequently today they also have an ANR capability. The most recent developments are a family of devices consisting of earplugs or of tight fitting moulds with a sound transmitter built-in connected to an external speaker/amplifier, radio, telephone or other communication devices as for example Bluetooth.. These devices are tightly peak limited so that they cut out the transmission of sound above a fixed level. These are helpful to people like firefighters in special circumstances where they work in a high noise levels such as airports [32, 33], to workers in heavy impact noise, motorcyclists and in a variety of military applications because they can be readily used with helmets.

How Much Protection Do HPDs Provide?

The Effectiveness of Hearing Protectors, Laboratory versus the Field

In the United States the noise reduction rating (NRR] was adopted in 1978 by the Environmental Protection Agency (EPA)[34] as a standard for HPD attenuation. This rates the optimal performance: tests are performed in laboratory conditions using new protective devices which are tester fitted. Whilst this might provide gold standard data, it bears little relationship to this actual attenuation achieved by the average worker in the field. When tests are repeated with user fitted devices on naïve listeners the results are much worse. In practical terms industrial hygienists halve the NRR to estimate the field protection. In addition, industrial sounds vary in their spectrum and the NRR is based on measurements made in A weighted sound levels, not adequate for all industrial sounds.

Decades of work by Elliott Berger frequently with his collaborator D. Gauger, and a group of Government scientists at NIOSH has ultimately led to a new American National Standard [35], published in July 2007. They test the attenuation of HPDs in industrial sounds in a variety of conditions measuring on subjects with minimal experience who fit their own after instruction by experts. For the first time the standard introduces a range of protection, and upper and lower boundaries of what might be expected in practice, the NRSa; it also includes a method to account for variations in the spectral noise requirement, NRSg, and finally a technique based on attenuation in the octave band method. The new methodology appears to be a great improvement over the NRR and will be much more realistic for use in the field. The differences between the two are well reviewed by Murphy [36]. EPA is expected to adopt this standard, hopefully in 2011. EU recommendations (directives) are in many ways similar to the new ANSI standard.

Problems Related to HPDs

These are:

Diminished directional hearing
Sense of isolation
Human factors issues:
- Interference from other protective devices
- Wrong size
- Incorrectly fitted
- Malfunctioning protector
- Too hot
- Ear canal infections
- Communication problems
- Conflict with pre-existing hearing loss

Directional hearing is impaired when wearing hearing protectors so that it is not always possible to tell from where the sound is coming, as for example a truck backing up or a shot fired [37]. Accident rates may be higher in certain occupations.

Interference from Other Protective Devices

To be effective there must not be a leak through which sound can enter the ear canal. To create a seal between the skull and earmuff is a challenge. The seals are made of soft material frequently filled with compressible foam or liquid. The use of safety glasses, particularly those with thick plastic temple bars (metal bars are sometimes forbidden for fear of electrocution) produces a slight sound leak where the temple bar passes between the muff and the skull. The problems faced by attaching earmuffs to a hard hat have already been dealt with. A respirator mask may also interfere with an earmuff [38].

Wrong Size

The anatomy of people's ears, skulls and ear canals varies and no one protector fits all people. The width of the skull, ear to ear determines the pressure produced by the spring on the muffs and therefore the comfort. If the skull is too narrow the pressure may not be sufficient, if it is too wide there is a strong temptation to deform the spring. While most plugs are now suitable for a range of ear canal diameter, not all eventualities are covered. The writer has large ear canals in which the standard foam plugs work well; tapered ones manufactured by the same company of the same material provided by one of the airlines for the comfort of its passengers are too small and sound leaks. Some people have very narrow ear canals and only custom plugs can be fitted. There are racial variations in the ear canal size which have led to the production of smaller Asian earplugs.

Incorrect Fit and Use

Even if HPDs are worn, it does not mean that they are working effectively. There are countless examples of protectors being improperly used: earmuffs upside down with the spring functionless below the chin; earmuff cups worn partially occluding the ear so that sound can enter and so forth. Earplugs are uncomfortable, until the skin of the ear canal adapts to their presence, which may take some weeks to occur. Too frequently plugs are worn ostentatiously in the outer part of the ear where they can be seen but are ineffective; proper seating is essential for good function. Moulded plugs should be fine but if there is a large plug of earwax or an extremely hairy ear canal the mould impression will be false.

Until recently it was not practical to demonstrate the effectiveness of protection to individual workers on a routine basis but now, with the various methods of Fit-testing [39] it is possible to do exactly that. Workers can be instructed in their proper use and at the same time have demonstrated how an effective fitting feels, which they can then replicate. There are several groups with techniques to undertake this including quite innovative ones which seat microphones deep in the ear canal and provide remote output of the attenuation. It cannot be over emphasized that hearing protectors are only part of a system of hearing conservation which must include instruction and supervision of its implementation including the way in which protectors are worn.

Maintenance

Hearing protection requires maintenance. This can be conveniently undertaken during annual hearing tests and should be checked throughout the year. A common problem is that the seals of muffs harden and become less effective; they should be replaced regularly; the springs may be deformed or just lose their spring, difficult to see by visual inspection only. The material of which the plugs are made alters with time and exposure to sweat: they become inflexible and tend to leak. These problems are dealt with in hearing conservation manuals and literature from the suppliers.

Micro-Environment

Wearing hearing protection in a hot humid environment is uncomfortable and may be unhealthy. This is common: some workplaces are extremely hot, think of metal smelting pouring and forming and much noisy work is undertaken in hot humid climates. Perspiration under a muff and may lead to skin irritation; the same is true of plugs and may result in external ear canal infection, otitis externa [40].

Communication Problems

It is difficult to communicate by sound against a background of intense noise; this may be worsened by wearing HPDs. Problems related to directional hearing are described above. A worker wearing HPDs will talk more softly because the level of speech depends on the level of the background sound heard by the speaker – they reduce the intensity of the external sound so the voice is dropped; the listener wearing HPDs requires the speech to be louder to overcome the protective action of the HPD. They also distort speech and damp out the all-important consonants. If communication is necessary then communication headsets should be provided.

The amount of attenuation provided should be suitable for the background sound, too much is isolating, too little is unprotective. In Germany there are regulations determining the amount of protection that is to be provided in different levels of noise [27]. Protectors should insulate for harmful noise but allow necessary communication, which vary from job to job. There are three different German requirements for hearing protectors, types S, V and W, each for different communication needs [41].

Matters are compounded if the listener is trying to communicate in a none native-language language; here discrimination of speech against a background noise is less successful even if not hearing impaired. This is a large problem in a workforce with migrant workers or workers with a different native tongue from management. There are also other problems of aculturisation including understanding instructions on how HPDsshould be used [42].

HPD Use in Hearing-Impaired Workers

An already hard of hearing person, usually with a high-frequency loss, may become quite isolated using HPDs, a common problem because so many workers already have hearing losses from prior noise exposure, military service and aging. Discriminating speech and environmental sounds is more difficult with a hearing impairment; if the hearing-impaired worker is wearing hearing protection those problems are worse. Hearing protectors should not interfere with necessary communication.

Needs of the Military

The hearing protection needs of the military are a special case. The intensity of military sound is an order of magnitude higher than anything that would be acceptable in the civilian arena. Fighting soldiers needs to be able to hear and sense from which direction sounds are coming at the same time as they may be using weapons or machinery which produce extremely high transient sound levels. Soldiers suffering from severe TTS from exposure to their comrade's gunfire may be sufficiently temporarily hearing-impaired not to hear battlefield sounds necessary for their own safety. Adequate earmuffs are difficult to fit under combat helmets, particularly as the lower portion of the cup must be thin to allow a rifle stock to sit against the cheek. Such muffs do not have enough internal volume to function properly. Many servicemen in the field require level dependent hearing protectors, with the ability to hear environmental sounds when times are quiet and appropriate protection when they are not, as for example firing a gun. Practical issues are succinctly and well-reviewed by Abel [43] who organised a focus group of soldiers to discuss these matters. The requirement is for hearing protection which can be easily turned on or off, else it is not used. The need to communicate is vital, a tank commander must be able to receive and give orders even if traveling inside an enclosed space with a sound intensity over 100 dBA. Much research has been expended on the development of sound excluding communication headsets and microphones. ANR headsets/ear muffs have been discussed above. The flight deck of an aircraft carrier,*"is perhaps the single most noise-hazardous work environment in the Department of the Navy. Dozens of personnel work in close proximity to multiple aircraft generating 140 dB(A) or more of recurring noise during workdays that may exceed 14 hours"* [44].

The cost of hearing protectors produced for the military is almost an order of magnitude more than the normal hearing protection used in industry: battle hardened electronics, specially shaped muffs and adjustable plugs. Soldiers on foot patrol or in firefights are still extremely reluctant to wear protectors. HPDs have been standard issue for US combat forces since 2002, but even so, one in four soldiers returning home, report hearing loss, dizziness or ringing in the ears, according to Army audiologists [45].

6. Establish Proper Monitoring

Regular hearing testing is an integral part of the hearing conservation programme, whether it be undertaken by an in-house Industrial Hygiene team or contracted out. The purpose of such hearing tests is to:

1   Establish a baseline for an individual worker and for the workforce as a whole;
2   Monitor that the hearing conservation programme is effective;
3   Identify workers whose hearing is worsening and particularly to identify those with 'tender ears'.

Regular analysis of annual hearing tests will demonstrate whether the hearing conservation programme is working; scrutiny of individual hearing test results will highlight workers who have a significant change. What is a significant change? In industrial practice the figure is frequently taken as greater than 10 dB change at two or more frequencies or a 20 dB change at one frequency. Practices vary between regions and countries; full details are available in local regulations and codes of practice.

7. Keep Adequate, Accessible Records

One of the features that has bedevilled large-scale hearing conservation has been record analysis and storage. Records were stored manually and except in the most devoted companies were difficult to retrieve, and ultimately were discarded. Now with microprocessors and direct data entry into computers from the audiometers, those who fail individual tests can be flagged; large-scale analyses can be undertaken both as a cross-sectional glimpse and over time. It is however imperative that the records be stored in an accessible manner which can survive change of personnel and of testing company. It is quite disappointing to see how few publications have been made of the effectiveness of the hearing conservation programmes which have now been undertaken by many larger firms for several decades.

8. Engineer Out the Hazards

This includes modifying machinery as well as limiting the spread of sound from the source to the listener. The techniques are outside the scope of this chapter.

9. Establish Proper Environmental Monitoring

It is important to note changes in the work environment so that it is possible to link changes in hearing of the whole workforce and of individuals, to events and changes which might have occurred at work. Examples include the relocation of machinery, the introduction of new or different types of machines, a change in the physical structure of the workplace itself and specific individual problems as for example a malfunctioning machine producing much higher sound levels than normal until the machine is repaired.

Problem Industries

Certain industries present exceptional problems throughout the world, industrialized and none industrialized alike; they include agriculture, construction, mining and oil and gas drilling.

Agriculture

This is a huge and heavily mechanized hearing damaging industry as hazardous to hearing health as heavy industry [46, 47]. In temperate climates work continues throughout the daylight hours, particularly when crops are ready to harvest, persistently exceeding the eight hour limit enshrined in tables of risk; the combine harvester may be driven from dawn to dusk. Modern agriculture makes use of heavy diesel powered equipment and many cabs are not soundproofed, so the noise exposure is high. There are many other sources of intense sound in this industry including grain drying fans, ventilation in poultry houses and the mass rearing of hogs were an individual squeal can exceed 100 dBA. Harvesting of many crops used to be quiet but backbreaking; now it is undertaken with the aid of noisy machines. The use of pesticides which by themselves may be ototoxic [11], combined with high levels of sound are a further risk to hearing [48, 49].

Migrant workers who make up a large part of the farm and horticulture labour pool in the US and by inference in other countries, are especially at risk for they work long hours and frequently have a language barrier in understanding regulations and safety measures [50, 51]

Educational programmes for high school children living in agricultural areas have been undertaken in the United States about the risks to their hearing of working in and around farms; this appears to be effective which augers well for the future [52].

Construction Industry

The construction industry is intensely noisy, produces significant preventable hearing loss and is almost universally exempted from normal industrial hearing conservation, although there may be specific statutes covering this industry in some countries. More than half a million are employed in the US, the numbers globally are huge. The full range of damaging sound is represented: explosions from blasting, impact noise from pneumatic equipment, and automatic nail firing machines; steady high level sound from the ubiquitous diesel engines, high-pitched sounds from circular saws, the list goes on. Frequently there is a combination of steady-state and impact noise. In many countries the workforce is transient, frequently ill-educated and quite often none resident.

Hearing protection in this industry, even when provided, is rarely worn throughout the work day. The comparison of self-assessment ("I wear it always") with observational studies shows HPDs are used for less than half the time exposed to noise. This reduces the shift long protection greatly and leads to an ineffective 3 dB shift long attenuation, even with well-fitting attenuators [53]. Workers worry about not hearing or locating warning signals. With the transient workforce efforts to monitor the effectiveness of hearing conservation programmes is missing. In the industrialized world these issues are slowly being addressed but they lag efforts to control industrial hearing loss [2]. The Canadian Province of British Columbia has a centralised programme to collect audiometric data in this industry, the only effective career long monitoring for construction workers known to the writer.

Mining

The mining industry is global, extremely loud and potentially chemo-toxic. Hard rock underground mining for minerals such as gold and nickel is noisy. Rock drills bore holes for dynamite which blasts the mineral seam to manageable pieces of rock which are then removed by heavy diesel equipment, taken to loud crushers and pulverized. The sound level is exceptionally high and the risks great. Opencast mining is equally loud whether it is for gold, copper, coal or oil (as in the Canadian tar sands). Chemicals are used in ore extraction.

Oil and Gas Drilling

Oil and gas rigs are loud and exposure lengthy. Workers live on offshore drilling platforms and oil rigs for prolonged periods, commonly two weeks at a time and the noise persists, TTS presumably reaching some asymptotic level. Hearing protectors are worn on the rig but there is no escaping noise during time off. The oil and gas drilling industry appears to be exempt from normal hearing conservation regulations, at least in the USA. There is concern that workers will develop significant hearing loss.

Police

Murphy et al [54] discuss firearms and hearing protection in the context of hunters, police and military. They point out that the sound pressure level from any firearm is usually sufficiently intense to warrant using an HPD even for one shot. Police practice regularly on firing ranges, frequently indoors and with multiple shooters. The peak sound level of small arms used by police vary, ranging between 157 and 170 dB. They recommend electronic level dependent ear muffs plus perhaps deeply seated earplugs.

Fishing Industry

Noise levels in fishing boats are high and exposure times long. Equipment used, often with auxiliary engines, is loud and the vessels' engines generate sound, from which crew are shielded in larger vessels but not in smaller ones [55]. Fishermen make long trips in small vessels for example off the coast of Senegal or Indonesia and their exposure to excessive sound far exceeds permissible industrial levels. The same may be true for tug boat crews employed pulling log rafts on the West coast of North America.

Newly Industrialized and Developing World

The existence of NIHL is well recognized, but preventative action lags Western Europe and North America by 40 years. Articles abound describing individual plants and instances of hearing loss in a wide range of countries in Latin America, South Asia, and Africa. Morata has worked extensively with Brazilian colleagues on aspects of hearing conservation in that country. They have reviewed toxic chemical exposure in oil refineries [13], chemical and noise exposure in printing plants [14] and the use of pesticides in agriculture [15]. Brazil like many rapidly industrializing countries is expanding its economy more quickly than regulations and the implementation of safety measures; meanwhile people lose hearing unnecessarily. The petrochemical industry seems to be better than others in safety compliance. Individual plants recognize the problems and work to prevent them; this however appears to be the exception.

Some of the problems of a Northern Indian plant are well described by Singh [56] and colleagues. They studied occupational exposure in small and medium scale industry with specific reference to heat and noise. They emphasise the importance of multiple co-existing hazards and the difficulty of dealing with them individually. Heat stress was more important than noise in the foundries and metal working shops; the majority of workers use protective devices but the difficulty of wearing HPD's during extreme heat exposure is very real. Hansia and Dickinson [57] reviewed hearing conservation practices in a South African gold mine.

16% of the workers did not appreciate that noise is a hearing loss hazard, 6% did not know that HPD's protected hearing, 3% believed they did not, 93% claimed that they used hearing protectors but only 50% were observed to. The workforce in South African gold mines is a relatively transient and workers disappear back to their homes in other southern African countries. There is neither the incentive nor the ability to undertake studies on hearing loss. The attitude there and in many developing world industries remains as it was in the UK in the early decades of the 20th century: some injury is part of the price of putting bread on the table.

Hearing Conservation Programme Costs

The economics of hearing loss are dealt with in Chapter 16. Sufficient to say, the costs related to occupational hearing loss are huge, in terms of compensation, rehabilitation (including hearing aids), sick leave, under-employment and un-employment. The US Veterans Affairs department pays almost $300 million a year for hearing testing and provision of hearing aids and a further $1.2 billion annually [59] in hearing loss compensation to almost 400,000 veterans! However the main costs are social isolation, and under-and un-employment, globally pervasive problems.

The cost of civil compensation usually includes the provision of hearing aids, their maintenance and replacement [1]. According to a study by Eurogip quoted by Schneider [1] the cost of hearing loss due to noise represents about10 % of the total cost of compensation of occupational diseases (period 1999–2001). It should also include increased absenteeism from stress [60] and lower quality employment and higher unemployment amongst the hard of hearing.

Are Industrial Hearing Conservation Programmes Effective?

There are disappointingly few reports. Daniell and others [25] reviewed programmes of 10 companies in the state of Washington, USA. They concluded that using the 5 dB exchange rate instead of 3 dB substantially underestimates the extent of worker overexposure, and that, in the region they studied, small and medium-sized companies gave limited or no attention to noise control; after 20 years of OSHA regulations, hearing conservation programmes were commonly incomplete and HPD use was inadequate. Hearing protectors were most used in larger companies with higher noise levels. Lee-Feldstein [61] published a five year follow up of the HCP at 5 separate locations of a large automobile manufacturer.She found it to be effective in 4 of the 5 locations, some of which were very noisy.

Suter [2] in 2009 reviewed the impact of the US hearing conservation amendment of 1981. She concludes that the noise-exposed workforce is more knowledgeable about hazards of noise, the use of hearing protective devices has greatly increased and that there have been significant strides in the technology for measuring noise and for protecting hearing. She states that there is much room for improvement; some of the noise regulation provisions are "embarrassingly out-dated", some in dire need of improvement and others such as engineering controls are not being enforced. There is little progress in reducing overall noise exposure. There is need for a major overhaul of the noise regulations with emphasis on engineering control, a reduction of the permissible exposure limit to 85 dB, and a shift to the three dB exchange rate.

The findings of Singh in small and medium sized industry in India has been described above [55].Hansia and Dickinson[56] give a stark review of hearing conservation practices in South African gold mines. Many did not appreciate noise as a risk factor, and a goodly number were unaware of HPDs and more did not use them regularly.

A Cochrane review in 2009 [62] of interventions to prevent occupational noise induced hearing loss included 21 studies. 14 of them, with more than 75,000 participants, evaluated hearing loss prevention programmes and six others evaluated hearing protection. There is low-quality evidence that legislation can reduce noise levels in the workplace and the effectiveness of HPD's depends on their proper use. There is no evidence that substantial reductions occur in practice although audiometric and knowledge management data are potentially valuable. In another Cochrane review of interventions to promote the wearing of hearing protection [24] only two adequate trials were found! In one, a computer-based intervention tailored to the risk of individual workers was found to be no more effective than a video providing general information. The other, a cluster randomized controlled trial, evaluated the effect of a school-based hearing loss prevention programme on pupils working on their parents' farms.. The intervention group was twice as likely to wear some kind of hearing protection as the control group that received only minimal intervention. The study itself was too short to determine whether there was less hearing loss in the active group.

Conclusion

Industrial and military hearing conservation programmes are designed to protect hearing and maintain the ability to receive wanted or necessary sound. It appears that globally they are poorly understood and implemented. In the end the question is philosophical: is not a healthy workplace the right of man?

References

[1]　Schneider, E., Paoli, P., Brun, E. (2005). Noise in figures, Luxembourg, European Agency for Safety and Health at Work.

[2]　Suter, A. H. (2009). The hearing conservation amendment: 25 years later. *Noise and Health*, 11: 2-7.

[3]　Council for the Accreditation in Occupational Hearing Conservation (CAOHC) UPDATE (2004). Ototoxicity: An Issue in Hearing-Loss Prevention. *The Workplace*, 16, 7-9.

[4]　Hodgkinson, L., and Prasher, D. (2006). Effects of industrial solvents on hearing and balance: A review. *Noise and Health*, 8, 114-133.

[5]   Campo, P., Gabriel, S., Gómez, M. D. S., Toppila, E. (2009). Combined exposure to Noise and Ototoxic Substances Luxembourg: Office for Official Publications of the European Communities.Available from: http://osha.europa.eu/en/publications/literature_reviews/combined-exposure-to-noise-and-ototoxic-substances/vie(Accessed 18 October 2011).

[6]   Sliwinska-Kowalska, M. (2007). Exposure to organic solvent mixture and hearing loss: literature overview. *International Journal of Occupational Medicine and Environmental Health*, 20, 309-314.

[7]   Kaufman, L. R., LeMasters, G. K., Olsen, D. M., Succop, P. (2005). Effects of concurrent noise and jet fuel exposure on hearing loss. *Journal of Occupational and Environmental Medicine*, 47, 212-218.

[8]   Morata, T. C. and Little, M. B. (2002). Suggested guidelines for studying the combined effects of occupational exposure to noise and chemicals on hearing. *Noise and Health*, 4, 73-87.

[9]   Prasher, D. (2009). Heavy metals and noise exposure: Health effects. *Noise and Health* 11, 141-144.

[10] Teixeira, C. F., Da Silva, A. L. G., Morata, T. C. (2002). Occupational exposure to insecticides and their effects on the auditory system. *Noise and Health*, 4, 31-39.

[11] Crawford, J. M., Hoppin, J. A., Alavanja, C. R., Blair, A., Sandler, D. P., Kamel, F. (2008). Hearing loss amongst licensed Pesticide applicators. *Journal of Occupational and Environmental Medicine*, 50, 817-826.

[12] Fechter, L. D., Chen, G., Rao, D. (2002). Chemical asphyxiants and noise. *Noise and Health*, 4, 49-61.

[13] Morata, T. C., Engel, T., Durão, A., Costa, T. R. S., Krieg, E. F., Dunn, D. F., Lozano, M. A. (1997). Hearing Loss from Combined Exposures among Petroleum Refinery Workers. *Scandinavian Audiology*, 26, 141-114.

[14] Morata, T. C., Fiorini, A. C., Fischer, F. M., Krieg, E. F., Gozzoli, L., Colacioppo, S. (2001). Factors affecting the use of hearing protectors in a population of printing workers. *Noise and Health*, 4, 25-32.

[15] Sliwinska-Kowalska, M., Zamyslowska-Szmytke, E., Szymczak, W., Kotylo, P., Fiszer, M., Dudarewicz, A., Wesolowski, W., Pawlaczyk-Luszczynska, M., Stolarek, R. (2001). Hearing loss among workers exposed to moderate concentrations of solvents. *Scandinavian Journal of Work, Environment and Health*, 27, 335–342.

[16] Mohammadi, S., Labbafinejad, Y., Attarchi, M. (2010). Combined effects of ototoxic solvents and noise on hearing in automobile plant workers in Iran. *Archives of Industrial Hygiene and Toxicology*, 61, 267-274.

[17] Schaper, M., Seeber, A., Van Triel, C. (2008). The effects of toluene plus noise on hearing thresholds: an evaluation based on repeated measurement in the German printing industry. *International Journal of Environmental Medicine*, 21, 191 -200.

[18] EPA. (2011). Environmentally Safe, No VOC Automotive coating.Available from: http://cfpub.epa.gov/ncer_abstracts/index.cfm/fuseaction/display.abstract. Detail/abstract/1568/report/0 (Accessed 18 October 2011).

[19] Henderson, D., Morata, T. C., Hamernik, R. P. (2001). Considerations on assessing the risk of work-related hearing loss. *Noise and Health*, 3, 63-75.

[20] Hamernik, R. P. and Henderson, D. (1976). The potentiation of noise by other ototraumatic agents. In: D. Henderson, R. P. Hamernik, J. Mills, D. S. Dosanj (Eds.), *The effects of noise on hearing*. (pp.291-307). New York: Raven Press. Facts.

[21] Kryter, K. D. (1985). The Effects of Noise on Man. 2nd ed. Orlando: Academic Press.

[22] (Anonymous) Case study: pneumatic impact press reduction. 59/ EN Facts. 2005. Available from: http://EW2005.osha.eu.int (Accessed 18 October 2011).

[23] Hetu, R., Getty, Y., Quoc, H. T. (1995). Impact of Occupational Hearing loss on the lives of workers. *Occupational Medicine: State of the Art Reviews*, 10, 495-512.

[24] El Dib, R. P. and Mathew, J. L. (2009). Interventions to promote the wearing of hearing protection. *Cochrane Database of Systematic Reviews 2009*, Issue 4. Art. No.: CD005234. DOI: 10.1002/14651858.CD005234.pub3.

[25] Daniell, W. E., Swan, S. S., McDaniel, M. M., Camp, J. E., Cohen, M. A., Stebbins, J. G. (2005). Noise exposure and hearing loss prevention programs after 20 years of regulation in the United States. *Journal of Occupational and Environmental Medicine*, 63, 343- 351.

[26] Lietdke, M. (2003). Selection of Hearing Protection. *Health and Safety International*, 3, 13- 21.

[27] Cavallaro, G. (2009). Army says new earplugs will save your hearing. *Army Times*, Sept. 9, 2009.

[28] Norin, J. A., Emmanuel, D. C., Letowski, T. R. (2011). Speech intelligibility and passive level dependant earplugs. *Ear and Hearing*, in press.

[29] Sound Advice Working Group.Note 5, 2007. Available from: www.soundadvice.info/ - United Kingdom. (Accessed 18 October 2011).

[30] Buck, K. and Zimpfer-Jost, V. (2004). Active hearing protection systems and their performance. RTO - EN- HFM – 111. Available from: http://www.rta.nato.int/pubs/rdp.asp?RDP=RTO-EN-HFM-111 (Accessed 18 October 2011).

[31] Berger, E. H. (2002). Active noise reduction (ANR) in Hearing Protection: Does it make sense for industrial applications? Available from: http://www.e-a-r.com/pdf/hearingcons/anr.pdf (Accessed 18 October 2011).

[32] Casali, J. G., Ahroon, W. A., Lancaster, J. A. (2009). A field investigation of hearing protection and hearing enhancement in one device: For soldiers whose ears and lives depend upon it. *Noise and Health*, 11, 69-90.

[33] Anonymous. (2010). Geneva airport fire fighters choose Phonak active hearing Protection. Available from: http://www.airport-int.com/article/fire-fighters-electronic-ear-protection.html(Accessed 17 October2011).

[34] Environmental Protection Agency.(1978). Code of Federal regulations 40 211B Hearing Protective devices. U.S. Environmental Protection Agency.

[35] ANSI/ASA S12.6-2008. (2008). American National Standard Methods for Measuring the Real-Ear Attenuation of Hearing Protectors. Available from: http://asastore.aip.org/general.do (Accessed 18 October 2011).

[36] Murphy, W. J. (2008). How to assess hearing protection effectiveness: what is new in ANSI/ASA S 12. 68. *Acoustics today*, 4, 40-42.

[37] Abel, S. M., Tsang, S., Boyne, S. (2007). Sound localization with communications headsets: comparison of passive and active systems. *Noise and Health*, 9, 101-107.

[38] Abel, S. M., Sass-Kortsak, A., Kielar, A. (2002). The effect on earmuff attenuation of other safety gear worn in combination. *Noise and Health*, 5, 1-13.

[39] Schulz, T. Y. (2011). Individual fit-testing of earplugs: A review of uses. *Noise and Health*, 13, 152-162.

[40] Davis, R. R. and Shaw, P. B. (2011). Heat and humidity buildup under earmuff-type hearing protectors. *Noise and Health*, 13, 93-98.

[41] Publications on signal audibility while wearing hearing protectors. Available from: www.dguv.de/ifa/en/fac/laerm/pdf/signal_audibility_engl.pdf (Accessed 18 October 2011).

[42] Rabinowitz, P. M. and Duran, R. (2001). Is acculturation related to use of hearing protection? *American Industrial Hygiene Association Journal,* 62, 611-614.

[43] Abel, S. M. (2008). Barriers to hearing conservation programs in combat arms occupations. *Aviation, Space and Environmental Medicine*, 79, 591-598.

[44] Rovig, G. W., Bohnker, B. K., Page, J. C. (2004). Hearing health risk in a population of aircraft carrier flight deck personnel. *Military Medicine*, 169, 429-432.

[45] Kennedy, K. and Anderson, J. R. (2004). War is hell — on your hearing. Available from: www.armytimes.com/news/2010/04/offduty_hearing_042310w (Accessed 18 October 2011).

[46] McBride, D. I., Firth, H. M., Herbison, G. P. (2003). Noise exposure and hearing loss in agriculture: a survey of farmers and farm workers in the Southland region of New Zealand. *Journal of Occupation and Environmental Medicine,* 45,1281-1288.

[47] Miyakita, T., Ueda, A., Futatsuka, M., Inaoka, T., Nagano, M., Koyama, W. (2004). Noise exposure and hearing conservation for farmers of rural Japanese communities. *Journal of Sound and Vibration*, 27, 633-641.

[48] Bell, E. M., Sandler, D. P., Alavanja, M. C. (2006). High pesticide exposure events among farmers and spouses enrolled in the Agricultural Health Study. *Journal of Agriculture Safety and Health,* 12, 101-116.

[49] Perry, M. J. and May, J. J. (2005). Noise and chemical induced hearing loss: special considerations for farm youth. *Journal of Agromedicine*, 10, 49-55.

[50] Castrogiovanni, A. (2008). American Speech-Language-Hearing Association Communication Facts: Special Populations: Migrant Workers in the United States.Available from:www.asha.org/research/reports/migrant_workers.htm (Accessed 18 October 2011).

[51] Rabinowitz, P. M., Sircar, K. D., Tarabar, S., Galusha, D., Slade, M. D. (2005). Hearing loss in migrant agricultural workers. *Journal of Agromedicine*, 10, 9-17.

[52] Ehlers, J. J. and Graydon, P. S. (2011). Noise-induced hearing loss in agriculture: Creating partnerships to overcome barriers and educate the community on prevention. *Noise and Health,* 13, 142-146.

[53] Neitzel R, Seixas N. The effectiveness of hearing protection among construction workers. *J Occup Environ Hyg*. 2005; 2:227-38.

[54] Murphy, W. J., Byrne, D. C., Franks, J. R. (2007). Firearms and hearing protection. Hearing review and hearing review products.Available from: www.hearing review.com/issues/articles/2007-03_06.asp (Accessed 18 October 2011).

[55] Neitzel, R. L., Berna, B. E., Seixas, N. S. (2006). Noise exposures aboard catcher/processor fishing vessels. *American Journal of Industrial Medicine*, 49, 624-633.

[56] Singh, L. P., Bhardwaj, A., Deepak, K. K. (2010). Occupational exposure in small and medium scale industry with specific reference to heat and noise. *Noise and Health*, 12, 37-48.

[57] Hansia, M. R. and Dickinson, D. (2009). Hearing protection device usage at a South African gold mine. *Occupational Medicine*, 60, 72-77.

[58] Morata, T. C., Dunn, D. F., Kretschmer, L. W.,Lemasters, G. K., Keith, R. W. (1993). Effects of occupational exposure to organic solvents and noise on hearing.*Scandinavian Journal of Work, Environment and Health*, 19, 245-254.

[59] Saunders, G. H. and Griest, S. E. (2009). Hearing loss in veterans and the need for hearing loss prevention programs. *Noise and Health*, 11, 14-21.

[60] Kramer, S., Kapteyn, T., Houtgast, T. (2006). Occupational performance: Comparing normally-hearing and hearing-impaired employees using the Amsterdam Checklist for Hearing and Work. *International Journal of Audiology*, 45, 503-512.

[61] Lee-Feldstein, A. (1993). Five-year follow-up study of hearing loss at several locations within a large automobile company. *American Journal of Industrial Medicine*, 24,42-54.

[62] Verbeek, J. H., Kateman,E.,Morata, T. C., Dreschler, W., Sorgdrager, B. (2009). Interventions to prevent occupational noise induced hearing loss.*Cochrane database systemic reviews*, July 8; (3): C D006396

Useful Resources

National Hearing Conservation Association.http://www.hearingconservation.org/
Noise and Health.http://www.noiseandhealth.org/

In: Prevention of Hearing Loss
Editors: V. Newton, P. Alberti and A. Smith

ISBN: 978-1-61942-745-7
© 2012 Nova Science Publishers, Inc.

Chapter XIII

Social and Community Noise

Peter W. Alberti[*]

Abstract

This chapter deals with social and community noise. Social noise is none occupational sound intense enough to be potentially damaging to hearing, community noise is any unwanted sound disturbing a community at large. Globally social noise is increasing while in the industrialized countries at least, occupational noise levels are reducing.

Social noise has a major impact upon age related hearing loss, some of which could be prevented if social noise was better controlled. Sources of social noise discussed include music, recorded and live which has been implicated as ototraumatic, the evidence for which is reviewed. Sporting activities, even being an audience member at a football or hockey game can harm hearing.

Sport shooting is particularly hazardous. The use of power tools and hobbies and of motor driven gardening implements is also ototraumatic. Motorcycles and other motorsports including hobby flying are reviewed as noise sources. Toys may also be damaging to hearing.

Community noise, the sounds that impact groups of people in their everyday life are important causes of the annoyance, diminished quality of life and they facilitate the development of stress related diseases such as hypertension. In the industrialized countries the main sources are transportation noise, principally road and air. In the megacities of the emerging world city noise dominates.

The specific sound sources are reviewed as are steps taken to reduce them. Aircraft noise is a nuanced issue: there are more but quieter planes and there is a delicate balance between the economic benefit derived from the establishment and expansion of airports and the impact on health. Finally some of the regulations are reviewed.

---

[*] Corresponding author: peter.alberti@rogers.com.

Introduction

Sound is all pervasive. It is an important distant alerting mechanism and a means of communication, totally complementary to vision. The ability to perceive sound is virtually universal in vertebrates, the receptors function over a significant range of frequencies, are sensitive to low intensity sound and yet rugged enough not to be damaged until the intensity is extremely high. Sound intensity is measured in a logarithmic scale; from just audible to damaging in humans is at least 80 dB, an enormous dynamic range.

Excessive sound exposure, whether it is acute acoustic trauma or chronic overexposure, produces hearing loss and some systemic disturbances. Because of the usual insidious nature of noise induced hearing loss [NIHL], concerns for, or unnoticed overexposure are realistic, although sometimes exaggerated. The impact of all noise damage to the ear, whether occupational or social is cumulative through life; there is worry that occupational and increasing levels of social noise exposure will precipitate troublesome hearing loss at a younger age than at present.

For the purpose of this chapter community noise will be taken to mean unwanted sound, annoying a community at large and social noise will be taken to mean intense, potentially hearing damaging sound of none-occupational origin.

Community noise is not new: two centuries ago straw was strewn on granite roadways to silence horse's shoes; some cities paved their streets with wooden blocks to abate noises from horses' hooves and carriage wheels. However our soundscape has changed. The world is rapidly urbanizing and city sound levels appear to be increasing, from sources as varied as traffic, airplanes, construction, horticultural equipment, music and advertising. These are difficult subjects to study. Let us look first of all at some of the problems and then examine possible solutions. A good overview is provided by the World Health Organisation [1].

Problems of Excessive Noise

Noise is more than just intense sound; it is unwanted sound however loud it is. Although the distant sound of an airplane might not be noticed in the city, it may be an irritating noise on a wilderness camping trip; even if a sound is not intense enough to damage hearing it may disturb sleep and also lead to other unwanted social and medical consequences. This is the field of community noise. Intense sound, whether experienced at work or in the social context may temporarily or permanently reduce hearing acuity and it may induce tinnitus. This chapter deals with noise in a community and social context, occupational hearing loss [OHL] is dealt with in Chapter 12.

Does all this matter? Unequivocally yes! Much human communication is by speech and hearing and the prevalence of hearing loss sufficiently severe to interfere with communication is high [see Chapter 2] and increasing. This is due to growing global industrialization and greater use of loud entertainments, such as amplified music [both listening and making], recreational shooting, motorsports, and home crafts .All sound, if sufficiently intense, may damage hearing, whether the exposure be social, occupational or military. Unwanted noise is also a classic stress inducing agent, and has been implicated as a possible cause of many stress related disorders, cardiovascular and psychiatric in particular.

Let us deal with hearing first. There is huge variation in individual response to excessive sound. Toppila et al. have recently attempted to unravel some of the causes for these differences [2]. They point out that under the International Standards Organisation (ISO) table of risk database, exposure to 100 dBA for an eight hour day for 30 years produces a median hearing loss at 4 kHz of 45 dB but the range is over 60 dB between the 10th and 90th percentile! Various factors have been suggested to explain these differences such as failing to measure total daily sound exposure including social and transportation noise, listening to personal music devices, concert going and the recreational use of tools and firearms, an inherited susceptibility and a synergistic action of sound with inhaled solvents used in the workplace or at home. Even when other factors are considered there is still significant variation. These factors are an important matter when attempting to legislate safe sound levels for all and explain why 'safe level's for social noise exposure are lower than for industrial noise. Social standards are designed to protect 100% of the population, industrial levels about 97%.

It is appropriate at this point to describe briefly the effect of intense sound upon the ear. Loud sounds initially produce temporary threshold shift [TTS]; most people have experienced this perhaps after being at a loud concert, a noisy work place or using a loud power tool: after the sound stops hearing seems dull but this recovers over a period of some hours.

With repeated episodes the recovery becomes less complete leading to permanent threshold shift [PTS]. The progress is usually insidious and the loss often first noted by others. By contrast, exposure to a very intense sound, known as acute acoustic trauma, may produce severe immediate TTS, a residual PTS, as well as tinnitus. This type of incident is most common in the military but in the social context may be caused by a gas cylinders exploding, a nearby firework or even a clicker toy too close to the ear.

What is unknown at this time is the relationship between minimal TTS which apparently recovers completely and long-term hearing loss. There is suspicion that ears which suffer from recurrent mild, totally reversible TTS, as for example from long term listening to personal music players [PMPs] at high intensity, repeated visits to disco, or occasional sports shooting with light weapons, develop PTS earlier than would be expected from presbyacusis alone. The mechanism involved may include a change of protein/genetic structure of the hair cell as a protective mechanism against acute sound which however alters the total viability of the cell itself. In addition Kujawa and Lieberman have shown damage to the afferent neurons in animal studies may occur even when TTS recovers completely which leads to earlier PTS [3, 4]. Cochlear hair cells in mammals do not regenerate. Chronic exposure to intense sound may mean hearing thresholds deteriorate at a more rapid rate than would otherwise be expected, producing difficulty in the workplace, socially, in the family and a lonely old age. It has been suggested that the incidence of hearing loss is more severe in those with a damaged cardiovascular system as for example atherosclerosis [5, 6]. Diabetes may also be a cause of hearing loss [7].

Noise induced hearing loss occurs more frequently in males than females and in terms of social noise teenagers and young adults appear to be most at risk. Discos and rock concerts are the haunts of the young; so are motor driven vehicles such as snowmobiles, fast motorboats and motorcycles. Loud mechanical noise is often equated with power, strength and virility. Young men compete in a variety of motor sport events, such as snowmobile, motor car or motorcycle rallies and hydroplane races. The engines used in competition are rarely adequately silenced, if at all, and can wreak havoc with hearing. TTS is virtually a normal accompaniment of these pursuits; if they are practiced excessively so are varying degrees of PTS. The operators of these devices should be advised to wear earplugs, or noise excluding communication devices.

Specific Causes of Potentially Harmful Social Sound

Sound exposure, even at harmful levels, deliberately sought as in music listening is technically not noise (an unwanted signal), so some write of socially induced hearing loss (SINL) and others of music induced hearing loss (MIHL). This is pedantic and for the purpose of this chapter, any potentially harmful sound will be described as noise.

Music

Music appears to be a fundamental need of mankind [8]. All peoples of the world make music and have done so back as far as records exist. It arouses emotions and gives great pleasure but as with any other sound, if listened to at too great intensity can produce unexpected damage to hearing. This risk has increased markedly with improvements in amplification and the development of personal music players (PMPs) such as MP3 players. Amplified live music is a product of the 20th century and can be harmful to musician and audience alike. Hearing loss of the musicians is a particular form of occupational disorder, that of the audience, a social one.

Almost from the start there has been concern that listening to PMPs will permanently damage hearing. The variables involved are the maximum possible sound output levels of the earpieces, the volume at which the device is played, the daily exposure and the susceptibility of the ear of the listener. The issue is a contentious one.

There was considerable media, professional and parental concern that the Walkman and portable CD players would damage hearing, although most studies found little of concern: the listening time was about an hour a day and the input to the ear between mid-70s and mid-80s dBA. The dynamic range of music played on the radio and cassettes is much less than the original performance or what is found on current CDs and digital recordings. Radio broadcasts and cassettes compressed the dynamic range between the softest sound and the loudest sound. Thus the range was not great and the likelihood of producing damaging levels of sound above an easily heard quiet passage was low.

Matters changed with the introduction of the MP3 players and the ear bud headsets. The dynamic range of the device dramatically increased and the output of the ear bud was potentially higher than its predecessors. Also the number of devices sold increased exponentially, more than 200 million in Europe between 2004 and 2008. Since then sales have continued to grow as have those of smart telephones which double up as an MP3 player. Thus many more are at risk. Studies have been undertaken to find out how much these devices are listened to on a weekly basis, of the headsets that are used and of the intensity of sound in the ear canal. It would appear the most are used for about 1.5 hours per day 6 to 7 days a week. The great majority listened to at intensity between 75 and 85 dBA but some are played much louder [9]. The ear canal sound intensity is higher in those wearing ear buds than in those using earphones. It is suggested but not proven that the louder the background noise, the higher the intensity at which they are played [10]; thus the intensity may be higher if the MP3 player is used inside noisy public transport than if it used in quiet.

Actual evidence for immediate hearing loss produced by these devices is not great, but there is concern that there will be long term damage to hearing. There is also concern, shared by the author that repeated sound insults to the ear, even if not provoking immediate PTS somehow change the hair cell and cochlear biology to make it less resistant to later age related degeneration.

However MP3 players are only part of the music environment; live music is important to many who attend discos, dances and pop concerts. There is a psychological energy related to listening at high sound levels which gives pleasure to many but puts hearing at risk. Disc jockeys may suffer from occupational hearing loss, their dancers from social noise exposure. Listening to disco music frequently produces temporary threshold shift and tinnitus, some of the audience when leaving having reduced hearing which gradually recovers. Efforts have been made to limit sound levels in discos and clubs but in reality in most communities have been ineffective. The sound levels vary but in general seem to be in the upper 90s dB range [12]. For most people this is fairly safe as long as the exposure is limited to a few hours a week and is not added to other intense sound exposure, as for example workplace and transportation noise. Tinnitus from sound exposure is generally considered to be a warning sign of an ear at risk for hearing loss; those who develop tinnitus should be advised to carry earplugs and wear them when exposed to such high sound levels.

Live concerts are frequently played at very high sound intensities, frequently over 100 dBA. Unfortunately if the music is too intense it can produce tinnitus, temporary threshold shift and in the most susceptible, permanent diminution of hearing [11]. Some bands are louder than others: The Who was notorious and their leader Pete Townsend became hard of hearing and then a major advocate for hearing conservation in rock music.

While much is written about the hazards of each of these pastimes individually, it cannot be over emphasized that it is the total amount of sound which is important. There is an extensive EU report raising concerns about music listening and making recommendations to diminish the risk of hearing loss [13].In Europe about 20% of young people are exposed to high levels of social sound, a figure which has tripled over 30 years. The average A-weighted a sound exposure level from listening to PMPsis 75 to 85 dBA. While recognizing that these levels produce minimal risk of hearing loss it is nonetheless recommended that the level be limited to 80 dBA.

There is urgent need to educate children, teens and young adults of the risk to hearing of excessive sound exposure and its contribution to later hearing loss. This is considered important enough that the U.S. National Institute of Communication disorders (NICD) [14] launched a new hearing protection campaign in 2008 targeting Tween's and their parents, entitled "it's a noisy planet, Protect their hearing. There have also been attempts to educate younger children about the risks of hearing loss. One such is "sound sense, save your hearing for the music!", a programme developed for grade 4 to 7 schoolchildren as a complement to the general health curriculum in Canada by the Hearing Foundation of Canada [15]. An independent study shows residual impact after six months [16].

When people are informed they are more often prepared to take preventative measures than if unaware of the risk they run. The goal of these programmes is to raise awareness of the hazards of excessive noise exposure and to change behaviour patterns. There are enormous practical implementation difficulties; teachers already carry heavy workloads and any further topic thrown into the health education mix, however important, is seen as a burden. To be really effective hearing conservation education should be built in to the curriculum *ab initio*; parents must also be informed to be helpful in reinforcing the goal. The 'tween group may well be best served by "self-help" groups utilizing the web where they can research and self-educate. These efforts too require significant support.

Sporting Activities

Sporting activities also raise the decibels and induce tinnitus. Studies at U.S. football stadiums, college and professional, showed peak sound levels well into the mid-90s dBA during events, [17] hardly surprising as some of them are enclosed spaces.(Figure 14.1). The cheers and whistles in a hockey stadium can exceed 100dBA [18, 19] and at a playoff in 2006 exceeded the permissible daily dose within 6 minutes. More recently, the Football World cup saw the introduction of the Vuvuzela, a trumpet like buzzer which was enthusiastically espoused by the spectators, buzzing at over 100dBA into the ears of fellow spectators [20].

Small Arms

Shooting guns is a widespread pastime both as a means of hunting and as an end in itself. In season, in France and Italy the fields and forests ring with the sound shots; in the United States alone there are said to be about 20 million hunters and a slightly larger number of target shooters. If these figures are extrapolated even prudently to other countries, the total amount of exposure is great. Firing weapons not only disturbs others, it frequently damages the hearing of the shooter. Murphy et al [21] indicate the muzzle intensity of sounds from a variety of pistols; large bore shotguns used for hunting game are equally noisy.

Table 13.1. Safe exposure levels, Leq and Losha

Safe exposure (hours)		
Sound level dBA	Leq	Losha
85	8	16
87	5	13
90	4	8
92	1.5min	6
95	47 min	4
97	30 min	3
100	15 min	2
102	9	1.5
105	4.75 min	1

Population studies have shown that those who engage regularly in shooting have a significantly higher prevalence of high-frequency hearing loss than matched peers who do not [22]. Target shooters are more likely to wear hearing protectors than hunters, who wish to be able to hear everything in the terrain around them although some wear "hunter's muffs", earmuffs with the electronic amplifiers for environmental sound which cut out when the gun is fired. Duck hunters are particularly at risk because they shoot from reverberating blinds and often with multiple shooters firing simultaneously [23].

Carpentry, Power Tools, Hobby Metal Working

The home handyman is at risk from hearing loss from power tools such as drills, saws and grinders, all of which may have sound outputs well above a hearing safe level [24], although not many are labelled as such. Those using them should wear hearing protection as they would if they were using them in industry. Some hobbyists wear HPDs but it is more often the younger ones [25]. This is a common cause of hearing loss. It should be an imperative that schoolchildren learning 'industrial arts' be instructed in the use of safety equipment including hearing protection and that their instructors should set a good example, something that is frequently forgotten.

Gardening, Horticulture and Agriculture

At first sight these pursuits may be thought of as havens of quiet. This is far from the truth: mechanization has brought new sound sources which are disturbing to the spirit and may even be damaging to the ear. There are many pieces of gardening equipment which use two-stroke motors and perhaps fans, as for example lawnmowers, hedge clippers, chainsaws, leaf blowers and edgers, frequently worn as a backpack when used as a leaf blower or at chest level using edging devices. Their use, leads to complaints about noise from neighbours and may lead to operator hearing loss as virtually all have a sound output in excess of 85dBA.

Studies of the hearing of those living in agricultural communities shows significant prevalence of noise induced hearing loss from teenage onwards [26]. Farming knows no time constraint except sunrise and sunset; in the summer months hours worked may be extremely long, much more than eight hours and OHL is common; general-purpose chores, using chainsaws, working in heavily ventilated and noisy bird breeding buildings [turkeys and chickens] exposes workers to high intensity sound and the squeal of pigs frequently exceed100 dBA. Much of this is OHL but in family farms where the teenagers 'pitch in' it is better described as community noise. Education of school aged population in farming communities has been some benefit. The use of hearing protectors appears to be increasing as it does with the landscape gardening crew.

Motorcycles and Light Aircraft

Motorcycles are widespread worldwide, a source of annoying community noise and sound intense enough to damage the hearing of the operator. In addition to the engine sound, the wind noise around many helmets is high; long-standing motorcyclists know of these risks and use a variety of ear protection [27]. It should be emphasized that the crash helmet on its own is totally inadequate as a hearing protector. There are strange issues involved with motorcyclists and hearing protection; those who wish to protect their hearing and wear earplugs do so illegally in certain U.S. states, notably California, for the legislators deemed that the earplugs interfere with communication. The cabin sound level in light aircraft when the engine is revving for take-off and the propeller pitched for this phase of the flight, frequently is close to 100 dBA. This is both potentially damaging to the hearing of the pilot, frequently a hobby flyer and interferes with communication from the control tower. Pilots have for many years worn sound excluding communication headsets, but in these circumstances the addition of active noise reduction is helpful.

Toys

Many toys are noisy and if used incorrectly may produce TTS or even PTS. Two classical devices are the cap pistol and the frog clicker, both of which produce very intense sound. Recent developments in cheap electronics have enabled the production of many sound producing toys [28]. These include toy electric guitars, toy dolls which sing, replicas of heavy construction equipment with the requisite sound and worst of all, some toy pistols, submachine guns and guns. This latter group is in a noisemaking category of its own and may reach more than 140 dBC close to the device; this was intense enough to give the tester tinnitus. The loudness of a toy depends upon its distance from the ear and testing microphone; clearly louder at 3 than 30cm although often enough toys are held close. Those with sound levels between 80 and 100 dB are probably safe if not used for too long but the parents should at least be alert to the potential for harm. Percussive devices detonating too close to the ear can produce ringing, as well as temporary or even permanent threshold shift. There are lists published annually pre-Christmas in the UK and in the USA of the noisiest [29].Fireworks are persistent source of acoustic trauma.

In Western countries firework displays are frequently produced under controlled conditions and are therefore supposedly safe; in many parts of the world they are used frequently and randomly and may produce acoustic trauma, tinnitus, transient and perhaps permanent hearing loss because of proximity to the explosion. The louder larger fireworks are prohibited for general use in the United States and Canada; this is not necessarily true in other parts of the world.

The Chinese in particular use firecrackers to celebrate feast days and weddings. They come in large rolls and are ignited and sound like automatic small arms fire. Occasionally a roll explodes producing hearing loss as well as other injuries. There are several reports in the literature of individual cases of hearing damage [30] from exposure to fireworks but there are also others which take a population approach and have shown that small percentage of young people exposed fireworks as for example the Norwegian national day or the Diwali festival in India [31] develop a permanent high frequency notch. The prevention of this type of injury is aided by limiting the amount of explosive allowed in an individual firework and by using them under controlled conditions.

Community Noise

As the population expands and its density increases road, rail and air traffic produce soundscapes both urban and rural which become ever more cacophonous. Add to transport sounds local sources, such as advertising, gardening, church bells, calls to prayer, public clocks, street vendors and neighbours and urban quiet is a remote memory.

Excessive community noise causes harm to health and wellbeing. Living in a high noise environment may disturb sleep, increase the prevalence of anxiety and depression, of hypertension and increase the risks of heart attacks. There are also economic consequences, residential property is worth less if it is in a noisy place such as a flight path of an airport or adjacent to a busy highway. There are educational sequelae to learning in noisy classrooms (see below and Chapter 15).

Aircraft and other noise sources interrupt conversation, interfere with hearing and diminish the ability to listen to music and the sounds of nature. Noise can have high nuisance value as well as possible health effects. It appears that excessive sound exposure, particularly if intermittent, and therefore more repetitively alarming than steady-state noise, inflicts stress on the exposed individual and the response is according to the general stress hypothesis proposed more than half a century ago by Hans Selye, an adrenergic fight, steroid flight response [32].

Community noise may be local, such as air-conditioning noise or excessive construction sound or more general, as for example wind farms and transportation noise. In developed countries, with lower urban population densities transportation noise is the major general issue; in developing country mega cities, general community noise including urban vehicle sounds takes pride of place. General construction projects, whether erecting new buildings or repairing infrastructure are frequent sources of complaint, but at least the 'project life' is finite.

Let us look at some of these sound sources. When window unit air conditioners were first introduced their noise irritated neighbours; they were followed by central air-conditioning units with larger outdoor compressors which raised a flurry of nocturnal noise complaints that have settled as the units have become almost universal, as sound insulation improved and because as more people install air conditioning, the noise of their own device is less irritating than that of the neighbours.

Low-frequency sound is more difficult to mask than high-frequency sound and to some is extremely irritating. There are many anecdotes about sleepless nights supposedly produced by listening to distant compressors or a new heat pump in someone else's backyard. The most recent and widespread iteration of this complaint is annoyance from the presence of wind turbines.

Wind Turbines

Wind turbines raise emotions, both positive and negative. Many people applaud their introduction because of the greener energy production but others complain about their aesthetics and disturbance from their sound, particularly at night. This has been studied fairly extensively in the EU, UK and the USA. The science is difficult. Wind turbines produce a slight thrumming low frequency sound which is more noticeable than a steady-state; this may be emphasised when several wind turbines are sited close to each other. The larger the turbine, the higher the noise production, presupposing similar design. Fairly straightforward reviews of the issues involved are given by Van den Berg [33] and in a report from the acoustic ecology Institute of Santa Fe, available on the web [34].

In general terms people become accustomed to a background noise which has been introduced into their basic soundscape. Wind farms are frequently in the countryside which is intrinsically quieter than an urban setting. If there is an intrusion more than 4 or 5 dB above the background sound, the intrusion is frequently perceived as annoying. The relative intensity required to produce annoyance is less at night than during the day and when this is coupled with a reduction of other night-time noise as for example less traffic sound, the turbine may dominate. Turbine sound also has higher intensity at night due to cooler air and probably higher wind speed.

Noxious stimuli irritate more when there is no personal benefit; when neighbourhoods have a financial stake in the wind turbines, the complaints tend to be very much less. Full discussion before turbines are erected is highly recommended so that the community has bought into their presence. It is recommended that in the absence of a background of masking sound, the nearest habitation should be about 1 km away from the turbines. This may be difficult to achieve in densely crowded EU countries, so more and more wind farms are being put out to sea but it should be noted that airborne and waterborne sound may be transmitted uninterrupted for long distances.

Transportation Noise

Exposure to high levels of sound is extremely common; The WHO estimates that 40% of the population of the EU is exposed to road traffic noise in excess of 55dBA and 20 % to levels in excess of 65dBA [1]; the numbers continue to grow as road traffic increases and airports expand. The proportions are higher in the UK [35] than the EU and the numbers exposed in developing world conurbations are higher again as are the sound levels. There have been many studies of annoyance produced by noise exposure but they all tell virtually the same story.

The main metrics used are 'annoyance' and sleep disturbance which are also the driving force in setting regulations for maximum noise levels. As far as community noise is concerned the most common annoying sound is road traffic followed by air-traffic and rail. Where air-traffic is evident, it becomes the major source of annoyance. One exception in Europe is Denmark where complaints about wind turbine noise dominate. There is relatively less air and rail noise compared to neighbouring countries and there are many more wind turbines.

Almost universally it appears that above 50 dBA complaints begin to rise quite steeply. A major German study [36] evaluated the difference in reaction to rail, road and air traffic. There are fewest complaints about railway noise and most about air traffic at the same intensity. At night the same levels of airport noise annoyed more than during the day; there was no day/night difference with road traffic and railway noise was less bothersome at night than during the day. Annoyance from air-traffic noise also rises more steeply as the sound intensity increases than for the other sources. Night-time noise may disturb sleep; as the ability to have uninterrupted sleep is highly valued, regulators in Europe placed a penalty of 10 dB for night-time exposure; noise regulations are frequently published with different daytime [L_{day}] and night-time [L_{night}] upper limits of acceptability.

In addition to being annoying, noise can be harmful to health and well-being. What levels of noise are considered harmful? Below 30 dBA, the sort of level found in quiet countryside, is totally safe; there is only evidence of harmless physiological response between 30 and 40 dBA. Above this level there is increased sleep disturbance and complaints. Above 55 dBA there may be significant cardiovascular issues. Building structure provides about 15 dB of protection even with the windows open. In addition the position of the bedroom is important: someone sleeping at the back of the house away from a highway or railway line is subjected to less intense sound than someone at the front.

In Europe, where it is assumed that people will sleep with a window partially open, the long-term goal for outdoor night-time sound levels is 40 dB but as an interim measure 55 dB is accepted.

This assumption is not made in the U.S. and further, the FAA has a programme to help insulate homes from sound produced within aircraft flight paths. This leads to slightly different acceptable levels of external sound, but in both cases are stricter at night than during the day. It should be noted that these levels are five dB lower than recommended by WHO in 1999 [37].

There are differences in those who complain about noise. The elderly complain least, it is suggested because they have other more important things to complain about; the writer suggests it may also be because the hearing is less acute, one of the few benefits of presbyacusis of which he has personal experience.

Those in poorer socioeconomic conditions seem to complain more; it is suggested this is because of frustration due to their circumstances being unlikely to change. While children are amongst the most vulnerable to the harmful effects of excessive sound they do not complain much.

What has been described so far pertains to the industrialized economies of Europe and North America. Many other countries are much louder and fewer controls exist. In the EU complaints about levels of urban environmental noise begin to escalate at 50dBA and above; in South Asia many cities regularly exceed 70dBA in residential areas.main sources are cars and truck engines, exhausts and pressure klaxons, music, religious institutions and marching bands associated with weddings.

Part of the reason for the difference is the much greater population density in the developing countries. The most densely populated city in the World is Mumbai, >29,000 people per sq. km; the most densely populated in Europe, 25th in the world ranking, St Petersburg (8500/sq. km).

There are 20m cities in Europe with population densities higher than the most densely populated North America city, 90th on the world list, Los Angeles (2750/sq. km) [38]. This explains the recent high interest in the EU in the matter of noise. There are several studies of sound levels in a variety of South Asian cities e.g. Karachi, Dhaka and Mumbai [39, 40, 41].As with the population of European cities, stress levels may be high [42]. These matters are dealt with further in Chapter (17).

The Impact of Excessive Community Sound

Environmental sound affects many facets of life including education, health and general well-being.

Education

Children learn better in a classroom in which it is bright enough to see and quiet enough to hear. The impact of environmental sound on learning is sufficiently great that the EU established project RANCH (*road traffic and aircraft noise and children's cognition and health*) to evaluate this. A major resulting multi country study by Stansfeld et al. [43] found that chronic exposure to aircraft noise could impair cognitive development in children and especially their reading skills. They found no impact from highway noise. They conclude that schools exposed to high levels of aircraft noise are unhealthy educational environments. Matsui and colleague evaluated children attending 19 schools around [44] London's Heathrow airport and also interviewed their parents. They found a significant dose-response relationship between aircraft noise exposure at home and performance on memory tests of immediate/delayed recall. However there was no strong association with other cognitive outcomes. Green et al [45] found that in New York City students in the schools most affected by airport noise were one full year behind their peers in other schools in reading ability. By contrast road traffic noise has been shown to impair reading speed (but not comprehension) and basic mathematics (but not mathematical reasoning) in Swedish schoolchildren aged 12-13 years [46].

The problems of learning in classrooms alongside the New York elevated railway are well detailed by Bronzaft [47]: children were doing so badly in classrooms facing the rail track that they were moved to the back of the school with great improvement in school performance. Her article summarizes years of work in the area.

Excessive environmental noise not only interferes with the children's hearing, it also increases the difficulty that teachers have in making themselves understood over a background sound. Teachers speak less, especially under the flight path of aircraft and suffer considerable vocal stress.

Open Plan Classrooms

Shield [48] and colleagues have recently undertaken a review of the effects of noise in open plan classrooms. They discuss methods of reducing unwanted sound and indicate that children with learning disability including those with hearing impairment do less well in this environment although others can thrive.

Health Issues

There have been major studies of annoyance and health issues related to airport, highway and rail traffic noise in the UK, EU, Canada and the U.S.. They are particularly relevant when planning new roads or airports and regulating operating times. Sleep disturbance is an important marker of health, which in Europe is measured by increased in motion during sleep, a sensitive measure. The U.S. uses a less sensitive but more robust measure, the number of awakening episodes. [49, 50]. Annoyance from noise increases the amount of sleep disturbance from highway and aircraft noise. After a while, people habituate to the sleep disturbance and wake less frequently. However their autonomic response to noise does not habituate and persists indefinitely.

An indirect link with the development of cardiovascular disease has been established: too much noise disturbs sleep and the sleep disturbance is related to the development of anxiety, hypertension, perhaps heart attacks and interferes with normal daytime performance including learning at school. As noise levels increase there is an increasing frequency of clinical hypertension and the risk continues to increase as the sound levels rise [51]. The prescription frequency of blood pressure-lowering medications is associated dose-dependently with aircraft noise from a level of about 45 dBA upwards, the results for antihypertensive use are not constant across countries; those for anxiolytics and antacids are.

Ndrepepa and Twardella [52] undertook a metadata analysis of the relationship between road traffic noise annoyance and cardiovascular disease. They found a positive relationship with hypertension and a weak relationship with ischaemic heart disease. There were statistically no significant associations between road traffic noise and the incidence of ischemic heart disease in the highway studies at Caerphilly and Speedwell in the UK [53], but there was a suggestion of effects when modifying factors such as length of residence, room orientation, and window opening were taken into account. The relationship with aircraft noise disturbance is more robust. In the Hypertension and Exposure to Noise near Airports (HYENA) [54] study, night time aircraft noise exposure (L_{night}) was associated with an increased risk of hypertension, in fully adjusted analyses. A 10-dB increase in aircraft noise exposure was associated with an odds ratio of 1.14 (95%CI, 1.01 - 1.29). As Babisch and van Kamp point [54] out,"Noise is a stressor that affects the autonomic nervous system and the endocrine system. It has been shown that excessive noise also leads to release of adrenal hormones: catecholamines and corticosteroids, chronic high levels of which may lead to cardiovascular disease. Under conditions of chronic noise stress the cardiovascular system may adversely be affected." He suggests that road traffic noise increases the risk of ischaemic heart disease, there is less evidence for this with airport noise, which however seems to lead to clinically significant hypertension. Kaltenbach et al [55] also suggest that in residential areas aircraft daytime noise in excess of equivalent of 60 dBA and 45 dBA at night are associated with an increased incidence of hypertension and that there is a dose response relationship between aircraft noise and inter-current arterial hypertension.

Psychiatric Disease

It was suggested many years ago that living in high levels of sound near airports produced excessive numbers of mental hospital admissions [56]. These studies are extremely difficult; the literature has some cross-sectional studies but no longitudinal ones. Frequently those living in insalubrious areas do so because that is all they can afford, perhaps because of pre-existing sickness. Stansfeldet al.[53] has reviewed this area quite extensively including a joint older study [57].They conclude that there is no evidence of community noise producing psychiatric disease, but it does increase symptoms of anxiety. There may be a greater use of hypnotics amongst adults and even some children living along aircraft flight paths in proximity to airports. Living alongside highways leads at most to a slight increase in anxiety, but not other psychiatric disease.The relationship between excessive noise and chronic disease is the subject of continuing difficult study. It is necessary to have detailed noise exposure measurements and epidemiological analysis to determine whether the prevalence of various disorders is greater than in the population at large, and then long term studies to see if the various disorders develop more rapidly in the population living in noisy areas than in matched population living in quiet. One of the confounding issues with population studies is that most are not matched with similar none noise exposed populations and they run the risk of having inappropriate conclusions drawn.

Transportation Noise

This section deals with highway, rail and aircraft noise.

Highway traffic is a major source of annoying noise in North America and Europe, the most significant in Canada [58] and the Netherlands [50] and by inference, elsewhere because it is so ubiquitous. Where airports operate at night they may overwhelm road traffic noise as the prime nuisance within their operational footprint. Highway sound is caused by engine noise, including intake of air for combustion and exhaust emission, by tires and highway composition. Tire tread design has changed in order to make them safer and quieter; road surfaces too are being altered to reduce sound. Untreated concrete surfaces are much noisier than asphalt. In warmer climates it is possible to make asphalt a little spongy so that it absorbs more sound than if it was solid; this is not possible on highways that are subject to snow and ice. Large commercial trucks are now much quieter than they were in the late 20th century although the use of older noisy vehicles (which are also more air polluting) in the developing world is a great concern. Barriers have been erected along highways in urban areas in order to divert sound upwards and disperse it more widely subjecting fewer houses close to the highway to excessive sound. These work mainly for homes within 100m of the highway, and must block line of sight from the noise source. For trucks this may be the exhaust, stuck in the air, so the barrier must be about 3m tall. For those in proximity, barriers reduce sound levels by 5-10 dB.

Rail noise is now much less of a problem than that from highways; welded tracks, rigid couplings and in many countries the adoption of electric locomotives has reduced sound levels significantly. The sound of trains increases slowly as the train approaches and diminishes slowly as it disappears so that there is no sudden change; humans adapt to this extremely well. Hundreds of thousands of people live alongside rail tracks with much less complaint than from those under the flight paths or along highways. In North America replacement of level crossings with bridges and underpasses has turned the iconic clanging of locomotive bells into distant memories.

The major exception is certain older above ground city rail transport systems as for example the 'El' (elevated rail track) in New York. This has been the subject of complaint about noise from riders and residents virtually since it was built in the 19th century. Bronzaft [47] has written extensively about this and especially its impact on education (see above). It seems likely that other elevated city trains produce similar problems especially if the trains run on elevated unshielded tracks and have tighter curves and thus more wheel squeal than faster lines.

Airport Annoyance

Airports are vital feature of 21st century urban commercial, economic and social life. They add immeasurably to the economy of the region which they serve and yet the noise that is created by aircraft and related road traffic is a constant concern to those residing within the vicinity or the flight path. How can this be minimized? There have been major efforts to reduce sound from aircraft. Aircraft have become larger and quieter. The current generation of jet engines is less noisy than its predecessor. However, the number of passengers flying is steadily increasing and air freight traffic is growing rapidly. Aircraft noise has been reduced by 20 dB in the past 50 years and in the U.S. there has been a 95% reduction in aircraft noise exposure since 1975 in spite of great growth in passenger traffic. This change is continuing as 747-200s and 767 jet liners are being phased out on economic grounds and being replaced by the quieter current jets. [59]

Nevertheless, aircraft noise persists and continues to disturb, a particular problem in densely packed conurbations as in Europe. Careful attention has been paid in some areas to the layout of runways and flight paths. However even when an airport is initially in the countryside it is often a magnet for developers; indeed Lindsay and Kasarda [60] suggest that airports are important economic drivers and attract industry around them which in turn spawns associated residential development (the Aerotropolis) and complaints about noise.

The economic benefit on a macro scale is real, but on a micro scale may be negative, particularly in terms of house values. Thus any efforts to build a new airport or expand existing ones are usually fiercely resisted and then only undertaken with significant prior study. The Germans have carried out extensive surveys of problems related to sound levels near airports, including studies both at Munich, Frankfurt and Cologne; there have been studies in London, Los Angeles and Atlanta and many others beside. When a plan to expand Frankfurt airport was unveiled in 1998 studies were initiated to identify the effects of aircraft noise in the vicinity of the airport and the final approval decision was not taken until all of the studies were available, more than 5 years later. Recent studies from Frankfurt which will serve as one model for others [61] showed that for equal amounts of sound exposure, aircraft noise was more annoying than that from trains or roads, it impacted the environmental quality of life, and to a lesser extent, health. There was a direct relationship between the equivalent sound level of aircraft and aircraft noise annoyance and it was higher than predicted from general exposure response curves. Citizens were concerned about their future environment and mistrustful of the authorities to reduce sound levels. Aircraft noise had an impact on noise specific stress reactions. People with pre-existing other morbid conditions showed more annoyance from noise than healthy ones. The relationships were not total; rather those with the most limited resources to cope with the noise were the most distressed by it. Longitudinal studies are required to assess these matters further.

If the predictions of the next generation of jet engines and planes are fulfilled, even with the addition of a third runway, the noise footprint at Heathrow airport may actually reduce. The development of quieter and more fuel efficient aircraft is an industry imperative [59]

The economic consequences of such evaluations are huge. In some jurisdictions airports close at night in order to combat problems and complaints about sleep disturbance and its resultant ill health. In others, operations are limited during the night time hour, which diminishes traffic, business and reduces some of the economic benefit of the airport.

There is also concern about the value of homes in the vicinity of airports which has been the subject of much study, under the general title 'hedonic property values'. A good meta-analysis published by Nelson [62] in 2004 of 20 studies in the U.S. and Canada shows a weighted discount value in property prices of 0.5 – 0.6% per decibel up to 75dBA in the USA and 0.8 -0.9% in Canada. However these are not simple situations; as aircraft become quieter, the noise footprint of airports may indeed be diminishing [59], always offset by traffic growth. Some estimates are given for the vicinities of Heathrow and east Midlands airports. On the other hand there may well be an increase in the value of commercial and industrial property because they are in the vicinity of new airports.

Regulation

In the 1960s community noise, which had been steadily increasing became the target of legislation in Japan in the 1960s and the UK in the early 70s. In 1969 the U.S. passed the National Environmental Policy act (NEPA) followed by the Noise Control act (NCA) in 1972. A system of highways had been developed, transportation noise had increased significantly, loud jet aircraft were proliferating and life in many people's communities was being disturbed. The environmental protection agency (EPA) worked assiduously to reduce noise and assumed much of the regulatory power. States and cities developed anti-noise laws and regulations; the U.S. became quieter. Then in 1981 the funding for this programme was withdrawn by Congress and the EPA programme shrank dramatically. The FAA has control of aircraft noise and combines its noise regulatory powers with the need to keep aircraft flying. Certain cities, notably Portland, Oregon have stringent noise rules which are applied; California attempts to implement community noise laws and regulations but in general anti-noise regulations in the U.S. have become a patchwork of rules frequently without much enforcement. It is no surprise that Europe is now being much more proactive in the regulation of community noise levels; the population density is much greater than in the U.S. and the supranational parliament, the EU has taken upon itself the need to regulate (frequently by directive) many things within Europe, including noise. There are extensive EU publications on noise, both industrial and community, to which the reader is directed [50, 63] often based on detailed research projects on noise levels around airports and the impact of noise levels on individuals. The European Parliament and Council in 2002 adopted a directive[63] the main aim of which is to provide a common basis for tackling noise problem. It contains three main points which underline the need for public involvement and initiative: Monitoring the environmental problem; Informing and consulting the public; Addressing local noise issues. This led a long-term EU strategy and corresponding deadlines to diminish noise problems. Many developing countries have anti community noise regulations including Pakistan and China [64, 65], but few have the means or the will to implement them.

Conclusion

Sound is a vital means of communication: it provides distant warning, enables complicated communication such as speech and provides pleasure. Many sounds are unwanted, frequently by-products of other activities and they can interfere with the reception of wanted signals as well as disturbing tranquility which is an important need for good health.

Much social sound is so intense that it damages hearing of individuals; community noise interferes with the whole populations and, continues to worsen as the world's population grows. It is important that communities recognize the problems produced by noise so that the levels can be reduced and so that legislation can be passed and most importantly, acted upon. These are import measures for global health which are not sufficiently widely recognized.

References

[1]   Berglund, B., Lindvall, T., Schwela, D. H. (2000). Guidelines for Community Noise. Geneva, World Health Organisation.

[2]   Toppila, E., Ishizaki, H., Pyykko, I., Starck, J., Kaksonen, R. (2000). Individual risk factors in the development of noise-induced hearing loss. *Noise and Health*, 2, 59-70.

[3]   Kujawa, S. G., Liberman, M. C. (2009). Adding insult to injury: cochlear nerve degeneration after "temporary" noise-induced hearing loss. *Journal of Neuroscience*, 11, 29:14077-14085.

[4]   Lin, H. W., Furman, A. C., Kujawa, S. G., Liberman, M. C. (2011). Primary neural degeneration in the guinea pig cochlea after reversible noise-induced threshold shift. *Journal of Associated Research in* Otolaryngology, 12: 605-16.

[5]   Cruickshanks, K. J., Wiley, T. L., Tweed, T. S., Klein, B. E. K., Klein, R., Mares-Perlman, J. A., Nondahl, D. M. (1998). Prevalence of hearing loss in older adults in Beaver Dam, Wisconsin: The epidemiology of hearing loss study. *American Journal of Epidemiology*, 148, 879-886.

[6]   Yoshioka, M., Uchida, Y, Sugiura, S., Ando, F., Shimokata, H., Nomura, H., Nakashima, T. (2010). The impact of arterial sclerosis on hearing with and without occupational noise exposure: a population-based aging study in males. *Auris Nasus Larynx*, 37, 558-564.

[7]   Kakarlapudi, V., Sawyer, R., Staecker, H. (2003). The effect of diabetes on sensorineural hearing loss. *Otology and Neurotology*, 24, 382–386.

[8]   Ball, P. (2010). *The Music Instinct*, London: Bodley Head.

[9]   Kahari, K. R., Aslund, T., Olsson, J. (2011). Preferred sound levels of portable music players and listening habits among adults: A field study. *Noise and Health*, 13, 9-15.

[10] Hodgetts, W. E., Rieger, J. M., Szarko, R. A. (2007). The effects of listening environmemnt and earphone style on preferred listening levels of normal hearing adults using an MP3 player. *Ear and Hearing*, 28, 290-297.

[11] Hohmann, B. W., Luy, D., Mercier, V. (2003). The sound exposure of the audience at a music festival. *Noise and Health*, 5, 51-58.

[12] Williams, W., Beach, E. F., Gilliver, M. (2010). Clubbing. The cumulative effect of noise exposure from attendance at dance clubs and night clubs on whole-of-life noise exposure. *Noise and Health*, 12, 155-158.

[13] Potential health risks of exposure to noise from personal music players and mobile phones including a music playing function Preliminary report, 2008. Available from: http://ec.europa.eu/health/ph_risk) (Accessed 18 October 2011).

[14] Its a noisy planet. Available from: www.noisyplanet.nidcd.nih.gov/Pages/Default.aspx NICDC (Accessed 18 October 2011).

[15] Sound Sense™ Available from: http://www.soundsense.ca/ (Accessed 18 October 2011).

[16] Neufeld, A., Westerberg, B. D., ~~Nabi~~, S., Bryce, G., Bureau, Y. (2011). Prospective, randomized controlled assessment of the short and long-term efficacy of a hearing conservation education program in Canadian elementary school children. *Laryngoscope*, 121,176–181.

[17] Engard, D. J., Sandfort, D. R., Gotshall, R. W., Brazile, W. J. (2010). Noise exposure, characterization, and comparison of three football stadiums. *Journal of Occupation and Environmental Hygiene* 7, 616-621.

[18] Behar A. (2007). *Hockey playoff noise.Canadian Medical Association Journal*, 176, 1462.

[19] Hodgetts, W. E., Liu, R. (2006). Research letter:Can hockey playoffs harm your hearing? *Canadian Medical Association Journal*, 175, 1503.

[20] Ramma, L., Petersen, L., Singh, S. (2011). Vuvuzelas at South African soccer matches: Risks for spectators' hearing. *Noise and Health*, 13, 71-75.

[21] Murphy, W. J. (2008). How to assess hearing protection effectiveness: what is new in ANSI/ASA S 12.68. *Acoustics today*, 4,40-42.

[22] Nondahl, D. M., Cruickshanks, K. J., Wiley, T. L., Klein, R., Klein, B. E., Tweed, T. S. (2000). Recreational firearm use and hearing loss. *Archives of Family Medicine*, 9, 352-357.

[23] Stewart, M., Borer, S. E., Lehman, M. (2009). Shooting habits of U.S. waterfowl hunters. *Noise and Health*, 1, 8-13.

[24] McClymont, L. G. and Simpson, D. C. (1989). Noise levels and exposure patterns to do-it-yourself power tools. *The Journal of Laryngology and Otology*, 103, 1140-1141.

[25] Nondahl, D. M., Cruickshanks, K. J., Dalton, D. S., Klein, B., Klein, R., Tweed, T. S., Wiley, T. L. (2006). The use of hearing protection devices by older adults during recreational noise exposure. *Noise and Health*, 8, 147-153.

[26] Ehlers, J. J. and Graydon, P. S. (2011). Noise-induced hearing loss in agriculture: Creating partnerships to overcome barriers and educate the community on prevention. *Noise and Health*, 13, 142-146.

[27] Motor cycle helmet noise. Available from: www.webbikeworld.com/motorcycle-helmets/helmet-noise.htm (Accessed 18 October 2011).

[28] Anonymous. Noisy toys. Health issue of the month. Sight and Hearing Association. Dec 2005. Available from: http://www.sightandhearing.org/news/healthissue /archive/hi_1205.asp29. (Accessed 17 October 2011).

[29] Anonymous.Hearing Loss in children: Annual Noisy Toys List (p3). Available from : www.healthyhearing.com/content/articles/Hearing-loss/Protection/47675 Accessed 18 October 2011).

[30] Segal, S., Eviatar, E., Lapinsky, J., Shlamkovitch, N., Kessler, A. (2003). Inner ear damage in children due to noise exposure from toy cap pistols and firecrackers : A retrospective review of 53 cases. *Noise and Health*, 5, 13-18.

[31] Gupta, D. and Vishwakarma, S. K. (1989). Toy weapons and firecrackers: a source of hearing loss. *Laryngoscope*, 99, 330-334.

[32] Babisch, W. (2002). The noise/stress concept, risk assessment and research needs. *Noise and Health*, 4, 1-11.

[33] Van den Berg, F., Pedersen, E., Bouma, J., Bakker, R. (2008). Project WINDFARMperception, Visual and acoustic impact of wind turbine farms on residents. Available from:www.windaction.org (Accessed 18 October 2011).

[34] Cummings, J. (2010). Wind Farm Noise: 2009 in Review (p4) Available from: www.acousticecology.org/srwind.html. (Accessed 18 October 2011).

[36] Stansfeld, S. and Crombie, R. (2011). Cardiovascular effects of environmental noise: Research in the United Kingdom. *Noise and Health,* 13, 229-233.

[36] Hoeger, R., Schreckenberg, D., Felscher-Suhr, U., Griefahn B. (2002). Night-time noise annoyance : State of the art. *Noise and Health,* 4, 19-25.

[37] Night Noise Guidlelines for Europe. Available from: www.euro.who.int/__data/assets (Accessed 18 October 2011).

[38] The largest cities in the world by land area, population and density Ranked by population density: 1 to 125. Available from: http://www.citymayors.com/statistics (Accessed 18 October 2011).

[39] Zaidi, S. H. (1989). Noise levels and the sources of noise pollution in Karachi. *Journal of the Pakistan Medical Association,* 39, 62-65.

[40] Chakraborty, M. R., Khan, H. S., Samad, M. A., Amin, M. N. (2005). Noise level in different places of Dhaka Metropolitan City (DMC) and noise-induced hearing loss (NIHL) in Dhaka City dwellers. *Bangladesh Medical Research Council Bulletin.* 31, 68-74.

[41] Ambient (p6). Noise Monitoring Metropolitan Cities December 2009. Available from: http://mpcb.gov.in/images (Accessed 18 October 2011).

[42] Suchday, S., Kapur, S., Ewart, C. K., Friedberg, J. P. (2007). Urban stress and health in developing countries: Development and validation of a neighborhood stress index for India. *Behavioral Medicine,* 32, 77-86.

[43] Stansfeld, S. A., Berglund, B., Clark, C., Lopez Barrio, I., Fischer, P., Ohrstrom, E., Haines, M. M., Head, J., Hygge, S., Van Kamp, I., Berry, B. (2005). Aircraft and road traffic noise and children's cognition and health: exposure-effect relationships. *The Lancet,* 365, 1942-1949.

[44] Matsui, T., Stansfeld, S., Haines, M., Head, J. (2004). Children's cognition and aircraft noise exposure at home-the West London Schools Study. *Noise and Health,* 7, 49-57.

[46] Green, K. B. and Pasternack, B. S., Shore, R. E. (1982). Effects of aircraft noise on reading ability of school-age children.*Archives of Environmental Health,* 37, 24-31.

[46] Ljung, R., Sorqvist, P., Hygge, S. (2009). Effects of road traffic noise and irrelevant speech on children's reading and mathematical performance. *Noise and Health,* 11, 194-198.

[47] Bronzaft, A. L. (2010). Abating New York city transit noise: A matter of will, not way. *Noise and Health,* 12, 1-6.

[48] Shield, B., Greenland, E., Dockrell, J. (2010). Noise in open plan classrooms in primary schools: A review. *Noise and Health,* 12, 225-234.

[49] Miller, N. P.and Schomer, P. D. (2009). How many people will be awakened by noise tonight? *Acoustics today,* 5, 26-31.

[50] Night noise guidelines (nngl)for Europe, (2007). World Health Organisation. Available from: http://ec.europa.eu/health/ph_projects/2003/action3/docs/2003_08_frep_en.pdf (Accessed 18 October 2011).

[51] Floud, S., Vigna-Taglianti, F., Hansell, A., Blangiardo, M., Houthuijs, D., Breugelmans, O., Cadum, E., Babisch, W., Selander, J., Pershagen, G., Antoniotti, M. C., Pisani, S., Dimakopoulou, K., Haralabidis, A. S., Velonakis, V., Jarup, L. on behalf of the HYENA study team. (2011). Medication use in relation to noise from aircraft and road traffic in six European countries: results of the HYENA study. *Occupationand Environmental Medicine*, 68, 518-524. Epub. 2010 Nov. 16.

[52] Ndrepepa, A. and Twardella, D. (2011). Relationship between noise annoyance from road traffic noise and cardiovascular diseases: A meta-analysis. *Noise and Health*, 13, 251-259.

[53] Stansfeld, S. A. and Matheson, M. P. (2003). Noise pollution: non-auditory effects on health. *British Medical Bulletin*, 68, 243-257.

[54] Babisch, W. and Kamp, Van I. (2009). Exposure-response relationship of the association between aircraft noise and the risk of hypertension. *Noise and Health*, 11, 161-168.

[55] Kaltenbach, M., Maschke, C., Klinke, R. (2008). Health Consequences of Aircraft Noise. *Deutsches Arzteblatt International*, 105, 31-32.

[56] Abey-Wickrama, I., A'Brook, M. A., Gattoni, F. E. G., Herridge, C. F. (1969). Mental-hospital admissions and aircraft noise. *The Lancet*, 294, 1275 – 1277.

[57] Stansfeld, S. A., Gallacher, J., Babisch, W., Shipley, M. (1996). Road traffic noise and psychiatric disorder: prospective findings from the Caerphilly study. *British Medical Journal*, 313, 266-267.

[58] Michaud, D. S., Keith, S. E., McMurchy, D. (2005). Noise annoyance in Canada. *Noise and Health* 7, 39- 47.

[59] Tam, R., Belobaba, P., Polenske, K. R., Waitz, I. (2007). Assessment of Silent Aircraft-Enabled Regional Development and Airline Economics in the UK. Available from: http://web (Accessed 18 October 2011).

[60] Lindsay, G. and Kasarda, J. (2011). Aerotropolis: the way we live next. New York, Farrar, Strauss and Giroux

[61] Schreckenberg, D., Griefahn, B., Meis, M. (2010). The associations between noise sensitivity, reported physical and mental health, perceived environmental quality, and noise annoyance. *Noise and Health*, 12, 7-16.

[62] Nelson, J. P. (2004). Meta-analysis of airport noise and hedonic property values: problems and prospects. *Journal of Transport Economics and Policy*, 38: 1-27.

[63] Environmental noise directive (2002/49/EC). Available from: http://ec.europa.eu /environment (Accessed 18 October 2011).

[64] Position paper for environmental qualityPakistan. 2003.Available from: http://www.environment(p10) (Accessed 18 October 2011).

[65] Law of the People's Republic of China on the Prevention and Control of Environmental Noise Pollution. 1996-10-29 From: The National People's Congress. Available from: http://www.epa.gov/ogc/china/noise.pdf (Accessed 18 October 2011).

In: Prevention of Hearing Loss
Editors: V. Newton, P. Alberti and A. Smith

ISBN: 978-1-61942-745-7
© 2012 Nova Science Publishers, Inc.

Chapter XIV

Building Design for the Hard of Hearing

John O'Keefe[*]

Abstract

Great strides have been made in recent decades to make buildings more accessible to the disabled. These improvements, although laudable, apply mostly to those whose handicap is visually apparent. Much more could be done for those with impairments which cannot be seen - the hard of hearing. People who have trouble hearing will often avoid situations that might embarrass them, for example a party in a loud room. In this sense, the built environment can act as a barrier to their integration with society. In most forms of verbal communication, a room and its natural acoustics is the channel between the talker and the listener. Some rooms are better than others. Good building design policy could easily encourage a design environment that is sensitive to the needs of the hard of hearing. This need not imply extra costs to a building, rather a re-focusing of design objectives encouraged by awareness programs and building code improvements. In this chapter, some of the challenges that buildings can impart to the hard of hearing will be presented and explained. Potential solutions will then be discussed.

Introduction

Building design can and does have an impact on the hard-of-hearing. Unbeknownst to most, acoustical design is now a mature and reliable science, as witnessed by the many successful concert halls built in the last quarter century. But this design knowledge, which could be so easily applied to the benefit of those with hearing difficulties, seldom is – if ever. The hard of hearing population have trouble with speech discrimination. In a noisy environment or an overly reverberant room, they have trouble picking out the words from the rest of the confusion. Intelligent building design can limit both of these problems.

[*] Corresponding author: johno@aercoustics.com.

In most parts of the world – certainly in the industrialised part of the world – local building codes require designers to accommodate the physically challenged in a myriad of ways. The concept of a "Barrier Free" building is now ubiquitous in construction. It's a concept of accessibility for all. Everyone should have a fair chance at enjoying the benefits of our built environment – without any barriers to that enjoyment. Wheelchair ramps, lifts and the like are obvious Barrier Free examples. The rewards of this policy are less obvious but no less cogent. Soon after it was formed in the 1960s, Wright State University in Dayton, Ohio, USA began to pursue a Barrier Free building philosophy, long before the idea made it into building codes. Walking the campus, one is first struck by the number of students with some form of physical challenge. Then, not long afterwards, comes the painful realization that before Barrier Free buildings, these people simply could not obtain a university education. Surely the Barrier Free ethos is good policy. Currently, however, the Barrier Free concept applies to those who are seen as handicapped. It could, and perhaps should, apply to those whose challenges can't be seen but are no less challenging.

With one exception, Barrier Free building codes do not yet extend to the hard of hearing. The exception being places of assembly in new buildings, for example a lecture hall, theatre or, in some jurisdictions, even a classroom. Most building codes dictate electronic hearing assist systems. These systems broadcast signals locally that can be picked up by the patrons' or students' hearing aids. Beyond that requirement – albeit an important one – building codes offer little other advantage to the hard of hearing. As a result, modern building design does not respond to their needs in the ways that it could. If a distilled version of the knowledge required to build a concert hall or opera house could be applied to a classroom, a lecture hall or, for that matter, any other room where people gather for social interaction, the hard of hearing of the next generation could reap the benefits afforded to the wheelchair bound community of today.

Let us first define the challenges that the hard of hearing might face in the built environment and then address how policy makers and designers might respond to those needs.

Perception of Sound in a Room

The Lombard Effect

Some rooms are louder than others. A natural response to a loud room is to speak louder in it. Everybody does this. The natural inclination of human communication is to speak loud enough to be heard. Thus, in a loud room, for example a room with mostly hard surfaces, the first conversation will begin at a louder than normal level. A second conversation will have to talk louder than that, the third even louder, and so on until one has to shout to be understood. We have all experienced this: it is something called the Lombard Effect [1]. As mentioned, the hard of hearing have trouble functioning in a noisy environment; with or without hearing aids. Many might want to avoid the embarrassment this situation would present them, so they do– and in so doing, cut off a normal mode of social interaction available to all others but themselves. A loud room which encourages the onset of the Lombard Effect is not a Barrier Free room for the hard of hearing. A properly designed room can avoid this problem.

We have all been to social gatherings, for example a party or perhaps a restaurant, where it was so loud that it was hard to understand anyone. This problem is exacerbated for the hard of hearing. We have also been to gatherings that might have the same amount of people but everything was fine. It was not too loud and conversations were easy to understand. The difference between the two gatherings is the room in which they were held. In the first example, the empty room was too loud to start with. When people started to gather, the Lombard Effect took hold of the crowd, the speech levels went up and soon enough, people had to shout to be understood. In the second example, the room was a naturally quieter environment. The Lombard Effect never materialised and conversation remained pleasant. The difference between the two examples was the room and, by inference, the decisions made by the room designers. We shall discuss, below, how these decisions might be more sensitively considered.

The Cocktail Party Effect

The Cocktail Party Effect [2] is often confused with the Lombard Effect – perhaps for obvious reasons! The two are not the same. People with normal hearing in both ears (so-called binaural hearing) can hear things that others cannot. An obvious test of audibility of a given sound, for example a sentence, is whether or not it is louder than other sounds that you might hear at the same time: a kettle boiling in the kitchen, a train going by or perhaps someone else's sentence heard at the same time as the one you want to hear. If it is going to be audible, it must be louder than anything else. That makes sense. It turns out, however, that our hearing perception is smarter than that.

With a pair of normal hearing ears people can pick out sounds that are actually quieter than the babble of noise surrounding the sound they want to hear. This is called the Cocktail Party Effect but it does not matter if you're trying to converse at a party in a crowded room or trying to pick out the sound of the cello in the orchestra at other end of a concert hall. Binaural hearing (i.e. hearing with two ears) initiates a neural process that can localise on the sound we want to hear and filter out the unwanted sound to provide cognition. One of the early researchers [3] made a comparison between a radio and our brain. Like a radio we receive a wide range of different signals but in the brain there is a form of audio filter that allows us to select which channel we want to listen to.

An example of sound without the advantage of the Cocktail Party Effect is a monaural recording of a conversation, i.e. on a single microphone recording device. Without the advantage of binaural hearing and, by extension, the Cocktail Party Effect, all the extraneous noise in the room becomes immediately apparent on the recording and conversations are much more difficult to understand. Think of the Nixon tapes in a Watergate documentary. Most of them can't be understood without subtitles.

Monaural (or single ear) hearing is not the only thing to compromise the Cocktail Party Effect. Loud rooms and hearing impairment can also defeat the Cocktail Party Effect.

Many of the hard of hearing have to operate without the advantage of the Cocktail Party Effect. For them, the sound of a large, loud gathering can be as bad as the sound on the monaural recording device (e.g. the Nixon tapes). Even for the normal hearing population, the Cocktail Party Effect can be negated at overly loud levels. Prudent building design can prevent at least part of this problem. A room designed to be naturally quiet will prevent the onset of the Lombard Effect (i.e. people shouting over one another to be heard) and thus prevent the need for the Cocktail Party Effect (i.e. trying to hear someone when everyone else is speaking louder).

Speech Intelligibility

So far we have been talking about communication over the distance of a few metres at most; conversational speech in a restaurant or at a party. The challenges at larger distances are more acute. For good speech intelligibility beyond a few metres two fundamental criteria must be satisfied; (i) the reflected sound that arrives at the ear within 50 milliseconds (1/20 of a second) must be louder that the sound that arrives after 50 milliseconds, (ii) the word or sentence that someone is trying to understand must be twice as loud (+10 dB) as other sounds that might interfere with it. We thus have the concept of so called Useful and Detrimental sound. For normal hearing listeners, the threshold between useful and detrimental sound is 50 milliseconds. For the hard of hearing it is shorter than this, probably in the range of 35 milliseconds or less. In short, for good speech intelligibility, the sound coming from the speaker and the first one or two reflections must be louder than anything else [Figure 14.1].

These discoveries were made as researchers were trying to build better theatres and concert halls but they apply equally to any space where people need to understand speech; a subway, a classroom, a cinema, a political rally. It would be very difficult for anyone to make it through their day where these fundamental concepts of communication between humans do not apply.

Multi-Modal Perception

In recent years, researchers have discovered that the understanding and appreciation of sound is a so-called multi-modal percept. That is, the neural process interpreting a sound employs both visual and aural stimuli. Other senses behave the same way; smell can influence taste, for example. Lip-reading has long been known to improve speech intelligibility – in both normal and hearing-impaired listeners. Other visual stimuli have a more nuanced influence on the appreciation of sound but they are, nonetheless, still important.

A long held credo for good acoustical design has been that "good sightlines make good sound lines". The reasoning is simple, if the head in front of a listener in a lecture hall is blocking the path between the talker and the listener's eyes; it's probably blocking the sound path between the talker and the listener's ears as well. What was not fully appreciated before, however, was what the listener sees plays a role in what he or she can hear.

Prudent building policy and design directives should respond to this. With one exception, good sightlines in a lecture hall or any other place of assembly are not currently mandated by building codes – but they could be. Ironically, the single exception is for patrons in wheelchairs. Surely, the advantage afforded to that sector of the population can be extended to the hearing-impaired.

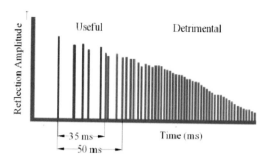

Figure 14.1. For good speech intelligibility early reflections are useful and late reflections are detrimental. For the hard of hearing, the threshold between the two is shorter, about 35 milliseconds (ms) rather than 50 ms.

Good sight lines can be achieved either by raising the talker on a platform or raising the seats towards the back of the audience. Often, both methods are employed simultaneously. A good designer will also stagger the seats from one row to the next, making sure that a listener is positioned between the two people in front. Another strategy or directive for classrooms would be to ensure that hearing-impaired students are seated at the front of the room with a clear line of sight to the teacher. This implies, by the way, a "front end" layout of the classroom where teachers are always facing the students.

Parenthetically, insofar as design policy is concerned, it would be advantageous to take a lesson from the nascent "green" building movement. Follow-up surveys have found that the way people use a green building is just as important as its design, perhaps more so. People using a room that, unbeknownst to them, has been designed to take advantage of natural light will, without thinking, flip on the light switch. They don't need to consume unneeded energy, and they probably wouldn't if someone had explained it to them. The problem is: nobody did. Likewise, in a room that might be used by the hard of hearing – the classic case being a classroom – the teachers need to be informed on how to use the room to its best advantage and to the best advantage of their students.

Acoustic Properties of Rooms

Reverberation

There are two components of any sound heard in a room, the direct sound coming straight from the sound source and the reflected or "reverberant" sound that has bounced off the different surfaces in the room; the walls, the floor and the ceiling. The direct sound terminates instantaneously after the sound source ceases. The reverberant sound will persist. The length of reverberant decay will depend on the room and the fittings inside it and is quantified by something known as the "reverberation time". In a small living room with soft furniture it could be as short as 0.25 seconds. In a large cathedral or atrium with hard surfaces, it could be as long as 8 or 9 seconds. The hard of hearing have trouble understanding speech in a highly reverberant space.

Reverberation times can be easily and reliably predicted. The reverberation time of a room is proportional to its enclosed volume and inversely proportional to the amount of acoustic absorption in the room (i.e. soft materials). So, if a room is too reverberant and it already exists, it is difficult to change the size (volume) but the reverberation time can be reduced by adding soft, acoustically absorbent materials. Conversely, if the room has not yet been built and the designers still have control over the volume but cannot use soft materials (e.g. a hospital room that must be kept clean), the reverberation time can be limited by keeping the volume small.

Some sounds benefit from reverberation, for example classical or choral music. Other sounds are often inhibited by reverberation. The reverberation in a large church or cathedral is an important embellishment to the sound of the organ or the choir but it makes speech difficult to understand. The more reverberation there is, the more difficult it is to understand speech. For the hard of hearing, this problem is exacerbated. For example, in America, the American National Standards Institute (ANSI) permits a maximum reverberation time of 0.6 to 0.7 seconds in a classroom. For the hard of hearing, research has found that it should be shorter, in the range of 0.4 to 0.5 seconds [4].

Loudness

As noted above, some rooms are louder than others. How does this happen and how can it be controlled? Three components control the natural loudness of sound in a room; the room's size (volume), its reverberation time and the distance between the sound source and the listener. Loudness is proportional to reverberation time and inversely proportional to both volume and distance. This simple concept – only reliably codified in the 1980s – makes sense on an intuitive level. Lively, reverberant rooms are louder than soft, non-reverberant rooms. Large rooms typically are not as loud as small rooms and, of course, the further away a sound is, the less loud it is.

So, once again, how is this applied in building design? In this example, consider a dining room in a home for senior citizens, many of whom might be hard of hearing. If the room is too loud, as public dining rooms can often be, normal hearing diners are going to have trouble understanding conversations, hard of hearing diners even more so. The designers of the room have three options to work with:

1   Distance, keep the diners close to each other; providing small tables for 4, maybe 5 people; avoiding large round tables for 10 or 12.
2   Keep the reverberation time short, i.e. include a lot of soft materials in the room. Placing carpet in a dining room can create health and maintenance issues and is therefore not a practical design option.
3   The ceiling should be soft and acoustically absorbent as should finishes on the walls.

Consider also the Lombard Effect, the situation where everyone is trying to talk louder than each other. In the dining room or, for that matter, any other room where speech is used, the Lombard Effect is initiated by the natural loudness of the room. Remember that people naturally respond to a loud room by speaking louder. The way to prevent the onset of the Lombard Effect is to control the room's natural loudness, and that is done by either making the room bigger (increase the volume) or making the materials softer (increase the acoustic absorption).

Ventilation Noise

Heating, ventilation and air conditioning (HVAC) systems are never noticed until they stop working, that is if the room is too hot or too cold. Ventilation noise, likewise, is one of those sounds that is never noticed until it is too loud. In almost all buildings, it forms the background or ambient noise that is ubiquitous but, if quiet enough, rarely ever noticed. The problem is in the grey area between where it really is quiet and where it is so loud that people complain. It is this grey area that affects speech intelligibility, more so for the hard of hearing. In this section we shall consider a room type where designers currently pay scant attention to ventilation noise, a classroom. Studies have shown that classrooms rarely satisfy the guidelines for normal hearing students, let alone the hard of hearing population. One study, in the early 1980s [5] found that classroom noise alone accounted for 50% to 75% of the variance of reading delays of one year or more in elementary school students – and that was for a normal hearing population. A more recent study has shown that hard of hearing children need to hear a word three times more frequently than a normal hearing child before that word can enter his or her lexicon [6,7].

Remember that to be understood, speech sounds must be heard at levels that are twice as loud (i.e. +10 dB) as any other sound. In a room, "any other sound" often means the ventilation system. Studies have shown that hearing-impaired need speech levels that should be at least 15 dB louder than other sounds [5]. This is true even when people are wearing their hearing aids. Modern hearing aids can distinguish between speech and noise – a very complex neural process – but only to a certain extent. So, for example, imagine a classroom with a noisy ventilation system and a teacher who is not talking loudly enough. The signal-to-noise ratio (i.e. how much louder the speech is than the ventilation noise) could easily be less than the 10 to 12 dB required by normal hearing students. A modern hearing aid can separate speech from noise to improve things but the improvement is limited to about 5 dB. The hearing aid cannot eliminate all of the ventilation noise. The result is a signal-to-noise ratio that is still often less than the 10 to 12dB that a normal hearing person requires.

Classrooms or other places of assembly for the hard of hearing need quiet ventilation systems. Recent studies have suggested levels in the range of 30 to 35 dBA[2] [4]. To achieve ventilation noise levels as low as these, an acoustical specialist will probably be required on the architectural design team – something that is rarely done. Low ventilation sound is especially important for the most challenged students, those in elementary school, the youngest of which are still forming language skills. There are some simple design practices that will help ventilation systems achieve this level of quietness. If the building has a central ventilation plant, recognise that this will probably be the noisiest room in the building. Classrooms should not be above, below or beside it; they should be separated across the corridor from the central plant. The plant should be located over washrooms, not classrooms. If the ventilation system is based on packaged air handling units located on the roof, these should not be located above a classroom. They should be positioned over an adjacent corridor or, preferably even further away, perhaps over a storage room. Air velocities should not be too fast, otherwise a hissing turbulence induced noise will be generated. Velocities should not exceed 2.3 meters per second (450 feet per minute).

---

[2] In the Heating Ventilation and Air Conditioning (HVAC) industry, background noise levels are quantified with a series of Noise Criteria (NC) curves. 30 to 35 dBA is about the equivalent of NC-20 to NC-25.

In the situation of an existing classroom, where it may not be possible to quieten the ventilation systems, teachers should use microphones. A typical application would have a teacher wearing a lapel microphone, which is then amplified through loudspeakers or, more likely, amplified then broadcast to the students' hearing aids.

Electronic Solutions

Buildings are no longer made of just bricks and mortar. Electrical systems, information technology (IT) and electronic communication play an increasingly important role in building design. Most of the hearing-impaired community wear hearing aids. As mentioned above, however, hearing aids aren't always the perfect solution, notably when speech is presented in a noisy environment. The solution, in that scenario, is to move the microphone closer to the talker. The microphone in a hearing aid could be 20 to 30 metres away from a talker. A microphone on a podium or on a lapel could be 200 to 300 mm away. Shortening the connection between the talker's microphone and the listener's hearing aid can be easily facilitated these days with electronic broadcasting systems. There are two popular systems; FM and infrared. Both have their advantages and disadvantages. Infrared systems usually sound better but require a line of sight between the transmitter and the hearing aid. FM systems don't require a line of sight but can have interference problems with other FM signals. FM systems are not appropriate in a building that might have privacy concerns as it is easy to eavesdrop on them.

In many jurisdictions these days, these so called Hearing Assist systems are required for "places of assembly" that seat 200 or more. A place of assembly is a lecture hall, theatre, concert hall, etc. Hearing Assist systems can, however, benefit other rooms, notably classrooms, as discussed above. If a school board cannot afford to install Hearing Assist systems in all of their classrooms, they can supply personal systems tuned to a broadcast frequency that a given student's hearing aid can receive. Hearing Assist systems can also be beneficial in residential buildings. A system, installed in the home, can allow hearing-impaired members of the family to hear voices coming from other rooms where they otherwise would not have the advantage of lip-reading. An FM system is required in this situation; infrared systems based on a line of sight broadcast will not work.

Public Address (PA) systems are another means of improving speech intelligibility but, again, the needs of the hard of hearing imply stricter guidelines when they are integrated into the building design. Remember that for good speech intelligibility, the useful early sound (i.e. direct plus 1 or 2 reflections) must be louder than the late detrimental sound and that the total sound must be twice as loud (+10 dB) as other sounds. The latter requirement is easily achieved by simply turning up the volume on the PA system. But that, in itself, is not always sufficient. Take the example of a subway or metro station, typically very reverberant rooms. A reverberant room has a lot of detrimental late reflections bouncing around. Sometimes these can be reduced with soft materials but these are difficult to keep clean and, over the years, form a build up of iron dust from the braking steel wheels. One solution is; rather than decrease the late detrimental energy, increase the useful early energy. This can be very easily done by increasing the number of loudspeakers on the platform. That way wherever a patron might stand, he or she is getting more early energy that late. Maximum distances between loudspeakers and listeners are in the range of 3 m for a normally hearing patron, slightly shorter for the hard of hearing. This implies that ceiling mounted speakers may not be a good option as they will be too far away. Speakers on the walls or, perhaps, hanging from the ceiling will work better.

Finally, staying with the example of a subway or metro, it is important to understand that the chain of hearing between a talker and a listener is as only as good as its weakest link. Good microphones and good annunciation are as important as anything else mentioned above. It is unlikely that the average train operator speaking from his cab into a telephone receiver will ever be understood in the rest of the car. Transit systems should have a centralised system of announcements where a train operator can call in, then have his or her message given by a trained speaker, into a good microphone in a quiet recording room or booth.

Examples such as this occur in all sorts of rooms where announcements might be made. In some cases, access to a trained speaker might not be available, for example on an airplane. Recognise however that video screens can be found in most public spaces these days. These combined with voice to text software could provide the hard of hearing with the visual cues they require.

Conclusion

The architectural design profession is a progressively minded, innovative community. Historically, they embraced the early 20th century concerns with fire protection. The conflagrations of London in the 17th century and Chicago in the late 19th century are unlikely to ever happen again. Building codes dictate against practices that would lead to conflagrations and, during building design, the code rules. Likewise, in the late 20th and early 21st century, both building code and other socially responsible guidelines have led to Barrier Free buildings that benefit not just the physically challenged but all of us.

Barrier Free building design requirements do not, however, currently extend to the hard of hearing. They could, very easily – and they should.

References

[1]   Rindel, J. H., (2010). Verbal communication and noise in eating establishments. *Applied Acoustics, 71*, 1156–1161.

[2]   Cherry, E. C. (1953). Some experiments on the recognition of speech, with one and with two ears. *Journal of Acoustic Society of America, 25*, 975–979.

[3]   Broadbent, D. E. (1954). The role of auditory localization in attention and memory span. *Journal of Experimental Psychology, 47*, 191–196.

[4]   Crandell, C. C. and Smaldino, J. J. (2000). Classroom Acoustics for Children With Normal Hearing and With Hearing Impairment, *American Speech-Language-Hearing Association, 31*, 362-370.

[5]   Valente, M., Hosford-Dunn, H., Roeser, R. J. (2008). *Audiology Treatment,* New York: Thieme Medical Publications.

[6]   Pittman, A. L. (2008). Short-term word-learning rate in children with normal hearing and children with hearing loss in limited and extended high-frequency bandwidths. *Journal of Speech, Language, and Hearing Research*, 51, 785-797.

[7]   Pittman, A. L. (2010). High-Frequency Amplification: Sharpening the Pencil. Available   from: http://www.phonak.com/com/b2b/en/events/proceedings/sound foundation_ chicago2010.html

In: Prevention of Hearing Loss
Editors: V. Newton, P. Alberti and A. Smith

ISBN: 978-1-61942-745-7
© 2012 Nova Science Publishers, Inc.

Chapter XV

The Use of Economic Analysis in Hearing Impairment Control

*Rob Baltussen**

Abstract

All over the world, people acquire hearing impairment, and all over the world resources are being consumed to support better hearing. This is what the process of economic analysis in health is all about: the connection between health and the resources that are utilized in promoting it. As health needs are almost infinite, but the resources available for their promotion are not, communities and individuals have to make choices. In particular, decisions have to be made about which needs are the most important and how available resources can be best used. Economic analysis can be an aid to making these decisions more clearly.

This chapter provides an introduction to the application of economic analysis to hearing impairment control (HIC). The aim is to provide an accessible source for those who are new to economics, with a view to enabling the reader to become more familiar with the use of economic analysis in HIC. The chapter discusses the importance of the economic analysis, and its main applications i.e. costing analysis and cost-effectiveness analysis. It thereby demonstrates that economic analysis should be seen as an essential planning and management tool for all of those who want to achieve better HIC in low and middle-income countries. It can help managers to run programmes which are more efficient. It has also shown how managers, by asking straightforward questions about how HIC services use resources, can obtain information that will help them improve their HIC programmes.

* Corresponding author: R.Baltussen@elg.umcn.nl.

Introduction

All over the world, people acquire hearing impairment, and all over the world resources are being consumed to support better hearing. This is what the process of economic analysis in health is all about: the connection between health and the resources that are utilized in promoting it. Here, the term 'resources' means not only money, but also the people, materials and time which could have been put to another use. As health needs are almost infinite, but the resources available for their promotion are not, communities and individuals have to make choices. In particular, decisions have to be made about which needs are the most important and how available resources can be best used. Economic analysis can be an aid to making these decisions more clearly.

This chapter provides an introduction to the application of economic analysis to hearing impairment control (HIC). The aim is to provide an accessible source for those who are new to economics, with a view to enabling the reader to become more familiar with the use of economic analysis in HIC. The chapter first discusses the importance of the economic analysis of HIC, and then discusses the main application of economic analysis, i.e. costing analysis, and the cost-effectiveness analysis of HIC. This chapter is a shortened version of a guide for programme managers on how to use economic analysis in hearing impairment control [1].

Why Is the Economic Analysis of Hearing Impairment Important?

Hearing Impairment Policy

The last decade has been one of rapid change in the international health arena. This is also true for HIC. In 1995, the World Health Assembly adopted a resolution on prevention of hearing impairment and deafness [2].Countries committed themselves to a comprehensive hearing impairment approach, including the preparation of national plans for the prevention and control of the major causes of avoidable hearing loss. The resolution also stressed the need for legislation on the proper management of important causes of deafness and hearing impairment, collaboration with non-governmental organizations, and for the provision of appropriate public information and education in particularly vulnerable or exposed population groups. In other words, the resolution indicated the need for countries to develop national HIC plans, and to include public health aspects within them.

Countries which are developing national plans face a number of challenges and choices when it comes to financing their programmes. Technological developments, rising expectations and aging populations fuel increased demand and consequently put upward pressure on costs. Concurrently, macroeconomic, demographic, and fiscal constraints limit the extent to which governments can simply allocate more public revenues to health and, more specifically, HIC. In addition, the UN millennium development goals[3]have drawn increasing attention at a national and international level to communicable disease control, meaning that resources are taken away from other (non-communicable) disease fields. The combination of upward pressure on costs and limitations within governments when it comes to increasing spending, forces managers to consider the way in which they establish their HIC programmes within their budgets.

There is no single answer to the question of how to best organize such programmes. Programme managers need to adapt constantly to this changing policy environment to ensure that hearing impairment needs are not neglected. In order for them to be successful in generating more resources for HIC, and to ensure that these are used optimally, they need skills and knowledge about not only hearing impairment, but also issues such as health care financing and economics.

2.2. Why Learn about Economic Analysis?

An understanding of economic analysis can help to both ensure that hearing impairment gets the attention it deserves, and that hearing impairment interventions are effective, efficient, equitable and sustainable. Economic analysis can help programme managers to address the questions set out in Box 1.

Box 1. Questions addressed in HIC with economic analysis

> 1. Should scarce resources be spent on HIC?
> 2. How should choices be made between different HIC programmes given the severe constraints on resources in most low and middle income countries?
> 3. Are HIC programmes being implemented in the least costly, and most efficient manner?
> 4. Will the choices made benefit the poorest and most vulnerable sections of the population?

In looking at the first question, one of the key tasks for most programme managers is to be an advocate for hearing impairment. At all levels – local, national, and international - economic arguments are increasingly being used to seek investment in different diseases and areas of health. To engage in these arguments, they first need to understand them. For example, programme managers should be able to explain why the treatment of chronicotitis media with antibiotics not only prevents hearing impairment, but is also a good use of limited resources. An understanding of economic analysis can provide programme managers with evidence-based arguments as to why investment in hearing impairment should be increased. These arguments will make sense not only to those decision makers working in health care, but also to those employed in public finance. A further example is given in Box 2.

When considering the second question, the reality is that programme managers often need to make difficult decisions about which HIC programmes to support. For example, they may have to choose whether funding should be used to provide subsidies for hearing aids, or whether the money would be better spent on increasing parents' knowledge of hearing impairment in childhood. Economic analysis can provide a systematic framework within which to make these tough choices. In simple terms, an HIC programme is efficient when it provides the greatest health outcome for the resources it uses. Economic analysis can help managers make difficult decisions by comparing the efficiency of different HIC interventions.

It can also assist in the measurement of the costs of services and the benefits they provide. Because economic analysis is conducted in a systematic way, it is possible to make comparisons between very different options, while still taking into account their multi-faceted benefits. A further example is given in box 3.

When looking at the third question, economic analysis can be used by managers to evaluate the performance of different service providers.

Box 2. Using economic evidence in support of HIC programmes: an example from the WHO

> The Unit of Prevention of Blindness and Deafness at the WHO is now using economic evidence to advocate for more investment in HIC. In its WHO-CHOICE project, WHO compares the costs and health effects of many different interventions in a wide range of disease areas. In African regions, most of the HIC programmes which have been subjected to economic analysis are providing good value for money, and a DALY averted costs between US$8 and US$1080 [4]. The economic attractiveness of these HIC programmes compares well to investment in other non-communicable diseases [5].

Box 3. Using economic evidence to choose between different HIC programmes: an example from the WHO

> The WHO-CHOICE project has evaluated three sets of interventions in HIC in Asia and Africa. In order of economic attractiveness, these are: treatment of chronic otitis media with antibiotics, treatment of meningitis, delivery of hearing aids, and screening for hearing impairment in combination with the delivery of hearing aids [3]. Obviously, and depending on: other interventions that may be candidates for implementation but have not been subjected to economic analysis; the epidemiology of hearing impairment in a given country; and other criteria which may be important for decision making purposes, country programme managers with limited budgets should give priority to scaling up the treatment of chronic otitis media and meningitis before starting to fund other programmes.

It can also help in the conducting of useful assessments of operational efficiency, by comparing the costs and service levels of different health facilities, thereby gauging which of them provides the best services at the lowest cost. This information can be used to help to define the most appropriate model for delivering HIC services in the future. A further example is given in Box 4.

However, economic analysis is not only concerned with efficiency; equity is also important. Looking at question 4 (see Box 1), economics is also concerned with the fair distribution of resources. In the same way that economists systematically examine the costs and benefits of services, they have also developed instruments with which to look at both who benefits from services and whether this is fair. Of course, people define fairness in different ways, but the tools can be applied to many of these. For example, one of the most critical questions that economists are concerned with is: which groups should benefit from the limited public subsidy of health, and which groups should finance their own health care? Should HIC programmes be free to all, or should they only be provided free to certain population groups? A further example is given in Box 5.

Box 4. Using economic evidence to assess operational efficiency: an example from Nigeria

In a city in Nigeria, an economic analysis compared a universal newborn hearing screening programme, as organized in a primary health care centre, versus one in a hospital (among other alternatives). Costs per child detected with permanent and early-onset hearing loss were lower for screening in the primary health care centre (US$602) when compared to in the hospital (US$2765) [6].This finding is of interest to low income countries where the percentage of hospital-based births is low. The authors argue that a gradual introduction of the former intervention is achievable in Nigeria within the framework of the newly established national health insurance scheme.

Box 5. Using economic evidence to assess equity: an example from India

A hearing impairment programme in Tamil Nadu, India, tested the use of active screening and the fitting of hearing aids in rural remote areas, versus the delivery of hearing aids to patients who present themselves to hospitals. The former appeared to be both cheaper and equally effective, and may also be a better way of reaching the rural poor [7]. This is a target group which was only marginally reached through the hospital delivery model. The screening approach is now being studied further for its long-term effects, and may then be considered for implementation in India on a larger scale.

Costing analysis

Why Analyse Costs?

There are many reasons why someone may require information about the costs of HIC programmes. Programme manager, for example, need to predict the costs when scaling up services while also staying within budget. In other circumstances, an analysis of costs may be necessary for programme managers to be able to compare the efficiency of different audiology clinics. They may also need to understand costs in order to prioritize between different HIC programmes. Cost information is a vital managerial tool, but it usually has to be interpreted alongside other data. For instance, being able to prioritize between different programmes not only requires information about costs but about the likely health effects. Costs are often the starting point of the process of investigation, but they are rarely the end.

Financial Costing Analysis

A first set of questions programme managers may face relates to financial housekeeping. Programme manages rare accountable to their employers – as they are, in turn, to the public – on the expenditure they incur or the resources they utilize. Expenditures are spendings made over a particular period of time to purchase the inputs required to produce products, services, or programmes. Being accountable means that they have to keep track of this expenditure, relate it to their budget, and take action if wide gaps between the two emerge.

They will also need to assess the use of personnel in delivering HIC services, as well as the efficiency of putting supplies, transport resources and other inputs to work. Moreover, for programme managers to be able to indicate the amount of funding likely to be required to continue their interventions, they will additionally have to make financial cost projections for the purpose of future budget planning. This is relevant at all levels of government, be it local or national. All of these issues, clearly, relate to financial costing and good housekeeping, i.e. being able to identify and control the money streams which are related to their health programme. This section outlines seven simple analyses that programme managers can use to assess costs and expenditure, set priorities, and appraise the performance, equity and financial sustainability of HICprogrammes.

Analysis 1 – Is Expenditure on Track with the Budget?

Keeping track of expenditure, i.e. money streams in a programme, is crucial and seems obvious, yet it is too often ignored: no-one can simply assume that budgeted funds have been spent exactly as planned, or that they have been used properly. The first step towards achieving accountability is through the budget. The budget provides guidelines on how resources should be used, and describes planned expenditure over a defined period of time – usually a year. If what has been spent exceeds the budget, programme managers will either have to look for additional resources, or -if that fails -the effectiveness of their programme may be seriously impaired. For example, a hearing aid delivery programme is unlikely to be successful if programme managers cannot afford to buy them. On the other hand, if they don't spend the entire funding that is available, the next year's budget may be automatically reduced. For all of these reasons, keeping track of expenditure and relating it to the budget is desirable. If spending on a particular item is delayed, or the budget allowance is, being consumed too rapidly, programme managers are able to take appropriate action.

If there is a mismatch between budget and expenditure, programme managers should be able to examine this in detail. It may be the case that the budget is badly prepared, or that the distribution of total resources is inadequate, e.g. too much money is being spent on personnel and too little on transport. Another explanation may be that the programme is being poorly implemented, in that resources are being wasted or used inefficiently. Look, for example, at the expenditure and costs related to a screening programme for hearing impairment in Box 6. The first column lists the capital and recurrent inputs, whereas the second reveals what the planned spending was. For instance, it was envisaged that US$21,000 would be spent on vehicles, and US$24,000 on equipment. The remaining columns show the actual expenditure on programme activities such as training, management, and delivery. For example, a total of US$26,000 was spent on vehicles (6th column), of which US$2,000 was for training, US$4,000 for management, and US$ 20,000 for delivery. The final column reveals that expenditure exceeded the budget on this particular input by 24%. Total expenditure exceeded the budget by 6%, with the greatest increase being for costs of building maintenance (47%). In absolute amounts, however, spending on vehicles was the most important cause of the problem. The regular monitoring of expenditure is one of the simplest ways for programme managers to develop an understanding of the link between resource use and the provision of services.

Analysis 2 – Is Money Being Spent on the Priorities in HIC?

A second simple costing analysis involves breaking programme costs down by different services. This can help programme managers to both establish how much money is being spent on different areas of HIC, as well as assess whether this is in line with priorities.

Table 15.1. Example: is expenditure in track with the budget? Budget and expenditure of a screening program (US$1,000)

	Budget	Expenditure				% (expenditure of budget)
		Training	Management	Delivery	Total	
Capital						
Vehicles	21	2	4	20	26	124%
Equipment	24	0	5	20	25	104%
Building	36	1	32	2	35	97%
Recurrent						
Personnel	96	34	11	62	107	107%
Supplies	34	3	12	11	26	77%
Building maintenance	1	1	1	0	1	147%
Total	20	41	65	11	220	

For instance, a costing analysis may reveal that a programme is spending an average of US$0.20 per capita on hospital care for hearing impairment, but only US$0.05 per capita on prevention activities. If the latter is considered to be a higher priority, an analysis of costs may encourage policy-makers and planners to take action. A simple example is provided in Box 7. Here, the breakdown of expenditure is compared to the population coverage of various HIC programmes in a hypothetical country. It reveals that antibiotic treatment of chronic otitis media is a first priority and relatively extensive coverage of the population in need is achieved. The second priority, hearing conservation at the work place, only covers 10% of the population in need, meaning that it is clearly not being met. With its low costs (3% of total budget), it seems that this programme is under-funded in comparison to e.g. ear surgery, which is a lower priority but receives more funding (50% of total budget).

Analysis 3 – Which Facilities Provide HIC Services for the Lowest Cost?

The assessment of both the quality and quantity of, for example, surgical services, is a standard element of the monitoring and evaluation of HIC programmes. Costing analysis can add a further dimension to this appraisal by placing the performance of services in the context of the resources they utilize. For example, if one ENT clinic performs better in terms of successful surgeries than another, but both use the same resources, then the second clinic may be able to improve its performance, without requiring additional funding. A comparison of costs could then identify the areas where the use of resources could be improved. A basic form of cost analysis is comparing the average cost of a service between facilities, or against a 'benchmark' cost.

Table 15.2. Example: Is money being spent on the priorities in HIC?
Assessing priorities in a hypothetical country

HIC programmes	Priority Ranking	Costs (in % of budget)	Coverage (in % of population in need)
Antibiotic treatment of chronic otitis media	1	15%	90%
Hearing conservation at work place	2	3%	10%
Ear surgery	3	50%	35%
Neonatal screening	4	4%	1%
Hearing aids to adults	5	28%	8%

The costs of different facilities could then be compared with this benchmark to assess whether they are efficient or not.

One of the most common causes of high average costs is the low take-up of services. For example, an ENT clinic with a capacity utilization rate of 50% is likely to incur considerably greater expenditure per surgery than a one where this rate is 90%. Another possible explanation for cost differences is variation in clinical practices. For instance, hospitals where expensive diagnostic techniques are used are likely to have higher costs. If this is the case, then an assessment needs to be made of whether this extra expenditure improves outcomes or not (see also the section on cost-effectiveness analysis).

Analysis 4 – Which HIC Programme Inputs Cost the Most?

Costing analysis can also be used to highlight the categories of expenditure to which attention should be paid: these are often the areas which require the greatest outlay, but the potential for cost savings is also more significant. The example in Box 6 shows that a 20% reduction in personnel costs - from US$107,000 to US$80,250 - would lead to greater cost savings than a similar reduction in the cost of supplies – from US$26,000 to US$19,500 - would. Breaking down the programme costs of different inputs can highlight areas of inefficiency. However, resources which incur the highest expenditure are not always the best candidates for cost-cutting: the money may indeed be well-spent.

Analysis 5 – Who Is Receiving the Most HIC Resources?

Costing analysis may also reveal the distribution of HIC resources across districts: if one area receives twice as many resources per capita than another, there may well be a case for their better distribution on the basis of equity concerns. There are many possible explanations if major differences are identified: e.g. more may be spent in remote districts because of higher transport costs. Alternatively, there may be differences in the efficiency of service delivery between districts, or perhaps authorities have decided to spend more in certain districts with the aim of striving for more equal hearing capabilities. Whatever the circumstances, it is important to identify a suitable explanation before any action is taken.

Costing analysis can also provide programme managers with an indication of who is benefiting from the resources being spent. For example, it can demonstrate the amount that both the poor and the rich pay for HIC services, as well as revealing how much the former benefit from exemption programmes. On the basis of this and other information, programme managers will then be able to assess whether interventions are reaching the poor and whether further action is required.

Analysis 6 – How Reliable Are the Sources of the Financing of an HIC Service?

Financial sustainability is an important factor when it comes to ensuring that HIC services continue after programme or project support has ended. Costing analysis can help managers to plan for the future by identifying the main sources of financing that are available to a hearing impairment service, as well as assess its stability. It can also provide an indication of the future financing requirements of services, and the level of fees or insurance required to ensure their continuation. Traditionally, financial sustainability has been assessed by examining the percentage of costs that are externally funded. Although this continues to be an important aspect of analysing sustainability, it is also important to consider the extent to which all sources of finance are reliable and assured in the medium-term. The reality is that some may be more dependable than others. In addition, the period of the financial commitment is also worth examining. High levels of financing, committed for a relatively short time from a limited number of sources can be a concern. Where funding is both promised for longer periods and institutionalized, then it may be more sustainable.

Analysis 7 – What Will Be the Costs of an HIC Programme in the Future?

Being responsible for a programme's budget and expenditure also means that a manager need to know what future costs are likely to be. To adequately estimate this, they may need to do cost projections, which are based upon knowledge of fixed costs (those that do not alter with changing output) and variable costs (those that do vary). Moreover, if they decide to extend the geographic coverage of their programme, they will need to have a detailed awareness of its cost structure, and knowledge of which costs are likely to change. For example, per person reached, the cost of supervision will be likely to increase if health centres in more remote areas are to be covered.

Economic Costing Analysis

This section explains that, for some policy questions, it is sometimes better to have a broader perspective than is the norm with simple financial analysis, i.e. economic analysis should be used. Economic costing attaches a value to all resource inputs in a programme, whether paid for or not. The basic idea is that since (free) resources used in one programme cannot be used by society in another activity, they have a value even when they do not have a price. This lost opportunity is the cost that society bears. For example, the volunteer labour which is employed in a HIC programme cannot be used by society for other activities. Economic costing attaches a value to these inputs, and can thus be seen as a more comprehensive and valid approach than financial costing when assessing HIC programmes from a societal point of view. Economic costing can be useful to programme managers for two reasons: to enable them to both assess the societal costs of an HIC programme as well as its sustainability.

Analysis 1 –What Are the Costs of My HIC Programme to Society?

To correctly estimate the societal costs of HIC programmes, all expenditure should be included, and not only that which has financial implications for the provider (typically the government). The value of 'free' resources should also be taken into account, since they cannot be employed for other activities and, therefore, have a societal cost. For example, consider that a programme manager has the choice between two options for providing hearing aids in a region: option A requires people to come to the hospital in the district capital; and option B includes outreach activities where the hearing aids will be delivered to health posts in villages.

Box 6. Example: Economic costing

> A study in Tamil Nadu, India, compared the costs of community-based screening of people for hearing impairment in combination with the provision of hearing aids at a secondary care level, to the provision of hearing aids to people who present themselves at the tertiary care level [7]. The research anticipated health care cost savings for the former programme as a result of the provision of services at the secondary rather than the tertiary care level. In addition, the study also anticipated that the former programme would reduce time and the transport costs of seeking and undergoing care, since the average distance to secondary care hospitals is generally less than to their tertiary care counterparts. Both types of costing information are relevant to the policy makers who have to make decisions about the implementation of such screening.

Assuming that both are equally effective, the programme manager will choose A because the budgetary (financial) implications will be less since no personnel, fuel, and vehicles are required for outreach-activities.

In making this decision, however, a substantial burden is placed on the population that has to travel to the district capital, and whose time cannot be used for e.g. productive labour. A programme manager should make the best choices from the point of view of society, which means that he/she should consider all (societal) costs, as well as the time costs of the population (i.e. economic costs). This may mean that the manager would choose option B rather than A. A further example is given in box 8. Deciding between interventions by comparing costs and benefits is discussed in detail in next section, which is concerned with cost-effectiveness analysis.

Analysis 2 – What Is the Sustainability of My HIC Programme?

Collecting information about all of the resources used in a health programme – both paid for and not – is important for its long-term sustainability. It provides programme managers with a better understanding of the future budgetary demands they may face in circumstances where donors will no longer support the programme. For example, if their hearing aid programme relies heavily on donated products, they may want to obtain a rough indication of how much it would cost to purchase these aids on the (international) market.

Cost Effectiveness Analysis

Why Perform a Cost-Effectiveness Analysis?

Programme manager are faced with the challenge of allocating limited resources between various programmes. Many factors come into play when making these decisions, including concerns about sensitivity, acceptability and equity. However, choices are also often related to money, and issues arise as to how they can best spend the budget available. CEA is a tool which helps programme managers to answer these questions. By comparing various options in terms of their cost (resource inputs) and their health effects, they will be assisted in designing the most appropriate and efficient HIC programmes. Programmes are said to be efficient when they lead to relatively large health effects for relatively low costs.

CEA can be used in several situations. It can help to establish the efficiency of the programmes that are currently in place, e.g. to convince the funding agency that its money is being well-spent. Alternatively, more resources may become available, and programme managers then have to decide how best to spend this money. In other words, CEA prevents them from overspending limited resources on less effective programmes, and under-spending on more effective programmes. The application of economics does not necessarily mean that less money should be spent, but rather that the use of resources could be made more effectual. A wide variety of issues can be examined in this way. CEA may guide decisions when programme managers need to choose between these of technology (e.g. cochlear implants versus hearing aids), the delivery site of interventions (e.g. hospital versus health centre for the delivery of hearing aids), or the target population (e.g. screening for hearing impairment among newborns versus school children versus adults).

Apart from assisting programme managers in making the right investment decisions, CEA may also shape programme managers' thoughts on related matters. For example, it requires them to clearly define all relevant policy options, which is something that is otherwise rarely done. Specifying desired outcomes (e.g. reduction of hearing impairment among children) can stimulate a new way of thinking about the best means to achieve these ends. Moreover, CEA takes differing perspectives into account. A programme may not be cost-saving or cost-effective from the point of view of a programme manager' budget, but may nonetheless be desirable from a societal position. This may shift the discussion away from a narrow budget effect to a broader assessment of societal good. Furthermore, it makes selections more explicit: rather than supporting a programme because it enjoys broad political support or appears to be effective, programme managers are required to think systematically about their choices and whether they are the best way of spending limited resources.

CEA is often used to indicate a broad array of analyses which compare costs to health effects. These are distinguished by how they measure the health effects of interventions or programmes. Depending upon the study question, one may choose from one of the following techniques:

Cost-minimization is used to describe and quantify the cost of a particular intervention, assuming that the health effects of the alternatives are equivalent. For example, an analysis which assumes that the effectiveness of community or hospital based treatment for hearing impairment is the same, might simply report the costs associated with each. Cost-minimization is, essentially, a 'costing analysis', as discussed above.

Cost-effectiveness analysis incorporates information about both costs and health effects to describe the value of a particular programme. It is relevant if the health effects of various interventions will be different. A CEA evaluates a programme through the use of a cost-effectiveness ratio in which all health effects are included in the denominator, and all costs or changes in resource use are part of the numerator.

$$\text{Cost-effectiveness ratio} = \frac{\text{changes in resources}}{\text{changes In health effects}}$$

This type of analysis can be utilized to compare the use of different types of technology (cochlear implants versus hearing aids), the delivery sites of interventions (hospital versus health centre for delivery of hearing aids), or the choice of the target population (e.g. screening for hearing impairment among newborns versus school children versus adults).This is the type of economic evaluation which is most commonly used and will be later discussed in detail.

Cost-benefit analysis differs from CEA in that it values both health outcomes and the costs of interventions in monetary terms, e.g. dollars. This overcomes the problem of comparing programmes which have different types of health effects. Because these are measured in money terms, net benefits or net costs can be calculated by subtracting the latter from the former. The health effects of an intervention can then be measured using the human capital approach in which it is assumed that saving the life of a working individual results in a health benefit equal to his (future) earnings. This approach may, however, undervalue the lives of individuals who are not employed in the formal employment sector, such as women, children and older adults.

Health effects can also be measured by the amount individuals would be willing to pay to avoid death or disability. There is, however, one limitation of this willingness-to-pay approach, namely that the responses to these questions are dependent upon the resources available to the individual; someone wealthy may be willing to spend more to avert death than someone poor.

Conclusion

Economic analysis should be seen as an essential planning and management tool for all of those who want to achieve better HIC in low and middle-income countries. It can help managers to run programmes which are more efficient. This chapter has focused on costing and cost-effectiveness analysis. It has demonstrated how, by asking straightforward questions about how HIC services use resources, managers can obtain information that will help them improve their HIC programmes.

References

[1]   Baltussen, R. How to use economic analysis in hearing impairment control. A guide for programme managers. 2009 (unpublished).

[2]   World Health Assembly. (1995). Prevention of Hearing Impairment, Resolution of the 48th World Health Assembly WHA 48.9, Geneva: World Health Organization.

[3]   United Nations.(2009). UN Millennium Development Goals. UN, New York. Available from: http://www.un.org/millenniumgoals/index.shtml. UN, New York.(Accessed 8 March 2009).

[4]   Baltusen, R., Smith, A. (2009).Cost-effectiveness of hearing impairment control in Africa and Asia. *International Journal of Audiology,* 48,144-158.

[5]   World Health Organisation. (2009). WHO-CHOICE database on cost-effectiveness. Geneva: World Health Organization. Available from:www.who.int/choice (Accessed 8 March 2009).

[6]   Olusanya, B. O., Emokpae, A., Renner, J. K., Wirz, S. L. (2009).Costs and performance of early hearing detection programmes in Lagos, Nigeria. *Transactions of the Royal Society of Tropical Medicine and Hygiene,* 103, 179-186.

[7]   Baltussen, R., Abraham, V., Priya, M., Achamma, B., Anand, J., Gift, N. Abraham, J. (2009). Costs and health effects of screening and delivery of hearing aids in Tamil Nadu, India: an observational study. *BMC Public Health,* 12,9:135.

In: Prevention of Hearing Loss
Editors: V. Newton, P. Alberti and A. Smith

ISBN: 978-1-61942-745-7
© 2012 Nova Science Publishers, Inc.

Chapter XVI

Access to Health Care

Abraham Joseph[*]

Abstract

The central theme of this chapter is the importance of universal access to health care. It is an important article of the Alma Ata declaration. The central focus of many National Health programmes has been the equity of access to health care. It can be inferred that equity and access are critical and also needs based. The discussion then leads to what defines needs - normative need, felt need, expressed need and comparative need. The factors that influence access, need and equity are many and in today's complex socio-political system interwoven in different ways.

This makes it difficult for the governments to comprehend it fully and evolve a meaningful strategy. The article then goes on list factors which are barriers to access and to highlight how access affects the three levels of prevention, namely primary (health promotion, specific protection), secondary (early diagnosis and treatment), and tertiary (disability limitation and rehabilitation). Policy makers would like to emphasise the first two levels which would decrease the burden considerably on care at the tertiary level which is the least cost effective of the three levels. Factors affecting hearing impairment have been taken to illustrate the importance of primary prevention and why, though simple and available, it has not been accessed by many especially in the low income countries. Maternal Child Health clinics though universally accepted as a basic health service even before the Alma Ata declaration are poorly utilised leading to preventable morbidity and deaths including hearing impairment.

Introduction

An important article of the Alma Ata declaration states that "Primary health care is essential health care based on practical, scientifically sound and socially acceptable methods and technology made universally accessible to individuals and families in the community

---
[*] E-mail: abrahamjosepha@gmail.com.

through their full participation and at a cost that the community and country can afford to maintain at every stage of their development in the spirit of self reliance and self-determination.

It forms an integral part both of the country's health system, of which it is the central function and main focus, and of the overall social and economic development of the community. It is the first level of contact of individuals, the family and community with the national health system bringing health care as close as possible to where people live and work, and constitutes the first element of a continuing health care process." [1].

Access to Health Care

Universal access to health care is the central message of this article. What is access to health care? There are several definitions: Academic leaders in the field have more carefully defined access to health care, at a general level, as entailing the ability to secure a specified set of healthcare services, at a specified level of quality, subject to a specified maximum level of personal inconvenience and cost, while in possession of a specified amount of information [2].

The concept of equity of access to health care is a central objective of many health care systems and has been an important buttress of the UK National Health Service since its inception in 1948.

Much has been written about equity of health care. Some of the important principles of equity discussed are [3].

- Equal access to health care for those in equal need of health care
- Equal utilisation of health care for those in equal need of health care
- Equal (or, rather, equitable) health outcomes (as measured by, for example, quality adjusted life expectancy

It can be inferred that access and equity are based on need. If so what defines a person's need? Bradshaw defined need along the following four dimensions:

1. Normative need, in which an expert, professional administrator, or scientist defines need by laying down their desired standard and comparing it with the standard that actually exists
2. Felt need, in which need is equated with want, and is assessed by simply asking a person or population if they feel they need a service
3. Expressed need, where felt need is turned into action
4. Comparative need, where the characteristics of a population who receive a service are ascertained, and where people with similar characteristics who do not receive the service are adjudged to be in need [4]. In order to meet these needs, access plays an important role. The WHO has recognized that poor access to health is an important reason for poor health utilization and thereby poor health status of a community.

Factors that Influence Equal Access for Equal Need

There are many factors which affect the access to health care and this differs from group to group. Many different factors potentially impact on differential access to health care across different groups. With current information, it is difficult to disentangle these, to form a fully comprehensive and coherent policy response. However, for illustrative purposes, some general comments can be made with respect to groups defined by income, geographical residence, and ethnicity. On the supply side, and with respect to groups defined by geographical residence, the geographical proximity to health care services varies quite considerably within many countries. On the demand side, which primarily refers to the individual's ability to pay for health care, user charges are increasingly being used or mooted in many countries as a method by which to attempt to quell the demand for health care, but there is some evidence that charges have a higher impact on the demand for health care in lower income groups than in higher income groups. Demand will also be influenced by factors such as knowledge, information, cultural beliefs, indirect financial costs (for example, travel costs), the opportunity cost of patients' time (for example, foregone wages), and their preferences. The concepts of access to medical care proposed by Aday and Andersen [5, 6,] were used as an initial framework for the identification of access barriers.

Enabling components define the resources patients or their communities may have available to facilitate (or in their absence, hinder) the use of services. In this study, the enabling factors we considered included health insurance status, family income, area of residence, and region.

Predisposing components are variables that describe or influence the propensity of individuals to use services. Predisposing factors that we examined included parental educational attainment, parental beliefs, use of home remedies, parental sources of advice when their child is ill, folk medicine practices, immigration status, age, gender, family size, parents' marital status.

Need components, which are primarily morbidity and health status measures, were not examined, because it is not always clear whether they are the products of access barriers, barriers in and of themselves, or a combination of both. The characteristics of the health care delivery system that were examined as potential barriers included provider practices and behaviours, lack of a regular source of care, type of practice setting, and excessive waiting times. Additional potential barriers that were examined and do not easily fit into the single categories of the Aday and Andersen framework include transportation problems, cultural issues, and language difficulties.

Literature Search

In a review of Latino children [4], a total of 27 out of 497 studies met the inclusion criteria for this review. Twelve (44%) of these studies used large, national, secondary data sets. Of the remaining 15 studies, most (60%) did not have relevant non-Latino comparison groups as part of the study design.

The above section clearly shows that access to health does have an impact on health status. What is the impact of access on those with hearing disorders and what can be done to address these factors? Preventive health care was defined by Leavell and Clark as primary prevention, secondary prevention and tertiary prevention [7]. Primary care has two components health promotion and specific protection. Secondary care is early diagnosis and prompt treatment, Tertiary care is disability limitation and rehabilitation which includes physical, social and psychological. Access does have an important influence at all three levels.

Table 16.1. Reference [4] Summary of Access Barriers to Health Care

Supportive Barrier Evidence

- Health insurance
- Poverty
- Geography; Area of residence or geographical area of residence
- Parent educational attainment
- Parent beliefs
- Use of home remedies
- Source of parent advice on child's illness
- Folk medicine practices
- Immigration status
- Provider practices and behaviours
- Inadequate communication/patient education
- Negative attitudes of staff
- Type of practice setting
- Excessive waiting times
- Transportation
- Cultural differences
- Language problems

Health promotion includes primordial prevention, healthy education, change in life style improved nutrition and better environment. Specific protection includes immunization, nutrients to prevent specific disorders such as anemia, avitaminosis such as keratomalacia and blindness and specific devices to prevent a disorder. The wearing of ear muffs is an example of this to prevent hearing loss. The vaccine against rubella is another example of specific protection against congenital rubella syndrome which includes hearing loss. These are simple low cost interventions which are not accessed by the most needy the poor and marginalized community.

Early diagnosis and prompt treatment is the second level. This is the level addressed by most national programmes. Screening for hearing loss beginning with neonatal screening is a good example. The screening which takes place at schools and work places are other examples. In hearing loss this plays a very important role as many of those with minor hearing loss are not aware of it especially if it is of gradual onset. A sudden loss of hearing loss following a blast is immediately recognized by the individual and they seek help. A mild hearing loss in children very often goes unnoticed by the child, the parents and even the teachers. Such students perform poorly in class and it is often attributed to poor intelligence. Such children are diagnosed only when screening for hearing is carried out. Many countries do not have this as part of the regular school health programme and so the child is permanently affected both in his scholastic performance and also stigmatised as a poor performer, a "mutt" by his teachers and class mates. Not only is it important to diagnose the child with hearing loss, it is also important to address their problem including access to hearing aids, their affordability and maintenance.

The third element of health care is tertiary prevention. This includes disability limitation and rehabilitation.

These elements are important in hearing loss and its management. This is best illustrated by understanding the disease process in otitis media. Health care should make it possible to diagnose a person with early signs of acute otitis media. This is specially so in infants and the preschool child. A missed otitis media may end as a perforation of the ear drum. If this too is not diagnosed and prompt treatment denied due to poor access to health care the outcome is chronic suppurative otitis media, CSOM. This is often neglected by the parents or may be poorly managed as seen in many poor income countries and hearing loss is the final outcome. In several studies the major cause in child hood of hearing loss is otitis media.

The second element of tertiary prevention is rehabilitation which includes physical, social and psychological support. A child with hearing loss if not diagnosed early does not learn to speak. If detected early it can be corrected and with the help of appropriate hearing aids, hearing can be restored Those with severe hearing loss will need special care which will include surgical intervention and if that too fails the child needs to be taught other means of communication . This is the physical rehabilitation –providing hearing aids and surgical correction with cochlear implants.

A person with hearing loss usually does not mingle with others, specially their peers which leads to social isolation. This leads to several problems including anti-social behaviour. To prevent this state of events social rehabilitation needs to take place with trained social workers. Those individuals who further deteriorate due to social isolation may develop psychological problems and need the help of psychologists and even psychiatrists.

Access to health care plays a very important role in this natural history of hearing loss and its progression. This needs to be understood well by health policy makers, health providers working at all levels of health care, the individual affected and the community at large as they play an important role.

A few conditions will be taken to illustrate the importance of access which was defined at the beginning of this chapter. Health promotion and specific protection play an important role in the natural history of disease or health conditions. Access to health care, especially primary care, depends on an individual's knowledge and attitude. Immunisation is a very effective specific preventive measure, especially rubella vaccine to prevent rubella syndrome. The last epidemic of rubella in the US was in 1964-65. Over 1 million cases of whom 20,000 had Congenital Rubella Syndrome (CRS). In 1997 there were only 5 cases of CRS of whom 4 were in Hispanics. Even though the effectiveness of the vaccine is undisputed the coverage globally is poor. Vaccination against rubella is not a national programme in many countries, a problem of lack of policy. In countries where it is provided access is an important factor for acceptance even if it is provided free. The vaccination programme must be conducted when mothers are free from home and farm work to attend the clinic. They must be convinced of the need and its benefits. Wrong beliefs, that vaccines can cause sterility, and are a means of effecting birth control, prevents mothers of certain religious groups from accepting the vaccine.

The Access Barriers to Health Care can be understood well by the analysis of poor acceptance of measles vaccine.

Poverty

This plays an important role if there is no national policy to include the MMR as a part of the national programme. The cost of the vaccine is beyond the purchasing power of the poor. Even if it is free there is a cost to travel to the immunization centre, such as travel cost or loss of wages for a daily wage earner due to the time taken to visit the clinic. Another aspect of poverty is that the poor do not seek health care till they become very ill. Especially in the farming community and during agricultural seasons they cannot afford to miss a day's work as it may affect the crops: perhaps transplanting, weeding, harvesting or storing. Early diagnosis is difficult in (such) some situations. Acute otitis media which proceeds to CSOM and hearing impairment demonstrates this well. A child with a painful ear is brought late for treatment and poor personal hygiene leads to infection which is not cared for as it is not thought to be serious enough to miss a day's work. This leads to hearing impairment, which is too mild in the early stage to be detected by the parents or teachers.

Geographic Area of Residence

Health care in remote mountainous and desert regions is poor. Access becomes a problem as individuals have to walk long distances to reach the clinic. When a place is remote health providers are also scarce. Even if the government provides a clinic and funds for staff such as nurses and health workers there will be few takers in such a terrain.

The reasons are valid - lack of facilities for children's education, lack of security especially for unmarried female workers, social isolation as houses are far and few between, to mention a few. Studies have shown that overall health coverage using vaccine as an indicator is always poorer in such regions.

In case of the person who needs a hearing aid, the person needs to make several visits to the health centre, once for the audiogram, next for taking the impression for the ear mould and another for the fitting of the hearing aid. If there is a need to change the battery or have some adjustments for the hearing aid the general clinic may not provide the services and the person will have to go to a secondary level health care centre or tertiary level centre where technicians are available.

Parent Educational Attainment

There is good correlation between parents' education and utilization of services. Education level is also related to the income of the family. Children of poor families drop out of school because the parents do not have money even to buy the books or because they needed an additional hand at home to work in the field or take care of a younger sibling, especially in the case of a female child. Because of poor education they are not able to understand the importance of prevention of disease or early diagnosis, nor the value of having hearing aids to improve school performance.

Parental Beliefs

Cultural beliefs and practices also contribute to poor access. This is more so in the rural rather than the urban districts. If the urban dwellers are first generation migrants from the rural regions they too are affected as much as rural dwellers as they come with the cultural beliefs that they grew up with. These are strongly embedded that it takes much effort to change them. It took several years of continuous education of the community leaders to motivate women to attend antenatal clinics or bring children for immunisation clinics which were held in their own village. Lack of awareness, along with superstitious beliefs are responsible for this.

To take a problem related to hearing impairment, a well- recognized complication of measles is otitis media. Another vaccine related disease is rubella. Both have very effective vaccines with minimal side effects compared to DPT vaccine. It was difficult to get parents to bring the children for the vaccination as they believed that measles, chicken pox and other exanthematous conditions are caused by the visitation of a god or goddess. Each disease is ascribed to a particular deity and so to do anything to prevent such a visitation will anger the deity and thereby cause more harm to the family or the child in particular. This is an example of poor access of health service due to cultural and religious beliefs and practices even if it is provided at their door step free of cost. The Muslim community in India refused vaccines for a long time thinking that vaccines caused sterility. . Even today many of the pockets where polio is occurring in North India are related to poor vaccine coverage among the Muslim community. Similarly there are certain Christian groups such as Jehovah's Witness which do not accept medical care especially blood transfusion in critical conditions and only believe in prayer for healing

Use of Home Remedies

The use of harmful home remedies can cause disease or worsen existing conditions. An example which leads to hearing impairment is the management of foreign bodies in the ear. If a foreign body especially an insect or a bean is found in the ear instead of seeking hospital services the mother or grandmother or the local healer will use traditional methods. This includes pouring of warm oil into the ear and then removing the foreign body with a hair pin or a locally made implement.

On many an occasions they succeed, especially if it is a small stone or slate pencil. By contrast, seeds absorb the oil and expand and also become friable and break into small pieces. In the attempt to remove a seed with a pin the ear drum is damaged ending with infection and perforation. This leads to CSOM.

Source of Parent Advice on Child's Illness

When a child is sick a decision has to be taken as to which health care to access. Usually it is the father or the grandparents. The decision is strongly influenced by previous experience and the environment in which they have grown up. The influence of parental education and beliefs has been addressed. The other is the experience parents have had in a hospital or with the health provider. This may be a doctor, nurse or community health worker. Quality of care takes precedence to proximity. Unfortunately not everybody can access the best care because of distance and cost. A mission hospital in Tamil Nadu India attracts many patients from the northern states because of past experience of some of their community members. The poor will have to access the nearest health facility.

Provider Practices and Behaviours

Studies have shown that access to a health care facility or provider depends on the attitude and practice of the health facility as well as the individual providers - doctors, nurses, therapists and technicians and support staff. Individuals prefer a centre which provides holistic care which includes the three levels, primary, secondary and tertiary. It also depends on the attitude and behaviour of the professionals. Access of a health care facility will also depend on acceptance and the affordability of the services provided. Acceptance will depend on quality of care, the attitude of the providers and their behaviour. A person is willing to pay more if the service is acceptable. In countries where health service is provided by the public system as well as private providers, those who can afford it, use private facilities. In the earlier section it was mentioned that access was influenced by proximity of service. To a person who pays for the services, quality of care overrides proximity. Other factors that influence acceptance are waiting time, attitude of staff and communication with staff especially related to language. In a country such as India which has over 25 official languages it becomes a problem when a patient moves from his home State to another where a different language is spoken. Some hospitals employ translators and guides to help such patients.

MCH and Hearing Impairment

Of the various promotive and preventive primary health care services, a good example to demonstrate the effect on prevention of hearing loss, is the maternal and child health programme. One of the components of the antenatal programme is screening for maternal infections. Often the pregnant mother is unaware of any subclinical condition affecting her. An apt example is of syphilis infecting the mother without her knowledge and where the fetus could be affected unless the mother is treated in the first trimester. Congenital syphilis can cause several abnormalities including impairment of hearing. Many mothers are getting rubella (German measles) in child bearing age, if they have not been infected in childhood. If a mother gets rubella in the first trimester there is a 20% chance that the fetus is affected and gets rubella syndrome. Rubella syndrome includes deafness, blindness, mental retardation and congenital heart disease. With the advent of the rubella vaccines the global incidence of rubella in the adults has fallen dramatically. This has resulted in the decrease of congenital rubella syndrome and deafness.

The other condition which can be picked up in pregnancy is HIV. If diagnosed before delivery, the newborn can be protected from acquiring the disease. The newborn is infected through the mother's blood during delivery or during parturition. Giving anti -retrovirus medicines to the mother before delivery and to the child for several weeks after delivery has decreased the mother to child transmission dramatically. Children with HIV are prone to various diseases which includes otitis media and consequent hearing impairment.

The third example of the effect of good antenatal care on the prevention of hearing impairment is the early detection of mothers with high risk factors. The factors include short stature, heart disease, poor obstetric history such as repeated abortions or still births, to mention a few. Such an individual is given special care throughout pregnancy and also admitted to the hospital well in time and not at the onset of labour pain. Such high risk pregnancies could end with premature rupture of membranes, premature delivery, fetal distress and consequently asphyxia neonatorum . This can lead to mental retardation and subsequent hearing impairment.

The Maternal Child Health service also provides preventive, promotive and curative service to the newborn till childhood. Growth monitoring takes place as well as screening for birth defects which includes hearing impairment. Early detection of hearing impairment makes a major difference in the outcome to hearing and speech. Early treatment for such conditions is described elsewhere in this book.

A second activity of the Well Baby Clinic is the immunization programme. The measles vaccines have contributed significantly to the decline of hearing impairment. Measles was once the major child killer among under fives. The introduction of measles vaccine, like rubella vaccine, has decreased the incidence of measles in childhood. In some communities the case mortality was as high as 20% especially in poorly nourished communities. One of the complications of measles is acute otitis media. In several communities, the traditional belief that measles is the visitation of a goddess is an obstacle to successful and early treatment of acute otitis media. Village folk were convinced that treating the ailment with injections and tablets would displease the goddess and the child would only get worse. Such cultural beliefs made it very difficult to get the community to accept vaccines. Measles is an interesting disease to demonstrate the influence of traditional beliefs and practices on the acceptance of a vaccine, the occurrence of a disease and its management and on the consequences which includes hearing impairment.

The MCH programme demonstrates the importance of availability, affordability, accessibility and acceptability of a programme. All countries provide MCH services especially in the poorer section of the community. However its utilization depends on the above factors. Infant mortality and morbidity including disability can markedly decline if the service is provided and the community can access it and also finds it acceptable.

Conclusion

When the factors leading to hearing impairment are analysed it is apparent that many conditions are preventable. The next obvious question is, then why is it not prevented. This chapter should help the reader to understand why simple preventive activities, though available universally, such as antenatal care and immunisation, are used by less than 50% of the population in many low income countries. It is also apparent that access and acceptance play an important part. Primary and secondary prevention are critical and needs to be effectively practised if hearing impairment is to be reduced thereby bringing about a reduction in the burden of disease.

References

[1]   Primary health care. Report of the International Conference on Primary Health Care: Alma-Alta, USSR, 6–12 September 1978. Geneva, World Health Organization (Health for All Series, No. 1, p.34).

[2]   Equity of access to health care services: Theory and evidence from the UK. Goddard M, Smith P. Centre for Health Economics, University of York, Heslington, York, YO10 5DD, UK

[3]   Oliver, A., and Mossialos, E. J. (2004). Equity of access to health care: outlining the foundations for action. *Epidemiology Community Health, 58*,655–658. doi: 10.1136/jech.2003.017731

[4]   Flores, G., and Vega, L.R., (1998). Barriers to Health Care Access for Latino Children: A Review. Family Medicine,30, 196-205.Thiede M. (2005). Information and access to health care: is there a role for trust? *Social Science and Medicine, 61*, 1452-62.

[5]   Aday, L., Andersen, R., Fleming., G. (1980). Health care in the U.S.: Equitable for whom? Beverly Hills, USA, Sage Publications.

[6]   Aday, L., and Andersen, R. (1975). A social indicator of access to medical care. *Journal of Health and Social Behavior, 16*, 39.

[7]   Leavell, H., Clark, E. (1979). Preventive medicine for the doctor in his community: An epidemiologic approach. (3rd ed.). R. E. Krieger, Huntington, New York, USA. ISBN 0882758152.

In: Prevention of Hearing Loss
Editors: V. Newton, P. Alberti and A. Smith

ISBN: 978-1-61942-745-7
© 2012 Nova Science Publishers, Inc.

Chapter XVII

National and Regional Programmes

Andrew W. Smith[*], *Maria Cecilia Bevilacqua, Xingkuan Bu,
Arun Kumar Agarwal and Shelly Khanna Chadha*

Abstract

Few of the low and middle income countries have national plans or programmes for prevention of hearing loss. WHO believes that strong national plans need to be aligned with its own programmes and policies in order to achieve people-centred care delivered through strong integrated health systems. It has followed up this ideal with the setting of indicators and targets to measure the number of Member States that are implementing comprehensive national plans on this subject together with relevant strategies recommended by the World Health Organisation (WHO).

The following three mega-countries have already taken the lead and developed plans to prevent hearing loss and commenced to implement them. All of them are different according to differing national needs, but all of them are attempting to reduce the burden of hearing loss in the most effective way possible. How they are doing this is set out in the following pages.

Introduction

Andrew W Smith

Prevention of hearing loss in countries is best coordinated and implemented through national programmes run by governments or large national or international NGOs. Unfortunately very few countries, particularly amongst the World Bank grouping of low and middle income countries, have such programmes.

WHO, in its recent *Global Status Report on Non-Communicable Diseases 2010* [1] stated that "NCD programmes and policies need to be aligned with strong national plans that strive

---
[*] Corresponding Author: andrew.smith@LSHTM.ac.uk.

to achieve people-centred care delivered through strong integrated health systems...Improvements in country capacity are particularly needed in the areas of funding, health information, health workforce, basic technologies, essential medicines, and multi-sectoral partnerships." WHO's 11th General Programme of Work for 2006-2015 entitled *"Engaging for Health: A Global Health Agenda"* [2] sets out the organization's six core functions. The fifth of these is "Providing technical support, catalysing change, and building sustainable institutional capacity". This is mainly done through providing technical support to countries, especially National Governments, and has been a central component of WHO's work since its inception. WHO is therefore uniquely placed to assist countries in developing and implementing their health agenda, and is now focusing increasingly on non-communicable diseases. Hearing loss is included in this group, but until recently there had been little recognition of the need to address this problem specifically in any of the top-level strategic plans of WHO. However, in its recent Medium-Term Strategic Plan for 2008-2013 [3], WHO has, for the first time, included indicators to assess progress in dealing with hearing loss. Strategic Objective 3 of the plan is "To prevent and reduce disease, disability and premature death from chronic non-communicable diseases". The following indicators have been included to address hearing impairment:-

- 3.2.4. Number of Member States that are implementing comprehensive national plans for the prevention of hearing or visual impairment
- 3.3.5. Number of Member States documenting, according to population-based surveys, the burden of hearing or visual impairment
- 3.5.3. Number of Member States implementing strategies recommended by WHO for the prevention of hearing or visual impairment

These indicators all have specified targets which are listed in the plan, but it is not clear at present whether WHO has the resources or technical capacity to assist member states to fulfil them. In the meantime several countries in the low and middle-income group have taken the initiative to set up national programmes to address the prevention and management of hearing loss. Amongst these are three of the so-called 'mega-countries', Brazil, China and India. The editors of this book were fortunate that they were able to obtain contributions from experts from each of these countries who were closely involved in the development of the programme in their own country. Each programme is unique in its own way, because each country has unique geographic, demographic and socio-economic characteristics. However, all have the goal of preventing and managing hearing loss in the most effective way possible. Readers who may be involved in setting up programmes to address hearing loss in their own country will find here much to learn from.

Brazil

Maria Cecilia Bevilacqua

Brazil is a country of continental size and many contrasts; 190 million inhabitants in a territory of 8.55 million square km (3.3 million square miles). The largest concentration of population is in the Southeast and Northeast; the GNI is US$8,040 GNI per capita (World Bank, 2009) [1]. Currently, 84% of the population is distributed in 5,565 municipalities with a highly varied population density, ranging from more than 10 million inhabitants, as is the case of São Paulo, to only 795 in the smallest municipality [2].

Moreover, a huge area of more than 500 million hectares, more than half of Brazil's territory, is covered by forests, such as the Amazon forest. It also has an extensive river system and an indigenous population of more than 800,000 distributed throughout the country but most concentrated in the State of Amazonas [3, 4]. This is the context in which the Public and Private Health System is structured.

The private insurance system covers about 20% of the population [5]. The other 80% of the population depend exclusively on the public health system. The so-called Unified Health System (SUS), funded by the Brazilian government, was created in 1988 to care for and promote the health of the entire population, thus improving the quality of life of Brazilians [6]. The SUS is one of the largest public health systems in the world. It ranges from simple outpatient care to organ transplantation [7], assuring full, universal and free access to the entire population. In addition to offering doctors' appointments, tests and hospital admission, the system also promotes vaccination campaigns, preventive actions and health surveillance initiatives such as food monitoring and drug registration – thus reaching the lives of every Brazilian [8].

The health care system is hierarchically structured: it consists of several interconnected units, each one of them offering a different kind of service. On the first level there are the community health centres that can be directly accessed by any person; for more complex services there are other facilities, such as the polyclinics and hospitals; and for urgent cases, people may go to the closest emergency unit [8].

Brazil is organized into 27 States, each having its State Health Department and in addition, the municipalities have their own Municipal Health Department. Sometimes the small towns organize themselves into health consortia and after considering medical assistance availability in the region, transfer patients from one city to another by bus, cab or ambulance, creating what is called an out-of-home treatment, which is funded by the municipality.

To meet the needs of the population, SUS implemented two projects that are considered a priority, and the expansion of which throughout Brazil is continually increasing in an attempt to provide the entire population with general care, namely:

1- Family Health, the main strategy of the Ministry of Health to redefine the public health care model, is redefining the handout model to a more self deterministic one, and is run through the implementation of multi-professional teams in primary health units. Multidisciplinary teams including one doctor, one nurse, one nursing technician or one nursing assistant and up to 12 community health workers assist families of a given region [9 - 11]. The community health worker is the professional in charge of disease prevention and health promotion activities in the communities, always under the supervision and coordination of a doctor or health worker [12]. Currently, there are about 32,000 Family Health Teams and almost 250,000 Health Community Workers throughout the country. The teams, in partnership with the communities, develop activities related to health promotion, disease prevention, diagnosis and treatment, recovery and rehabilitation [2].

2- To better meet the needs of the population, SUS created the Family Health Support Center (NASF), an organization that is under the responsibility of the municipal health departments. Currently, these Centers are classified in types I and II. Type I must have, at least, 5 health professionals with higher education and cover more than 7 Family Health teams. NASF II must have 3 health professionals with higher education and cover, at least, 3 to 7 Family Health teams, regardless of the population density of the region [13]. In line with the guidelines of the Unified Health System and the National Health Policy for People with Disabilities, the National Policy for Hearing Health Care highlights the importance of access, equity, completeness and social control in hearing health care. It also reaffirms the importance of continuing education for professionals as a way to qualify the service and the need of information about hearing health.

The core objective of this policy is to restructure a *regional* and *hierarchical* service network that implements an integrated care line to address the main causes of hearing loss and establishes guidelines for the accreditation of *primary, secondary* and *tertiary care* provided to hearing-impaired individuals.

How the Programme Has Been Implemented

It is a real challenge for any country to organize a nationwide programme that meets the needs of hearing impaired. Brazil is a country that can claim to have implemented such a service. A lot of progress is still needed, especially in reaching the hinterland of this large country, yet this service has improved every year. The so-called National Policy for Hearing Health Care is unquestionably considered an achievement of the whole society. Pressure of hearing-impaired groups on the federal government and the support given by the scientific communities of Audiology, Speech and Language Therapy and Otolaryngology were essential to bring this policy to life. It is also important to mention the political will of the government, without which everything would have been more difficult.

Before the implementation of this policy there were many initiatives in place to try to meet hearing-impaired people's needs, but all of which had a handout policy approach, i.e. they considered the person a poor thing instead of a common citizen with rights and duties.

It was only in the early years of this millennium that a different proposal started being discussed to approach this issue from a legal rights perspective, i.e. people with disability seen as active citizens in the Brazilian society. The experience of groups of professionals from other areas of the Brazilian health system also contributed to bring this proposal to the hearing impairment field.

In 2004, the federal government issued the National Policy for Hearing Health Care with a series of regulations detailing how to provide this service to hearing-impaired individuals. In order for the National Policy for Hearing Health Care be effective it is critical, among other measures, that each of the three care levels, *primary, secondary* and *tertiary care,* available for hearing-impaired individuals, develop their own activities and articulate among themselves to ensure appropriate referral and counter-referral between units of different care levels, to fully benefit the user. The effectiveness of the policy represents progress in health care quality, efficacy in preventing damages and health promotion, coupled with optimization of budget allocation for this area [14]. Municipal administrators must create conditions so that health administrators have access to information and learning that may contribute to the planning of *ACTIONS* focused on hearing health.

Primary Care Centres (PHC)

Organized primarily in the Health Units throughout the city or countryside, the PHC is the most visited place by local people in search of health care. It is the place where people go for vaccines, where elderly people go for general care or for some free medicines provided by the public health network. Health community workers and family doctors already in this system must be supported by secondary and tertiary level audiology services regarding the prevention of hearing loss and other aspects related to hearing disorders [15]. Primary care includes activities related to promotion and protection of hearing health, prevention', and the earliest possible identification of potential hearing loss or disorder and referral to specialized services, and rehabilitation. Another relevant aspect of Primary Care is the Continuing Education of health professionals, which may happen during team meetings or be developed through discussions and/or specific activities. Continuing Education should always be considered when planning the activities of the team responsible for hearing health in the health units so that the consolidation of practices change the team's manner of working in relation to aspects of hearing health. The Hearing Health actions of Primary Care include preventive actions, in general, such as:

– health education (information, education and Family guidance);
– hearing disorder prevention;
– early identification of hearing disorders;
– share of cases that require other care levels (secondary and tertiary levels);
– rehabilitation actions aiming to reduce disabilities and facilitate user access to rehabilitation as close to home as possible.

These actions are added to other types of service provided by the Unified Health System [16] such as care for:

a) Pregnant women:

– control of factors that affect the developing fetus (hypertension, diabetes, use of ototoxic drugs among others);
– immunization and control of diseases that can lead to congenital infections (rubella, syphilis, toxoplasmosis, cytomegalovirus);
– advice such as raising the baby's head during feeding to prevent alterations of the middle ear.

b) Children and teenagers:

– early identification of newborns that should be referred for specialized evaluation, based on clinical history, of diseases that compromise hearing health and risk factors for hearing loss;
– immunization and control of childhood diseases like mumps, measles, meningitis;
– monitoring of sensorimotor, psychological, cognitive, visual, hearing and speech development by observing children/babies behaviour;

- family guidance on speech and hearing development considering parent's concern and/or suspicion regarding hearing skills of their children;
- guidance to prevent accidents caused by the introduction of objects and cotton swab into the ear, which can hurt and damage the natural lubrication of the canal (cerumen);
- attention to upper airway disease (recurrent otitis and others);
- guidance on the risks of exposure to non-occupational noise (electronics, toys, leisure environments with high level of noise, etc.);

c) Adults:

- guidance to prevent accidents caused by the introduction of objects into the ear, which can hurt and damage the natural lubrication of the canal (cerumen);
- guidance on risk factors for hearing in the work environment (noise, vibration, chemicals) and use of personal protective equipment (PPE);
- guidance on the risks of exposure to non-occupational noise (electronics, toys, leisure environments with high level of noise, etc.);
- identification of adults, including the elderly with complaints about alterations in hearing, vertigo, tinnitus or wheezing, who should be referred for specialized evaluation;
- guidance and monitoring on the use of medications for hypertension, diabetes and kidney diseases;
- actions aimed at workers' health, or occupation-related hearing loss, are given specific attention, regardless of hearing health.

Secondary Care

Specialized care is structured as referral services for diagnosis, selection and provision of hearing instruments, speech therapy and monitoring of hearing function, use of the hearing aid and its benefit for the quality of life of the users.

Secondary Care units are the first place for referral from primary care and referral back from the Hearing Health Care Service of Tertiary Care. The units must be coordinated and integrated with the local and regional systems, providing specialized care to people with ear diseases, particularly people with hearing impairment.

The Hearing Health Care Services of Secondary Care and their specialized professionals work in a comprehensive manner and shall:

- assist the development of actions promoting hearing health and preventing hearing disorders in joint actions with the primary care teams that will be coordinated by local administrator;
- provide otolaryngological care, hearing evaluation and speech-language evaluation;
- screen and monitor hearing in newborns, preschoolers and school children and in workers with frequent exposure to high sound pressure levels referred by primary care;

- perform diagnosis of hearing loss in 3+ year old children, young adults, adults and elderly with hearing loss, considering the evaluation and rehabilitation specifications required by each of these groups;
- ensure rehabilitation through clinical otolaryngology treatment; selection, adaptation and provision of individual hearing aid, monitoring of speech service and therapy for adults and 3+ year old children;
- ensure psychological assessment and therapy, social work service, guidance to family and school;
- refer children under 3 years old, patients with diseases related to unilateral hearing loss and those experiencing difficulty performing hearing evaluation for diagnosis to Hearing Health Care Service of Tertiary Care;
- provide general otolaryngology care and secondary care otolaryngology exams;
- train and educate primary care professionals for hearing health through trainings, workshops, conferences, seminars and local or regional meetings;
- provide technical support to primary care teams to identify cases that need referral to other service levels;
- visit primary care health units to discuss clinical cases.

Tertiary Care

Hearing Health Care of Tertiary Care provides for the diagnosis of hearing loss and its rehabilitation in children under 3 years old and in patients with related diseases (neurological, psychological, genetic syndromes, blindness and low vision), unilateral loss and those experiencing difficulty in hearing evaluation in lower care service level. It provides specialized multiservice assistance to people with otology-related diseases especially to hearing-impaired people. The centres require special equipment, physical infrastructure, specialized human resources and have to be duly accredited by the Unified Health System. For this level of care the policy requires a team composed of at least two otolaryngologists; one neurologist and/or neurologist-pediatrician; one pediatrician and/or neurologist-pediatrician; six speech therapists (three with experience in hearing rehabilitation and three specialized in audiology), one social worker and one psychologist. With this team the service must ensure comprehensive care to patients (diagnosis, clinical treatment, selection, adaptation and provision of individual hearing instruments - hearing aids, monitoring and treatment).

To ensure health completeness and the purpose of the National Policy for Hearing Health Care, these three levels of care need to be integrated in a network, with co-responsibility of all involved. The actions should be planned in order to meet the core objective of the National Policy for Hearing Health of People with Disabilities, which is social inclusion.

The regulation, control and evaluation of actions focused on hearing health care shall be within the three spheres of government (municipal, state and federal). Each municipality, in compliance with guidelines and principles of universality, equity, regionalization, hierarchy and completeness of health care, must include Prevention, Treatment and Rehabilitation of Hearing as part of their Municipal Health Plans and States and Federal District Regionalization Master Plans.

Another aspect to be considered is the Newborn Hearing Screening (NBS) programme. Today, the country is making big efforts to better structure this intervention for the Brazilian population. On August 3, 2010, the government approved Law No. 12.303/10, reference, which mandates the implementation of Newborn Hearing Screening throughout the country but evidence showed that the tertiary care services had no structure to meet this demand. To guarantee the NBS, two professionals are critical: the community health worker and the family doctor. Groups of professionals in Audiology and Otolaryngology have suggested that these professionals monitor babies who fail the newborn hearing screening, yet this is still under discussion and in the implementation phase.

Using the scheme of the national health system that is well structured in Brazil [2], the hearing health services were organized by regions and states. Noteworthy, each of these levels and services corresponds to what we call *Hearing Health*.

Structuring of Hearing Health Services

To implement this policy the federal government funded the creation of Centers of Hearing Health Services, determining one center for every one and a half million people, totaling 146 services currently (see distribution in Table 17.1). These 146 services are distributed in the five regions of the country (North, South, Northeast, Southeast and Central-West), as shown in Table 17.1.

There are 146 accredited Audiology services at the Ministry of Health as shown in Table 17.1 and the team requires a minimum of six Audiologists per service totaling at least 876 professionals working in these centers.

Additionally, there are 24 hospitals that perform cochlear implant surgery through the Unified Health System (Figure 17.1).

Table 17.1 and Figure 17.1 show a lack of audiology services and cochlear implant centers mainly in the North and Central-West regions, even considering a lower population density.

SUS enables the Brazilian population access to electronic devices such as hearing aids or cochlear implant (CI) free of charge. The number of devices provided by the Unified Health System has increased year after year - in 2010, a total of 176,821 hearing aids were granted at a cost of US$ 81,529,890.61 and 626 CI surgeries were performed at a cost of US$17,347,353.31, including the hearing device and surgical costs (Table 17.2).

Table 17.1. Distribution of authorized cochlear implant (CI) centres and audiology services accredited by the Ministry of Health (DATASUS, 2011)[16]

Region	Number of CI Centres	Audiology Services		
		Secondary Care	Tertiary Care	Total
North	1	1	5	6
Northeast	6	16	20	36
Southeast	13	25	35	60
South	3	21	14	35
Central-West	1	2	7	9
TOTAL	24	65	81	146

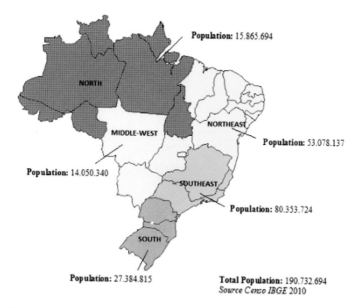

Figure 17.1. Distribution of Brazilian population per region.

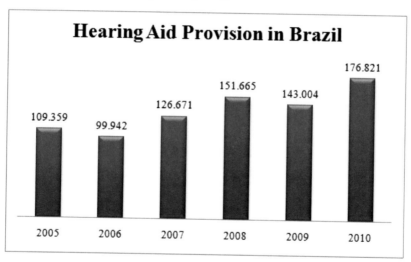

Figure 17.2. Distribution of hearing aids during the last 5 years. (DATASUS, 2011)[16].

Table 17.2 shows the distribution of audiological procedures per age group during 2010. It is worth mentioning that these procedures also refer to all the tests related to audiological diagnosis and hearing aid provision. The universal hearing screening and the procedures related to workers' health, which are occupation-driven, have not been included in the system and results have not been tabulated here. Therefore, the investment made by the government is much higher than that reported and it is not possible to track all the information given the way they are organized.

According to production data (Tabwin/Datasus, 06/21/2011), in 2010 a total of 55,737,867 procedures were conducted and 176,821 hearing aids were granted. (Table 17.2).

Table 17.2. Distribution of number of procedures, number of hearing aids, and budgeted authorized by the Ministry of Health. (Tabwin/Datasus, 06/21/2011) [16]

		Procedures (n)	Hearing Aid
0 - 3 years of age	Frequency (n)	128.868	2.705
	Cost (US$)	2.644.367,81	1.495.906,25
4 - 7 years of age	Frequency (n)	188.924	3.445
	Cost (US$)	2.129.411,80	1.797.390,62
8 - 15 years of age	Frequency (n)	287.159	9.777
	Cost (US$)	3.560.872,16	4.858.937,50
16 - 60 years of age	Frequency (n)	587.426	60.290
	Cost (US$)	11.687.187,41	27.932.828,12
61 - 110 years of age	Frequency (n)	626.030	100.604
	Cost (US$)	12.938.784,71	45.444.828,12
Additional data	Frequency (n)	1.182.462	-
	Cost (US$)	25.824.676,65	-
TOTAL	Frequency (n)	55.737.867	176.821
	Cost (US$)	58.785.300,56	81.529.890,61

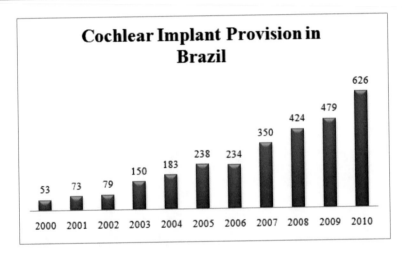

Figure 17.3. Distribution of cochlear implant surgery perform during the last 10 years (DATASUS, 2011)[16].

Table 17.2 shows most of the hearing aids were granted to elderly persons, that represents 20% of the total Brazilian population. Although hearing loss is more common in the elderly, SUS has yet to have more access to other age groups that need hearing aids, such as the children. It is important to understand how the Brazilian government allocates the budget. Table 17.2 shows that spending on procedures is high - US$58,785,300.56 - and some saving could be achieved if there were professionals with better training regarding hearing aid fitting and a protocol with–fewer procedures for this area. However, the government databank reports total procedures, not distinguishing hearing aid fitting from diagnosis-related procedures. Figure 17.3 shows data on cochlear implant surgery. This is an alternative in expansion for the treatment of hearing impairment.

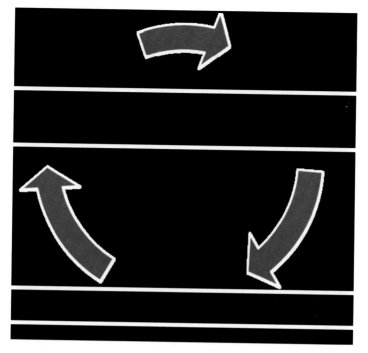

Figure 17.4. Diagrammatic Summary of the Brazilian National Policy for Hearing Health Care.

Practical Issues That Occurred in Initiating and Running the Programme, Failures and Successes

The Brazilian health system is a mixed system, including public and private institutions whose regulation is determined by SUS. Thus, a private institution may provide public service to the population where there is no public service available, provided the institution is registered with SUS to perform such service.

According to this proposal, the services that could be enrolled should be preferably in public, charitable (non-profitable) and finally private institutions. All universities and training centers for Otolaryngology and Audiology professionals have signed up and became part of the public health system. Yet these institutions were not sufficient to provide coverage for the whole country and many private institutions have signed up too.

One of the most difficult aspects in the deployment of the services was the lack of knowledge by local administrators about normal and impaired hearing. Numerous meetings were held and Otolaryngology and Audiology professionals had to strive to make booklets to explain each diagnosis tool and their functions, audiological diagnosis, hearing aid adaptation and so on. This was very important because those people had decision power over funds and auditing services and they lacked the basic knowledge to perform this function in the auditory field. Gradually, this knowledge has been acquired by health professionals from other fields of knowledge (medical, nursing, psychology, etc.), but some issues still arise in more distant regions of the country.

1) definition of evaluation and monitoring criteria of auditory rehabilitation services;
2) improvement of assistance by means of qualification and education of those professionals.

In recent years, electronic devices related to hearing impairment have achieved some technical breakthroughs. In the field of sound amplification, strategies for digital signal processing have brought more flexibility to devices, which also acquired a multitude of algorithms that process the incoming sound in a different way. Particularly, the cochlear implant has brought radical change to the treatment of severe and/or profound bilateral hearing impairment, since it provides greater efficiency in the perception of speech sounds, thus enabling linguistic sophistication for most children with such disabilities. Despite this progress, the use of hearing aids or CI alone does not eliminate the reduction in the processing capacity of the sound signal caused by sensorineural hearing loss, hence the importance of the rehabilitation process.

Given the technological advances, it is necessary to recycle and adapt prior knowledge of traditional methods of hearing intervention for the establishment of a new therapeutic model aimed at stimulating auditory skills. Brazil is characterized by significant socio-economic contrasts, heterogeneity of infrastructure distribution and differences in the education level of professionals, which, coupled with the geographical difficulties, create differences in the quality of hearing health service from one region to another. From a total of 1833 speech therapists specialized in audiology, 67% reside in the Southeast. The difficulty of access to continuing education in other regions is one of the causes of this scenario. Continuing education of these professionals should be understood as a strategy to increase service efficiency and reduce service costs by adding value and greater flexibility to work processes, reducing mistaken practices and increasing problem solving cases.

3) decentralization of services with the implementation of the referral and counter-referral system that can reach the most distant regions not being restricted to big centres. This is a big issue for the whole Brazilian heath system and is also seen in hearing impairment care. As much as the government strives to facilitate the transfer of population to big cities for specialized care, that does not happen satisfactorily;

4) the system is still not widely known by the population so the demand for service among infants, children, youth and young adults is low. It is indeed pretty much sought by the elderly, probably because this population has more free time to go for the health system service, besides the higher prevalence of hearing loss in this group.

5) improvement in the use of those public resources for auditory rehabilitation, as a result of the proposed technical regulation;

According to the Constitution of Brazil, every citizen is entitled to free health care (without costs). The Federal Government funded the Audiology Services and Cochlear Implants Centers with their own money without taking money from the budget of the states and municipalities. After a few years, the government transferred to the states and municipalities the responsibility for managing funds and allocated 250 million Reals for this area (about US$156-million American dollars).

After approving the budget for the Ministry of Health there is still the need to establish collaboration among municipalities and states to discuss money allocation. Consensus was reached about the total budgeted for Hearing Health. The question is "Is it enough?", and the answer is "No". Now it all depends on Brazilian society pushing the government to release more funds for this area. On the other hand, it is mandatory professionals offer a high quality service at lower costs. Thus, the cost of procedures may decrease and the number of people served by the system may increase. Summarizing, the Brazilian National Policy for Hearing Health Care (Figure 17.4) is a very important step to the treatment and social inclusion of the hearing impaired person but it is necessary to improve the system. In 2012 there is going to be introduced a new proposal for a National Program of the Disabled Person. This new program is hoped to provide more equity in the health system in Brazilian society.

China

Xingkuan Bu

Hearing disability not only harms impaired individuals and their families, but also places a heavy burden of social development. Since the WHO general assembly made resolutions for prevention of deafness and hearing impairment (PDH) in 1985 and 1995, countries responded actively to the WHO calls. Many national, regional and global programmes were drawn up and implemented, [1, 2].

China's government is highly concerned about prevention of deafness and hearing impairment (PDH). Relevant laws, statutes and regulations such as "women and children's care law", "safeguard law of handicapped people", "clinical criteria of ototoxic drug use", "regulation of hearing protection in industry" etc were issued in the past twenty years. There are PDH systems including vaccination, newborn hearing screening, control of ototoxicity and genetic hearing loss research programmes. Advances are focused on raising public awareness, initiating the national plan of prevention and rehabilitation of hearing impairment (2007-2015) and enhancing prevention and rehabilitation activities - "Hearing the Future", newborn hearing screening programmes, hearing aids and cochlear implant services , for example.

Raising Public Awareness of PDH

In 2000, China's government designated March 3rd as the annual "National Ear Care Day. The themes were "Prevention of ototoxic hearing loss (2000)", "Early identification and intervention of hearing impairment in children (2001)", "Helping hearing disabled people – saving poor deaf children (2002)", "Enhancing health quality, reducing congenital hearing loss (2003)", "Hearing health care goes to districts (2004)", "Concerning ageing hearing loss – better hearing, happy life (2005)", "Preventing deafness and hearing impairment, enjoying healthy ear and better hearing (2006)", "Protecting youth's hearing - combination actions from urban to rural (2007)", "Wonderful Olympic - I can hear (2008)", "How to use hearing aids correctly (2009)", "Cochlear implantation - a new hope for hearing reconstruction (2010)" and "Hearing habilitation starts from early detection - promoting the newborn hearing screening program (2011)" respectively.

Large consulting activities were held in almost all main cities throughout the whole of China on a single day. This annual public campaign plays a great role in raising awareness of PDH and spreading scientific knowledge about hearing. Especially, it made more people know the risk of ototoxic damage from the abuse and/or improper use of ototoxic drugs. It also made more people conscious of the importance of early detection and early intervention for hearing impairment in children.

Awareness was also raised in the media by TV shows, radio broadcasts and publishing stories, which showed hearing aids and/or cochlear implant providing successful rehabilitation from a deaf-child to an excellent university student.

These awareness activities encourage more and more hearing impaired people and their families to accept modern treatment for their hearing problems.

Initiating the National Plan of Prevention and Rehabilitation of Hearing Impairment (2007-2015)

In order to reduce the social and economic burden from hearing impairment, China's government issued "China's national plan of prevention and rehabilitation of hearing impairment (2007-2015)" in 2007 [3]. The plan consisted of five parts summarized below:

Present Status and Problems

According to the second China national sample survey on disabilities in 2006, there were 27.80 million hearing disabled people. Because the criteria of disability were more strict, the figure was lower than international societies' data, particularly comparing with developed countries [4].

It should be noted that this was a questionnaire based, rather than an audiometric survey. Hearing impairment hurts affected individuals both in physical-physiological and psychological spheres; in addition, it impacts the family and even society. China's government is highly concerned with prevention and rehabilitation of hearing impairment and has had great achievements. But because of its huge population, particularly the fast increasing ageing segment and complex causes of hearing loss, China is facing severe challenges in this field. The main problems are how to control and reduce hereditary and noise induced hearing loss, how to develop good newborn hearing screening programmes, how to improve hearing aids services and how to balance development both in urban and rural areas.

Policies

a) Prevention first, then combination with treatment and rehabilitation
b) Community- based policies with priority for children
c) Multi-resources integration.

Aims

General aim: Everyone has the rights to obtain hearing health care and rehabilitation services. Detailed aims by 2015:

a) Coverage rate of primary ear and hearing health care will reach 80 % (county level);
b) Coverage rate of hearing and speech rehabilitation services will reach 80 % (county level);

c) Compared with 2006 data, the incidence of ototoxic, infectious and noise induced hearing loss will all be reduced by 10% respectively;

d) Comparing with 2005 data, the coverage rate of newborn hearing screening will increase 30 %;

e) Coverage rate of hearing aids and/or cochlear implants for children will reach 90%;

f) 60% of the hearing impaired population will know how to deal with hearing loss scientifically.

Management

a) Enhancing the government leadership role. Local plans were made and issued by local government in 2008.

b) Enhancing manpower development, particularly focusing on primary ear/hearing health care and NHSP training and completing services' network.

c) Promoting PDH by multiple approaches such as women and children's health care, vaccination, drug monitoring, noise control, OME treatment, injury prevention systems etc.

d) Promoting hearing rehabilitation system; setting up connecting networks between diagnosis-and, medical treatment services, and hearing aids fitting, cochlear implant, rehabilitation and special education services.

e) Promoting public awareness, increase activities around national ear care day, distributing hearing care leaflets and providing public hearing health education.

Evaluation

a) Annual evaluation should be made by local government itself and spot-checked by the central government.

b) An interim evaluation will be made in 2010 and the final assessment will be in 2015.

Enhancing Prevention Activities

Hearing the Future (HTF) project was based on "China's national plan of prevention and rehabilitation of hearing impairment (2007-2015)"; it is a 5-year nationally implemented plan aiming to improve hearing health care through prevention, early detection, treatment and rehabilitation, and thus reduce the socio-economic burden of hearing impairment. It was initiated in 2005 by three partners including the China Ministry of Health (CMOH), China Disabled People's Federation (CDPF) and GN ReSound. The Memo was signed on January of 2006 by 3 partners and the legal common agreement was signed on September of 2008 [5]

The project mainly works in three cooperative areas: 1) Hearing screening, diagnosis and treatment infrastructure build up; 2) Audiology training/education and hearing health regulation. 3) Hearing rehabilitation and public awareness. GN ReSound provides financial, technical and management skills support and China Advanced Hearing Advisory Board (CAHA) and the project office support the overall instruction and detailed plans. A CAHA meeting will be held annually to make sure there is a systematic approach at the national level.

The project was first implemented in 2006; the executive team (CAHA) took the leading role in the project to unify the different opinions, the project was implemented by diversified events with full involvement of CAHA national wide. By the end of 2010, 7 annual CAHA meetings had been held. In 2008, CAHA 5 was developed to an international event, 'China Audiology Summit (CAS)', which is the highest level conference and drew great attention from professionals and hearing industry.

Table 17.3. HTF 2006-2008 Main events and achievement

Year	The training/education for professionals					the benefit for stakeholders	
	Total activity	international	national	Provincial	participants	Serviced patient (indirect)	Awareness for stake holder
2006	21	0	18	3	1,936	8,554,000	965,000
2007	25	4	15	6	5,768	9,945,500	1,750,000
2008	17	5	12	0	2,670	9,600,000	500,000

The events, conducted in near 30 provinces, can be divided into international, national, provincial, city, district and community initiatives. Participants included representatives from the MOH, CDPF, institutes, private sector, NGOs and manufactures.

The project acted as a bridge connecting government, professionals, funding agencies, research institutes and commercial entities; it connected people in different geographic and economic areas and China hearing health care to international institutions. So far, there have been about 150 Chinese and 50 international experts in CAHA.

Up to 2008, the project conducted a total of 63 major events with nearly 10000 professional people involved. The events provided indirect benefit to 26 million hearing impaired people and increased public hearing awareness about hearing loss (Table 17.3).

1. Action in Hearing Screening, Diagnosis and Treatment

a) The project covered the audiological clinical service, training/education events and research fields. Especially, it covered comprehensive audiological training in screening, diagnosis, hearing aid and rehabilitation. Most trainees were from hospital and CDPF channels, they built the strong audiology work force for the field.

b) The project utilized 3,000 professional faculty through organizing the systematic audiological training course and conferences at different levels, they were the backbone of the field. These people facilitated development of audiology in China; also they opened the communication to international colleagues in hearing healthcare. The project built a systematic Chinese audiology training resource.

c) The project plays an active role on setting clinical/technical standards/ regulations and reports to policy makers on a regular basis. It accelerates field development and insures the quality of the health service, especially hearing aid services.

d) The project published 20 HTF white papers to promote hearing health development.

2. Action in Audiology Training/Education and Hearing Health Regulation

a) The project supported establishment of approximately 2,800 centers including hearing screening, diagnosis, hearing aid fitting and rehabilitation, enhanced hearing healthcare basic infrastructure in China. These centers provide related services to around 20,000,000 patients.

b) To set up a standard HTF-International Audiology and Training Center (IATC) as a practice model in Asia

3. Action in Hearing Rehabilitation and Public Awareness

a) With CDPF/CRRCDC, conducted hearing network build up- pilot programme in Aging.

b) The project supported the setting up of approximately 800 rehabilitation centres.

c) The project built a series of HTF communications including HTF brochure, newsletter, white paper, training material for professional, brochure for patients.

d) The project organized diversified awareness events on hearing prevention, diagnosis, rehabilitation and healthcare, targeting officials, doctors, hearing impaired people and the public.

4. HTF Routine

So far, HTF has established resources and regular activities such as CAHA group (national and international) and the annual meeting, international audiology and training center (IATC), professional training seminar series, China national database of hearing health care service provider, website: www.hearingthefuture.com (Chinese and English version), newsletter (Chinese and English version), brochures for public, hearing mobile service car (Hearing Express), community-based hearing care activity series, marketing and communication package and HTF Foundation (in construction).

Newborn Hearing Screening Programmes (NHSP)

Approximately 19.5 million babies are born every year and at least 20,000 hearing impaired newborns are added annually [6] in China. Such large numbers of those hearing impaired newborns create a severe public health and social problem. NHSP has been strongly recommended by China's government since 1999. A series of documents such as regulations, national plans, technical criteria and training books have been issued and implemented. National and local training courses and conferences have been held every year since 2000. Staff have to pass the examination and be certified before they can work in this field.

Up to now, more than 20 provinces and/or municipalities (three fourths of China) have implemented the programme at different levels. There are screening centres, usually located in a Women and Children health care centre, responsible for administration connected with newborn PKU and CH screening, diagnostic centres, usually located in Otolaryngology/Audiology departments, and (re)habilitation centres in each province.

Because of the huge population and developing economy, manpower and technical resources, it was impossible to use one model for all of China. Instead, a "Tri-basic sustentation" strategy for NHS was used.

First, hospital-based universal screening (US) was essential and strongly recommended by government and professionals. The first screening tool was otoacoustic emission screening in well- baby units and automated auditory brainstem response tests in newborn intensive care units (NICU). A re-screen was organized for infants who failed and is conducted within 42 days. Diagnostic procedures are available between 3-6 months. After diagnosis, (re)habilitation was undertaken in rehabilitation centers for hearing impaired children.

Secondly, targeted screening (TS) is recommended in rural and remote areas; newborns with high risk factors should be referred to a screening centre within one month after birth.

Thirdly, community screening (CS) was performed. Every child's hearing should be monitored by children's health care system with a questionnaire and simple tests at the community level. Targeted hearing loss screening revealed congenital permanent bilateral or unilateral hearing loss (30-40 dB above, 0.5 – 4 K Hz in average). Auditory neuropathy in NICU, or conductive hearing loss are included. There is still no accurate incidence data of hearing impairment of newborns; results varied from 2.35 ‰ to 5.90 ‰ in different reports [7,8] Current problems are:

1. There is a lack of manpower, especially audiological professionals.
2. Screening is usually conducted quite well, but diagnosis and follow up are difficult.
3. There is a lack of national and provincial databases.
4. There is unbalanced development. In the capital and coastal cities such as Beijing, Shanghai, Nanjing, Jinan etc. the screening coverage rates are between 95-98 %. In addition, hearing screening was not only for newborns, but also extended to 6-year old children in these cities. Since 2002 there has been simultaneous screening for hearing and ocular diseases in over 20,000 newborns cases in Jinan Maternal and Children hospital. There were pilot studies on NHSP plus screening Mt.12SrRNA 1555G, GJB2 and SLC26A4 genes' mutations conducted in a few hospitals. By contrast in a few remote areas, most deliveries are at home and the screening rates were very low.

In order to enhance the programme, the Ministry of Health China issued "Administration of newborn screening" and updated the national NHSP plan and the technical criteria in 2009.The updated plan showed that by 2012 the screening rate of UNHS in WBN should be 80%, 40% and 30% in east, middle and west region of China respectively, and the screening rate in NICU would be 90% in all regions by 2012. By 2015, the NHSP plan would be completed at national-provincial-city-county levels (data base included) and all indices would be increased. NHSP provides the earliest opportunity to identify and remediate hearing impairment in one's life and has precious value. In such a network, multidisciplinary cooperation is the key-point for success. The government played a significant role in the public health programme.

Hearing Aids and Cochlear Implant Services

China's government issued an official document to set up hearing aid dispensing as a formal career in 2008. In consequence, people have to pass the national examination and be licensed before providing hearing aids to hearing impaired persons. In order to fit "China's national plan of prevention and rehabilitation of hearing impairment (2007-2015)", the government initiated a "National rescue programme of cochlear implant and hearing aids services for poor deaf children, 2009-2012". 1500 deaf and 9000 hearing impaired children from poor families would receive cochlear implants and hearing aid services as appropriate free of charge including (re)habilitation training. The Government of China provided special funds – 400 Million CNY for the programme. It was the largest fund for cochlear implant and hearing aid services in Chinese history. Besides the government programmes, there were, and are still, private donations in this field. In addition, since 2009 free hearing aids have been provided for poor children, and also for poor hearing impaired aging people in Shanghai; hopefully, this service will soon be extended to other places. Medical rehabilitation devices and services will be covered in the national basic medical insurance in Jiangsu province by 2012. China has made great progress in prevention and rehabilitation of deafness and hearing impairment. The WHO designated three WHO collaborating centres for PDH in China (two in Beijing, one in Nanjing) 2008-2009.

More work for the national PDH plan will be carried out; more and more hearing impaired people in China will have their lives improved as a result.

India

Arun Kumar Agarwal and Shelly Khanna Chadha

As per WHO estimates, 6% of the Indian population [1, 2] suffers with moderate or higher degrees of hearing impairment, termed as Disabling Hearing impairment [2]. As per the National Sample Survey Organisation (NSSO), India [3] in 2002, 3,061,700 persons in India are afflicted with a hearing disability. This is 16.56% of the total number of 18.49 million disabled persons in the country. The rural population has been shown to be affected more often than the urban population. Poor economic background has also been held partially responsible [4]. The common causes accounting for hearing loss are ear wax, chronic otitis media, otitis media with effusion, dry perforation of the tympanic membrane, congenital hearing loss, noise induced hearing loss and ototoxicity. The lack of health awareness and education has also played a significant role in the high incidence of hearing impairment across the nation.

The Launch

Taking cognisance of these facts, the Ministry of Health and Family Welfare, Government of India, constituted a task force in 2005 to work out the modalities and strategies for Prevention of Hearing impairment in the country. The National Programme for Prevention and Control of Deafness (NPPCD) was launched on a pilot basis in August 2006. It was initially implemented in 25 districts, over 10 states, and one union territory in the country. In 2008, this project was given the shape of a fully- fledged National Programme and is to be gradually expanded to include 200 districts by the end of the 11th Five year plan of

India in 2012. The programme has also been integrated with the National Rural Health Mission, which is an overarching initiative of the Ministry.

The Programme Concept

The programme is based on the concept of the 'HEALTHY EAR DISTRICT' promoted by the Society for Sound Hearing. As per this concept, each district, comprising a population of approximately one million, is to be the functional focus of the programme. All the activities and capacity building are centred on the district. This is to ensure that the services and facilities reach where they are most needed. This concept ensures the presence of an Ear, Nose and Throat (ENT) surgeon and audiological manpower at the level of the District hospital along-with suitable diagnostic and therapeutic resources.

Aims and Objectives of the Programme

1)   To prevent the avoidable hearing loss on account of disease or injury
2)   Early identification, diagnosis and treatment of ear problems responsible for hearing loss and deafness
3)   To medically rehabilitate persons of all age groups, suffering with deafness
4)   To strengthen the existing inter-sectorial linkages for continuity of the rehabilitation programme, for persons with deafness
5)   To develop institutional capacity for ear care services by providing support for equipment, material and training personnel

The Focus of the Programme

The focus of the programme includes both hearing impairment and ear diseases that can lead to hearing loss and/or have serious health consequences for the sufferer. The main priorities under the programme include:

- Otitis media
- Congenital and childhood hearing loss
- Presbyacusis
- Noise induced hearing loss
- Wax impaction
- Ototoxicity

The Health Care Delivery System

India has a well developed health care delivery system right down to the grass root level. The concept is depicted below from grass root level upwards. The size of population each centre caters for is written in parenthesis and the relevant manpower (NPPCD) deployed at each level is represented in italics:

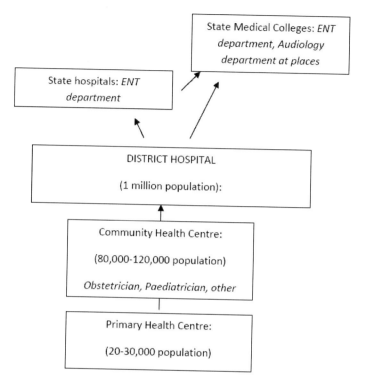

The National Programme for Prevention and Control of Deafness utilizes the existing health care system and focuses on capacity building and service provision within this system. Each level has its designated role, as outlined below:

The *State Medical College* is a centre of excellence which supports the programme in the state with provision of expertise for training as well as patient care and referral. This function overlaps with the State hospitals at certain places.

The *District Hospital* is the nodal point for the implementation of the programme. The ENT doctors and audiologists at the district hospital are involved. However, the programme also looks towards the involvement of private practitioners practising within these districts. The district hospitals have been strengthened with the provision of suitable manpower and equipment to enable diagnostic as well as therapeutic and rehabilitative procedures to be carried out here. The Capacity building measures include:

- Posting of two persons at the district hospital: one audiological assistant and one teacher for hearing impaired children
- Provision of audiological diagnostic equipment including a pure tone audiometer (along with a sound treated room), impedance audiometer, handheld oto-acoustic emission machines.
- Provision/upgrading of surgical equipment including the operating microscope, micro-drill and micro-ear surgery instruments.

The Primary Health Centre (PHC) and Community Health Centres (CHC)

The General duty medical doctors at the PHC/CHC level and school health doctors are being trained in order to reorient them to ear problems and they are provided with the basic diagnostic equipment. The obstetricians and paediatricians at the Community Health centres as well as the State level hospitals and Medical Colleges are being giving a reorientation in early identification of common ear problems and hearing impairment.

Multi-Purpose workers (MPW), and the grass root functionaries, Accredited Social Health Activist (ASHA) and Anganwadi workers(AWW) have been sensitized to the programme and to their specific roles in the programme, through sensitization programmes. The School Health system also plays a very important role in the programme.

The *Roles and Responsibilities:* of each level of manpower have been defined and can be stated in

Box 1.

STATE MEDICAL COLLEGE ENT DOCTORS & AUDIOLOGISTS: Their main role is to serve as resource persons for trainings of all levels and also to provide support and guidance to the District level manpower in the handling of difficult cases and sophisticated investigations.
DISTRICT LEVEL ENT DOCTORS & AUDIOLOGISTS: They are to serve as the reference centre for the lower levels. They have to provide all modalities for audiological diagnosis as well as surgical expertise for management of common ear operations. They are also the resource peoples for training lower levels of manpower, while being the main coordinators for the programme. In most districts, it is the District hospital ENT surgeon who plays the role of the District Nodal Officer for the programme
OBSTETRICIANS & PAEDIATRICIANS: They have to play their part in the early identification of the deaf child. They can also guide the community towards proper ear and hearing care practices and preventive modalities for deafness and ear diseases. The paediatricians are also expected to diagnose, treat and, where required, refer the children with ear diseases.
PHC Doctors: Are the first level of contact of the community with formal health care. They have to diagnose ear diseases, treat the cases which they are competent enough to handle and refer the rest to an ENT surgeon for an expert opinion.
SCHOOL HEALTH DOCTORS: Have to carry out ear and hearing screening activities at the local schools within villages.
MPWs: The MPWs are expected to carry out hearing screening of all children brought to the sub-centre for immunization, with the help of a questionnaire and behavioral tests and to refer them to the district hospital for formal testing, when indicated.
AWW, ASHA: They are expected to carry out screening at the doorsteps with the help of a family based questionnaire provided to them. They also perform the important role of awareness creation at the grass root level.

ADDITIONAL MANPOWER UNDER THE PROGRAMME:

AUDIOLOGICAL ASSISTANT: has to perform the tasks of carrying out the diagnostic tests at the district hospital and assisting the Nodal officer and audiologist, where one is available.

TEACHER FOR HEARING IMPAIRED: has to cater to the preschool educational needs of the identified hearing impaired children along with suitable treatment provision. They also have to maintain the records and prepare the reports for the programme and also organise the screening camps in consultation with the NGO.

SCHOOL TEACHERS: of the Primary section are required to conduct a survey based on a predesigned questionnaire. Children who are suspected to be suffering with any ear disease are examined by the School health/PHC doctors.

Activities [5]

The various activities being carried out under the programme include:

1. Manpower Training: Training and re-sensitization of existing human resources in the concepts of primary ear and hearing care is an essential component of the programme. Seven levels of trainings included are:

   a. Sensitization of the district level ENT doctors and audiologists
   b. Sensitization of the district level audiologists
   c. Obstetricians and paediatricians working at various centres under the programme
   d. PHC doctors and school health doctors
   e. Multi-purpose workers
   f. Anganwadi workers and ASHA
   g. Parents of disabled children within the community

Standardised and field tested training manuals and lectures have been developed for use throughout the country.(Figures 17.5- 17.7)

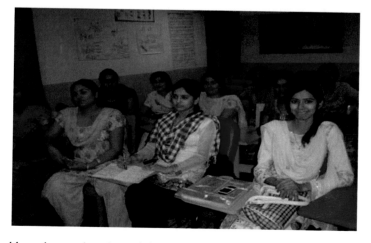

Figure 17.5. Health workers undergoing training.

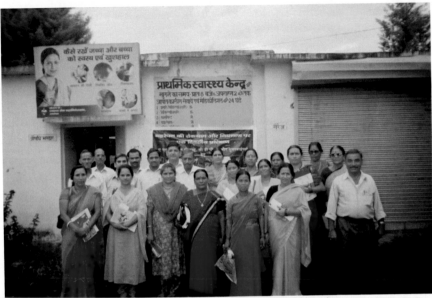

Picture courtesy Dr. Saurabh Varshney, State Nodal Officer, Uttarakhanad.

Figure 17.6. Training of grass root level workers in Uttarakhand, North India.

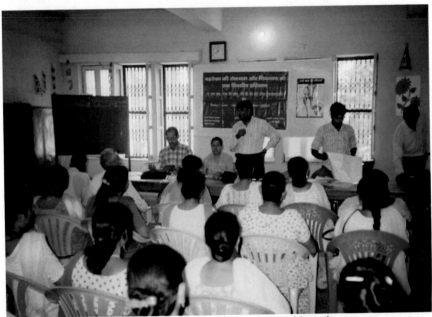

Picture courtesy Dr. Saurabh Varshney, State Nodal Officer, Uttarakhanad.

Figure 17.7. Training of Multipurpose Health workers underway in Dehradun, Uttarakhand, North India.

2.   Capacity Building of the institutions through:

   a.   Manpower deployment at the district hospital
   b.   Provision of equipment

3. Development of innovative and indigenous 'IEC' (Information, Education and Communication) material for creation of awareness within the community. Material such as posters, flip charts, handouts, TV clips, audio- clips have been developed and translated into the relevant regional languages.
4. Service provision is the most important aspect of the programme.

Service Provision [5]

Services provided include:

Screening of Persons for Ear and Hearing Diseases

This is carried out through:

- *Community based camps* that are held in different parts of the district every month. These camps are coordinated by the staff at the district level including the audiological assistant. The purpose is to identify persons with ear diseases as well as hearing loss. Suitable therapy can be started at the camp, when possible or the patient be referred to the district hospital for investigations and treatment. It also helps to create awareness within the community. The camps are held in collaboration with local non-governmental organisations (NGOs).
- *School Screening camps/activities* carried out by the teachers and school health doctors, where available. Where such a person is unavailable, the screening can be done by a trained person such as the Primary Health Care (PHC) doctor or an ENT surgeon. (Figure 17.8)
- *Infant hearing screening.* With the help of the hand held OAE machine, the audiological assistant is expected to screen all babies born at the district hospital or admitted there at any time during the first year of life. The MPWs carry out community based screening for those not reaching the hospital.

Diagnosis and Medical Treatment

Patients can seek treatment at the PHC as well as the district hospital. At the PHC Centre, the primary level physician can examine the ear of the patient with the equipment provided under the programme. They can provide or start the treatment when possible. Those patients who cannot be treated at the PHC, or who require investigation or special treatment can be referred to the district hospital.

Audiological Investigations

Most audiological diagnosis will be carried out at the district hospital with the help of the equipment provided, by the audiologist as well as the audiological assistant at this centre. Referral to tertiary centre will be required only for the purpose of special investigations such as brainstem evoked response tests.

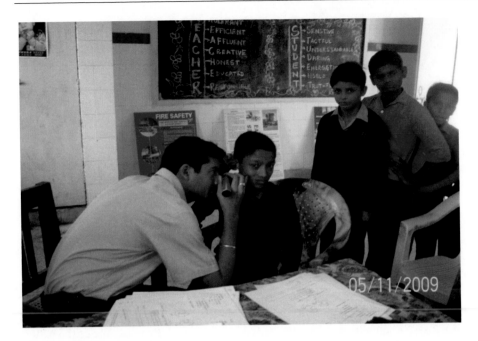

Figure 17.8. School screening.

Surgical Treatment

The district hospitals have been equipped to provide all possible surgical options that are commonly required by a patient suffering from common ear disease. All common ear surgery is now carried out at the equipped centres. However, certain surgical procedures, which may be beyond the competence of the surgeon at present, such as cochlear implantation or surgery for complications of otitis media including intracranial problems, have to be referred to the medical college for management.

Hearing Aid Fitting

Children under the age of 14 years who are identified under the programme and adjudged by the ENT surgeon and audiologist/ audiological assistant to be in need of a hearing aid are fitted with a hearing aid free of cost at the district hospital. This facility is available in limited numbers only (100 hearing aids per district per year). The hearing aid will be fitted with a custom made mould and maintained (other than batteries) free of cost by the identified hearing aid supplier under the programme. The same benefit can also be extended to other beneficiaries (above 14 years) under the programme at the discounted cost as per the government rate contract.

Hearing and Speech Therapy, Rehabilitation

These are provided to those needing it at the district hospital. The ultimate objective is ensure prompt and suitable rehabilitation in order to mainstream these children into regular schools at an early age in life.

Monitoring and Evaluation

is a very important aspect of the programme as it allows judgement of the progress made by the programme in various districts, states and the country as a whole. For this purpose, monitoring proformas for all levels have been developed.

Current Status of the Programme

The programme is being implemented through the National Rural Health Mission initiative of the government of India. The programme is currently running in over a quarter of the districts of the country. It is planned to expand the programme to the entire country over the next 5 years.

Other Initiatives

There is a variety of other programmes running and under consideration within India, at the sub-national levels. Significant amongst these are the:

1. Less Noisy City programme
2. School Screening Programme

Less Noisy City

The Government of Delhi is considering the launch of the Less Noisy Delhi programme. The concept has been developed and promoted under the Sound Hearing 2030 programme.
The activities proposed under this programme are as follows:

1. Create and publicize an Anti-Noise Cell, so that people know where to complain about noise related problems and have the problems addressed at the earliest.
The composition of the Anti-Noise Cell should be:

- Technical advisors:
  o ENT Doctors
  o Audiologists
  o Environmental health expert
- Public health expert
- Representatives of Pollution Control Committee of the city
- Representatives of the Central pollution Control Board
- Representatives of the administration
- Environmental scientists
- Representative of police force and the traffic police
- Legal representative
- Representatives of the Resident Welfare Associations (RWA)
- Project managers

The scope of this Cell would be to receive noise-related complaints through phone and mail. The complaints should be verified by the environmental scientists and suitable action would have to be taken against the offender/s where the complaint is found to be valid. The nature of the action would have to be in keeping with the existing legislation in this regard.

In order to ensure the successful implementation of this concept of Less Noisy City, this cell has to be the key point so that people in the city can make any noise related complaint to this cell and be assured that the same will be addressed in a proper manner. At the same time, frivolous or baseless complaints must not be encouraged to prevent the misuse of this cell.

2. *Awareness campaigns.* As prevention is the main key, it is important to create awareness about the harmful effects of noise on the body.

    a.   Campaign through advertisements on city buses, train or metro
    b.   Television programmes
    c.   Radio programmes
    d.   Pitch stories to newspapers and magazines
    e.   Write magazine articles
    f.   Speak to school students
    g.   Speak to civic groups e.g. RWA
    h.   Produce and distribute brochures / put up posters at public places including hospitals
    i.   Locate and promote a celebrity spokesman for the anti-noise cause.

3.   Make the implementation of a *Noise Conservation Programme* mandatory in all factories and industrial houses. A Noise Conservation Programme is recommended by OSHA (Occupational Safety and Health Administration) and consists of:

    a.   Hearing screening of all employees at time of joining
    b.   Sensitization and awareness programmes
    c.   Use of hearing protectors
    d.   Reduction of noise level by engineering and architectural measures
    e.   Regular surveillance of workers by annual audiological check up.

Besides the industry, this programme should also be implemented for other high risk groups such as:

- Traffic policemen
- Workers at busy intersections
- Disc jockeys at discotheques/ bars/ restaurants
- Workers in business process outsourcing organisations who might be at risk

4.   Strict implementation of existing legislation with respect to
    - Traffic noise e.g. no horn zone,
    - 10 pm time limit for loud speakers etc.

5. *Recommendations regarding development of new legislation pertaining to:*
Monitoring and regulation of noise levels in various urban areas including:

- Cinema halls
- Restaurants and bars
- Discotheques
- Malls

This is essential as these places are often noisy and habitual or prolonged exposure to this is a potential cause for auditory and extra-auditory effects of noise.

6. *Noise labels.* It has been observed that many items of daily use, such as household equipment, children's toys and firecrackers emit high levels of noise.

Noise labels would consist of labels on each of these items regarding the levels of noise that they emit. Wherever, the levels are above the permitted levels, it should be accompanied by a warning regarding the potential side effects. Even I-Pods, Walkmen and MP3 players should come with a warning about the harmful effects of playing the music at loud levels and be fitted with noise limiters.

This would serve a two-fold purpose:

- It will generate greater awareness about noise.
- May motivate some of the manufacturers to lower the emission levels by using better quality material and better engineering techniques.

7. *Provide guidance and guidelines* to the city developers regarding development of new roads and housing in a manner that is environment friendly and makes use of noise absorbent material and various natural and artificial noise barriers. This should be done in consultation with the local Ministry of Environment. Guidelines developed should be valid, practical and affordable.

8. *Create active anti-noise groups in schools, colleges and in RWA,* that will make it their job to identify noisy elements within the community and who will have the linkage to convey the same to the authorities from where the requisite action can be taken.

9. Issue *"Noisy dozen" awards* to major noise polluters

10. Promote *Noise Awareness Day*

11. Promote an annual *Noise Free Week.*

School Screening Programme

In keeping with the principles of school health, the Delhi government has an elaborate School Health programme. The School Ear and Hearing Screening Programme has been run in various parts of the city since the last three years. This programme has been facilitated by the Rotary Club in parts of the city.

The activities undertaken as a part of this programme include:

1. *Development and field testing of a Screening Proforma*
2. *Introductory visit to the school.* On the day prior to the screening, a visit was made to the school and a meeting was held with the teachers of the primary sections. They were instructed regarding the objective and methodology of the survey to be carried out. They were informed about the common ear diseases that are prevalent among children and the need to identify these. They were then introduced to the Screening Proforma. They were informed about how they had to fill it for each of the children in their respective sections.
3. *Screening Camp* On the day of the camp, a team of four doctors visited the school.. The activities for the camp included:

   a. Awareness creation through

   - Promotional talk: A brief talk was held in the morning, prior to the actual screening. This talk included: importance of healthy ear care habits and principles of good ear and hearing hygiene.
   - Display of awareness material

   b. Screening of all the children through

   - Ear check- up: by otoscopy/headlight
   - Hearing check- up: with tuning forks and behavioral observation
   - Impedance audiometry: with a hand-held screener, in order to identify secretory otitis media.
   - Wax removal: Wherever required and if possible, removal of wax/foreign body was done at the time of the clinical examination.

   c. Once the screening check-up had been completed, the list of children found to be suffering with any ear problem was prepared. This list was handed over to the school principal as well as the section teachers. The problems were coded as:

   - Require attention: to be sent to the ENT department at a nearby referral hospital for treatment. Children with problems such as wax, or diagnosed secretory otitis media and foreign body in the ear fell into this category
   - Require special attention: to be sent to tertiary referral hospital for investigations and treatment. Children with a safe type of otitis media or mild- moderate hearing loss fell in this category.
   - Require URGENT attention: to be sent to a tertiary hospital, at the earliest possible for suitable treatment. Children suffering with an unsafe type of chronic otitis media or severe hearing loss of any nature were included in this category. A referral slip was also handed over to them, to facilitate their visit to the referral hospital.

d. Linkages to suitable referral centres in the area where the school was located, were developed prior to the initiation of screening activities. This is an essential component of the programme, in order to ensure proper service provision to the children requiring investigations and management.

Acknowledgments

Figures 17.6 and 17. 7 are by courtesy of Dr Saurabh Varshney, State Nodal Officer, Uttarakhanad, India.

Conclusion

The three large countries that have reported their national plans for prevention of hearing loss in detail here all believe that they have made significant progress in setting them up and in starting to implement them.

All believe that they still have a long way to go. In Brazil the National Policy for Hearing Health Care is an important step towards the treatment and social inclusion of hearing-impaired people. It will be enhanced in 2012 by a new proposal for a National Program for People with Disabilities which is intended to bring more equity to the health care system in Brazil.

However there remain many challenges to improve this part of the health system because of the country's socio-economic contrasts, variable infrastructure, and differing professional education overlaying its vast size and varied geography.

China has made great progress recently through the National Plan of Prevention and Rehabilitation of Hearing Impairment (2007-2015), and its implementation has been strengthened recently by inputs from the three newly designated WHO Collaborating Centres in China for prevention of deafness and hearing impairment.

There are still serious problems to be faced in its increasing and ageing population, especially in reducing hereditary and noise induced hearing loss, developing newborn hearing screening programmes, improving hearing aids services and balancing development in urban and rural areas. In India, the National Programme for Prevention and Control of Deafness looks at all levels of prevention.

There is a particular focus on awareness creation and capacity building with the help of WHO training materials adapted to local needs. The programme commenced in 2006 and continues to be expanded to reach more districts and different states. However much work still remains to be done in order to reach the current goal of reducing the burden of disease by 25% by the year 2012.

The ultimate goal is complete coverage of all districts in India by the programme over the next few years. These 3 large countries have set a huge example to the rest of the world to follow suit and set up national plans and programmes in this neglected field. It will be interesting and exciting to see how other countries take up the challenge.

References

Introduction

[1]   Global status report on non-communicable diseases 2010. WHO, Geneva 2011. Available at: http://whqlibdoc.who.int/publications/2011/9789240686458_eng.pdf (Accessed 2 October 2011).

[2]   Engaging for Health: Eleventh General Programme of Work 2006-2015 A Global Health Agenda. WHO, Geneva 2006. Available at: http://whqlibdoc.who.int /publications/2006/GPW_eng.pdf (Accessed 2 October 2011).

[3]   Medium-Term Strategic Plan 2008–2013 (Amended), WHO Geneva 2010. Available at: http://apps.who.int/gb/ebwha/pdf_files/MTSP2009/MTSP3-en.pdf Accessed 2 October 2011).

Brazil

[1]   IBGE.(2011). Instituto Brasileiro de Geografia e Estatística. Available from: http://news.bbc.co.uk/2/hi/americas/country_profiles/1227110.stm (Accessed 25 July 2011).

[2]   Paim, J., Travassos, C., Almeida, C., Bahia, L., Macinko, J. (2011). The Brazilian health system: history, advances and challenges. The Lancet [Periodico on line] DOI:10.1016/S0140-6736(11)60054-8. Available from: http://www.thelancet.com/ series/health-in-brazil (Accessed 9 May 2011).

[3]   3.Carvalho, R.M.M.A., Soares, T.S., Valverde, S.R. (2005).Caracterização do setor florestal: uma abordagem comparativa com outros setores da economia. *Ciência Florestal, Santa Maria, 15,* 105-118.

[4]   Pagliaro H.(2010). A revolução demográfica dos povos indígenas no Brasil: a experiência dos Kayabí do Parque Indígena do Xingu, Mato Grosso, Brasil, 1970-2007. Caderno de Saúde Pública [online]. 2010, vol.26, n.3, pp. 579-590. ISSN 0102-311X. Available from: http://www.scielo.br/pdf/csp/v26n3/15.pdf (Accessed 25 July 2011).

[5]   Zucchi, P., and Ferraz, M.B. (2010). Economia e Gestão em Saúde. (1ª edição). São Paulo, SP: Manole.

[6]   Guanais F.C. (2010). Health equity in Brazil. British Medical Journal, 341:c6542

[7]   Guanais F.C. (2010). Health equity in Brazil. British Medical Journal, 341:c6542

[8]   Bevilacqua, M.C., Alvarenga, K. de F., Costa, O.A., Moret, A.L. et al. (2010). The universal newborn hearing screening in Brazil: From identification to Intervention. *International Journal of Pediatric Otorhinolaryngology 74,* 510–515.

[9]   Bevilacqua, M.C., Novaes, B.C., Morata, T.C., (2008).Audiology in Brazil. *International Journal of* Audiology, 74, 45–50.

[10]   10 Harris, M., Haines A. (2010). Brazil's Family Health Programme. *British Medical Journal, 341:*c4945.

[11]   Rocha R, Soares, R. (2010). Evaluating the impact of community-based health interventions: evidence from Brazil's family health program. *Health Economics, 19,* 126–158.

[12] Sossai, L.C.F., Pinto, I.C., Mello, D.F. (2010). O agente comunitário de saúde (ACS) e a comunidade: percepções acerca do trabalho do ACS. *Ciência, Cuidado and Saúde, 9,* 228-237.

[13] Molini-Avejonas, D.R., Mendes, V.L.F., Amato, C.A.H. (2010).Speech-Language Pathology and Centers for Supporting the Family Health: concepts and references. *Revista da Sociedade Brasileira de Fonoaudiologia, 15,* 465-474.

[14] Brasil (a) Portaria GM/MS nº 2.073 de 28 de setembro de 2004. Institui a Política Nacional de Atenção à Saúde Auditiva. Diário Oficial da União. 29 set 2004; Seção 1:34.

[15] 15.Victora, C.G., Barreto, M.L., Leal, M.C., Monteiro, C.A., Schmidt, M.I., Paim, J., Bastos, F.I, Almeida, C., Bahia, L., Travassos, C., Reichenheim, M., Barros, F.C., and the Lancet Brazil Series Working Group. (2011). Health conditions and health-policy innovations in Brazil:the way forward. www.thelancet.com Published online May 9, 2011 DOI:10.1016/S0140-6736(11)60055-X. Available at http://www.thelancet.com /series /health-in-brazil

[16] DATASUS. (2011). Available from: http://www2.datasus.gov.br/DATASUS/index.php

China

[1] Bu, X. (2004). WHO prevention of deafness and hearing impairment and the work in China. *Chinese Journal of Otorhinolaryngology, 39,* 316-318 (In Chinese).

[2] Ku, Y-A. (2009). Introduction of WHO prevention of deafness and hearing impairment. *News and Reviews of Otolaryngology, 24,* 16-17. (In Chinese).

[3] Chen, Z. (2009). Introduction of China's national plan of prevention and rehabilitation of hearing impairment (2007-2015). *News and Reviews of Otolaryngology, 24,* 7-8. (In Chinese).

[4] Runping, Y. As population grows older, number of disabled soars. News item on Chinese Government's Official Web Portal, dated Friday, December 1, 2006. Available from: http://english.gov.cn/2006-12/01/content_458783.htm (Accessed 24 October 2011).

[5] Lassen, J.G., Feng, M., Fan, M. (2009). Introduction of hearing the future – a five years plan of prevention of hearing impairment in China. News and Reviews of Otolaryngology, 24, 24-27. (In Chinese).

[6] Audiology Division, ORL-HNS Branch, Chinese Medical Association. (2009). Guidelines for newborn and infant hearing screening. *Chinese Journal of Otolaryngology, Head and Neck Surgery,*44, 883-887 (In Chinese).

[7] Wu, H., Shen, X., Li, Y.,Tao, Z., Zhang, F., Chen, X., Jin, X. (2007). Universal newborn hearing screening and effect of early intervention. *Journal of Shanghai Jiaotong University (Medical Science), 27,* 10-13(In Chinese).

[8] Nie, W., Gong, L., Liu, Y., Xiang, L., Lin, Q., Qi, Y., Nie, Y.(2003).Results of newborn hearing screening in 10501 cases. *National Medical Journal of China, 83,* 274-277 (In Chinese).

India

[1]   Situation review and update on deafness, hearing loss and intervention programmes.(2007). Delhi: World Health Organisation, Regional Office for South East Asia.

[2]   WHO-SEA multi-centre study on the magnitude and aetiology of hearing impairment using the who ear and hearing disorders survey (WEHDS) protocol, survey results from four sea countries, submitted by Ian Mackenzie at a meeting in Delhi, South East Asian Regional Office Headquarters, World Health Organisation, in May 2001.

[3]   National Sample Survey Organisation. (2003). Disabled Persons in India, NSS 58th Round (July-December 2002), Available from: http://mospi.nic.in/rept%20_%20pubn /485_final.pdf (Accessed 24 October 2011).

[4]   Chadha S.K, Agarwal A.K, Gulati A, Garg A. (2006). A comparative evaluation of ear diseases in children of higher versus lower socioeconomic status. *Journal of Laryngology and Otology. 120*, 16–19.

[5]   Garg S, Chadha S, Malhotra S, Agarwal AK (2009). Deafness: burden, prevention and control in India. Natl Med J India 22:79–81.

In: Prevention of Hearing Loss
Editors: V. Newton, P. Alberti and A. Smith

ISBN: 978-1-61942-745-7
© 2012 Nova Science Publishers, Inc.

Chapter XVIII

Global Prevention of Hearing Loss: Achievements and Future

Peter W. Alberti, *Valerie E. Newton*
and Andrew W. Smith

This book attempts to identify and summarize important areas related to the prevention of hearing loss and deafness. It reflects to a large extent the application of general advances in science, technology, medicine, psychology and sociology to this field. No discipline however large exists in isolation. The sense of hearing, connecting the listener to the external environment, people and things, straddles these disciplines. Advances in medicine, including the development of antibiotics brought about a dramatic reduction in life-threatening ear infections; advances in psychology and neural imaging are bringing about a greater understanding of hearing and listening; the first application of the transistor was to produce a hearing aid and the cochlear implant would not have been possible without the implantable cardiac pacemaker. The huge strides in the understanding of genetic disease are being applied to congenital deafness so at least now the causes of these problems are better understood and parents and hard of hearing individuals can be better counselled. The aging of society brings with it cognitive problems which have become central to large parts of hearing science. The recognition that more than 50% of hearing loss can be primarily prevented has produced a paradigm shift in attitudes to the management of this disorder. Work related to the prevention of hearing loss spans an area from molecular biology to the social structure of communities. Much has been achieved; even more need be undertaken, both in research and the application of current and future knowledge to this area.

Without knowledge of the size of a problem it is unlikely that action will be taken. In the 1980s the WHO suggested that there were 40 million people worldwide with disabling hearing loss; this appeared to many to be an underrepresentation of the facts. There was minimal evidence available; very few studies of prevalence had been undertaken although the US public health and the UK provided figures by the late 1980s, which if extrapolated, were

---

* Corresponding Author. E-mail: peter.alberti@rogers.com.

far in excess of this. By the mid-1990s the figure had been raised to 125 million people worldwide with an unequivocally disabling hearing loss, which was again revised upwards in the last decade to 275 million. The increase in numbers resulted from better epidemiological data and the significant growth in world population, especially the aging population.

However, it is quite clear is that, in spite of the excellent surveys undertaken in the past 15 years, much more work is needed. There have been no studies reported from Eastern Europe and Central Asia and there are only limited South Asian studies. It is of note that in those areas where the regional WHO office was interested in hearing loss, surveys have been undertaken; where regional WHO offices had other priorities, as for example in the European office, which includes all the old USSR and therefore Central Asia, little has been done. It is only in recent years that the Pan American Health Organisation (PAHO), the name for the WHO Regional office for Latin America has taken an interest and only now is information coming from that region. There is urgent need for continuing surveys of hearing levels so that a more accurate idea can be obtained of global prevalence. It is highly likely that it is even higher than currently described.

This begs the question what is a "disabling hearing loss"? A figure of 40 dB in the better hearing ear was selected by WHO because it was unequivocally disabling; many thought this cut-off point was too severe. Stevens and others working on behalf of the global burden of disease (GBD) project have now accepted that a 35 DB, four frequency average, in the better ear is a point where a hearing aid is necessary and now estimate that almost half a billion people worldwide have this degree of hearing loss They also identify, fairly unequivocally, that the prevalence increases with poverty, it is much lower in the industrialized nations than in the rest of the world. When the life span increases in developing nations, the prevalence will grow again, due to presbyacusis, hopefully offset by improved health and less early HL. This is an extremely dynamic situation.

Why are prevalence figures so important? If individuals and society are to invest money and resources in all levels of prevention of a disorder, there must be evidence that the condition is common enough and important enough to initiate action. Governments are more likely to spend money to prevent something with a 4% prevalence than a 0.4% prevalence. The disorder should have significant social and economic consequences. Further it should be amenable to prevention and management. Hearing loss fits these criteria. The primary, secondary and tertiary prevention of hearing loss have all improved in quality within the last two decades and its debilitating social and economic consequences are being revealed.

It is important to know the cost to the individual and to society of a particular condition; costs to society of inaction as well as of remedial action. How much revenue is lost by hearing-impaired person being unable to work and earn income at the same level as an otherwise equal normal hearing person? How productive are they, on average compared with their normal hearing peers? How much additional funding is required to educate the hearing impaired? How much additional funding is required in sheltered accommodation and other aid for the hearing impaired? What is the cost of prevention and treatment? There are limited funds available for healthcare, habilitation and rehabilitation. In order to prioritize hearing loss a good case must be made that the expenditure is cost effective. To this point, very little hard economic evaluation has been undertaken. The book includes a chapter on some aspects of cost analysis in the developing world; what is now required is that these analyses are applied and extended globally. Evidence from the industrialized economies is extremely soft, an Australian study and estimates from the US suggest that overall costs seem to be extremely high but there is an urgent need for serious economic evaluation of all degrees of hearing loss, from the mildest to the most severe; from childhood to old age, as well as the cost benefit of intervention. This has been undertaken in several parts of the world for cochlear implantation, but has not occurred for more common procedures such as hearing aid fitting and industrial hearing conservation! The costs for hearing compensation amongst veterans are known in the USA and are huge. Without this basic information, prevalence and cost, efforts at prevention, individual, regional and international will falter.

Much has been learned about the mechanism of hearing; the function of various parts of the cochlea has been discovered as well as the types of hearing loss which occur with specific malfunctions. This has led to novel preventative measures and treatment for certain types of hearing loss, albeit many still experimental. The use of antioxidants to prevent hearing loss from acute noise injury appears promising, although it is unlikely that it will become a substitute for other hearing conservation measures in industry. Targeted delivery of drugs is a general need especially in oncology; this will lead to new methods of delivering medication specifically to the inner ear. In avian models it has even been possible to demonstrate regeneration of hair cells and there is hope that this may be possible in the mammalian cochlea. Stem cell therapy will come into its own, in the cochlea as in other parts of the body, although many challenges remain, not least of which is the connection of new hair cells to the brain.

It is wrong to think of the sense of hearing in isolation. Hearing is only one of the sensory inputs which connects the brain to the environment. Like vision, touch, balance and smell, auditory signals are integrated by the brain and become important information to allow a person to function. The role of hearing or the lack of it, in the cognitive functioning of the elderly, is now being better recognized. To hear may be easier than to listen. Labelling someone as cognitively impaired without testing their hearing and vision is doing them a disservice; a hearing aid in an elderly person may bring them back into contact with the external world and an apparent cognitive deficit, disappear. The relationship between hearing, listening and cognition is currently an area of intense study. Equally important, attention is moving from hearing, a peripheral function, to listening, a central function. This will lead to improved communication techniques with and by, the hearing impaired, especially the elderly. As a rapidly increasing proportion of the population is aging and the dependency ratio worsens, anything which will lead to more independent living is both welcome and necessary.

The sense of hearing is part of a communication system: sound source, transmission medium and reception (hearing). For example, the acoustic conditions in which communication is attempted play an important role in how effective it is, particularly for someone with hearing loss. The acoustic environment in transportation hubs such as bus stations, airports and railway stations are almost uniformly poor as are most of the auditory messages transmitted within buses, subways, trains and planes. To the writers' knowledge there are no regulations about fire alarms in homes for the elderly, such as flashing lights or vibrating signals which would bypass auditory deficits; this need not be, but until those who design these spaces are obliged to improve the conditions, they will remain poor.

The prevalence of hearing loss diminishes with the severity of the loss; most hearing-impaired people have a slight loss which interferes somewhat with their lives but which is only troublesome in poor acoustic conditions. Indeed the interface area between hearing loss which requires a hearing aid and does not require one is often dictated by the acoustic conditions in which listening is attempted. Better attention to acoustics in public places would significantly help all people, whether hearing impaired or not as well as diminishing markedly the number of hearing aids which are required. Dining halls or cafeterias in general, and specifically those used by the elderly, deserve better attention to their acoustics than they usually receive. A little sound deadening by rugs, wall hangings and ceiling acoustic tiles can turn an auditory 'Tower of Babel' into an environment where it is possible to distinguish what is being said. Perhaps the worst example is classrooms where it has been unequivocally demonstrated that poor acoustic conditions interfere markedly with learning. All too often classrooms have hard surfaces, no sound- absorbing areas and poor isolation from adjacent rooms and the exterior. This is a global issue and one where a certain amount of expenditure in the educational system will have a huge positive effect on learning. Pioneering work in the United States has produced a model standard which could well be adopted elsewhere.

Much has been done in recent years to provide access for the disabled; in reality that is mainly for those with mobility problems, so wheelchair access is common, those with visual loss are helped by braille imprinted on elevator buttons, and auditory signals in elevators and street crossings, and ridges in the pavement in all Chinese cities, but little has been done for the hearing impaired. One of the great problems with long-term preventative measures is that they are costly up front without immediate payback. As an example, universal newborn hearing screening is relatively expensive but the benefit to society comes later when those who were identified and habilitated are able to earn a better living than they might otherwise have done, but that cost benefit is years after the initial expenditure on screening.

There is likely to be considerable debate over the need for and use of the standard childhood vaccines in the next decade. A major, and perhaps unexpected, benefit of vaccination has been the reduction of hearing loss produced by these diseases. Vaccination has been extremely efficient in eliminating many disorders, such as measles, mumps and rubella so that fewer parents now know the havoc that these disorders may create; all they see are possible side effects; the rate of vaccination continues to diminish so that ultimately herd immunity may again be lost and the diseases will re-emerge. The risk of a future epidemic of rubella, and its consequent devastating impact on the foetus of pregnant rubella sufferers is real. The recent emphasis on vaccination in developing countries will help reduce the prevalence of hearing loss, important for they often do not have the resources to manage hearing losses when they occur.

Otitis media is a major burden in childhood, pain, transient hearing loss, visits to physicians, parent's time off work to look after the children when taken to the physician, cost of treatment; all add up to billions of dollars annually in the United States alone. Vaccines to prevent otitis media are an attractive idea but at present this seems to be a chimera because of the many different organisms involved. Yet it seems probable that vaccines for otitis media will play an increasing role in preventing this disease and its sequelae, as will vaccines against meningitis, a minor cause of hearing loss in the industrialized nations but a major cause in the meningitis belt of central Africa; vaccination is affordable in that region, the management of the disease and the subsequent deafness experienced by up to 25% of those who survive, is not.

There is an increasing understanding of the genes involved in a considerable amount of congenital hearing loss. Hopefully this will lead to the development of treatment. It is well known that Connexin 26 is associated with many forms of congenital hearing loss; what is now needed is some means to prevent the mechanism whereby this association leads to the problem in the first place. Many genetic aberrations have already been discovered, and many more will be, as will means of modifying their action. To date advances in genetics have significantly improved the taxonomy of deafness; what are now needed are mechanisms to modify or repair the causative genes. Again, advances on the broad front of genetics are likely to provide means of prevention as will the further development of pharmaceutical agents aimed at preventing apoptosis.

The past quarter century has seen the establishment of programmes of newborn hearing screening for hearing loss, a welcome advance. This occurred both because of the demonstrated beneficial outcome of early management and because the technology for testing improved: the rather unspecific noisemakers used in the 1970s and 80s to attract the attention of newborns have given way to oto-acoustic emission testing and automated ABR. Successful trials of Universal Newborn Hearing Screening (UNHS) have been undertaken and its widespread adoption has been seriously advocated. And yet the number of complete national programmes of UNHS is still very limited. In the United States some states have the programme, others do not; in Canada some provinces have a programme, some do not. The UK has a well-established national programme and recently Germany mandated it for the whole country, which is far ahead of most other nations. Still too many countries base their newborn hearing screening on limited hospital programmes or on high risk registers, both of which miss a high proportion of those born deaf. National UNHS programs are required in most countries of the world, but they are only worthwhile if matched with appropriate habilitation resources. That is a major problem, screening and identification without concomitant management resources is hardly ethical and certainly economically wasteful.

Cochlear implants have had a dramatic effect's on habilitation and rehabilitation of the profoundly hearing-impaired. But they are too expensive for global use, the devices are costly, so is the surgery and habilitation that is required to fit them properly. In general when electronic devices become widespread, their price drops. This has not been the case with cochlear implants although by now the development costs must have been well recouped? Devices costing thousands of dollars are unaffordable in countries where the median incomes are a small fraction of the cost of the devices and the total individual annual health expenditure is measured only in tens of dollars. The same was true of lens implants; their price dropped massively when manufacturing started in India; as it is of medication for HIV AIDS, which with significant public pressure, has become much cheaper in many poor countries. There is a similar need with cochlear implants.

What is true of cochlear implants is even truer of hearing aids. In the past 20 years hearing aids have dramatically improved. Analog devices have now given way to digital ones almost all of which can be programmed for different listening situations. The fitting paradigms have improved and it now seems we may be on the threshold of devices which automatically adjust themselves to the acoustic environment and the need of the user. However, costs remain extremely high, so high that they are out of reach for many. Twenty years ago there were many manufacturers of hearing aids so that the economics of developing digital circuitry was out of reach of most the small manufacturers. There has now been a significant consolidation in the industry; the number of manufacturers diminished dramatically while the number of instruments produced has increased. The cost of a digital circuit design can therefore be spread over more devices and the price should come down. And yet they sell for thousands of dollars each in North America and Europe even though, when purchased in bulk, similar devices may be obtained for very much less from the manufacturer.

The main problem with hearing aids remains how little they are used. The penetration rate for hearing aid sales, even in wealthy nations is low, and still far too many that are purchased are not worn. Better economics of hearing aid provision mean little if the devices, once provided are not of help.

Some of the reasons which prevent their more widespread use include the human factors of their fitting and daily wearing. They are difficult devices to fit properly to the ear if, as is common, a custom-made mould is used, although it is debatable whether one is needed for most mild losses, where a standard open plug is probably sufficient, but not yet widely used. Major changes in fitting practice are needed. When a mould is required, at present an impression is taken and the client must return for later fitting, impractical in many places. There is need for a one- stage mould making process, which appears to be being developed but has not yet been widely adopted. Current hearing aids are run on zinc air-batteries because the amount of power that can be stored is more than can be stored in a rechargeable battery of the same size. However they are too costly in many parts of the world and even in the industrialized nations, the cost of batteries may be a burden to the elderly. Work on solar cells has been ongoing and some are in use, but mainly on a trial basis. Unfortunately the rechargeable batteries, to date, do not hold the same amount of energy as the zinc oxide air battery. Cheaper and longer lasting power supplies are urgent needs; these may be rechargeable batteries, solar cells or some yet to be discovered mechanism. There is much work in this area for portable phones; batteries are close to being charged by body heat and motion with enough power for modern circuits. Perhaps we will see hearing aids fit in the ear canal and left undisturbed for months. The interface between the hearing aid and the user is also difficult. Small controls and little battery boxes are difficult to manipulate, particularly for the elderly with diminishing dexterity; what is required are better means of changing batteries and inserting the devices. But most of all, hearing aids do not restore hearing well enough for many users; expectations are high, the results less appealing. There is need for a systems approach to aural rehabilitation, which will include the hearing aid, but not rely totally upon it. Such programmes have been demonstrated to be effective but are not widely available, even though they are almost certainly more cost effective than merely proving an aid.

As life expectancy increases in all parts of the world, hearing loss in the aged will play a much greater role than it has in the past. Without adequate hearing and vision, independent living is difficult and many will require sheltered or at least assisted accommodation who could manage on their own if they could hear and see better than they do. A mild cognitive impairment, which in a normal hearing person is just a nuisance, may be a severe problem when combined with a hearing loss. Hearing losses should be identified, if possible, before cognitive decline occurs, so that a timely hearing aid fitting may be undertaken. Counselling associated with hearing loss in general and specifically with a new hearing aid, should include discussion and education of other family members.

The social anthropology of hearing loss is extremely important but does not yet seem to play a role in the mainstream. How do the hard of hearing interface with society, and society with them? Some work has been undertaken in the interaction between deaf parents and deaf children, and normal hearing parents and deaf children; there are distinct differences in communication ability and family dynamics; communication between a deaf parent and a deaf child may be better than if the parent is normally hearing.

Some studies have been undertaken about the family interactions of hard- of- hearing working age adults. Intra-family roles can be reversed and tension may occur between family members because of the apparent lack of attention to the family by the hard of hearing person, usually occasioned by the hearing loss. Intra- family irritation is common. Hearing loss leads to social altercation, alienation and isolation, within the family as well as without. It should not be so. How should normal hearing staff react to the hearing loss of their normal hearing colleagues? It is likely that they will be huge changes in what is possible resulting from the widespread use of portable electronic devices where the smart telephone and the tablet computer are just the beginning.

It is not clear that the disability level for hearing loss should be set at the same in all societies. Customs at home and the need for aural communication at work vary so that a level of 35 dB may be too stringent in some areas and not stringent enough in others. The way the hearing-impaired act, react and function across cultures has been somewhat evaluated; where speech is not much used, hearing loss is less of a problem What in fact is a disabling hearing loss in the villages of central Africa, a rural setting in South Asia or urban China? The places are chosen at random. Likewise in the workplace.

Occupational noise is the tobacco of hearing loss. Noise induced hearing loss is the single, most preventable cause of a massive amount of hearing deficit, entirely preventable but far too infrequently dealt with. Like tobacco, it has been known for more than a century that excessive sound exposure produces significant problems, in this case hearing loss and yet for too long this was accepted as part of the price of earning a living. Only recently, and then in limited segments of the global population, have serious steps been taken to prevent this happening.

There remain several important unanswered questions about the impact of noise upon hearing. It is conventional wisdom that if hearing recovers completely from the temporary threshold shift (TTS) produced by noise exposure, the ear will not be at any greater risk for future damage from noise. This is a particularly important question with regard to the long-term effects of social noise exposure in the younger population, from sound sources such as a disco, loud band or even a personal music player. It may also be a question with industrial noise and certainly is one with military noise when many people who fire small arms, even on a training range, develop a TTS. Recent animal experiments suggest that there may be long term damage to the ear even after complete recovery from TTS. There is need for long-term human studies in this area. Hard evidence to support (or deny) this hypothesis is urgently required. If it is so, the ceiling of acceptable levels of social and industrial sound may have to be lowered.

The EU has recommended social sound levels should be below 80 dBA to protect all, including the most sensitive ears. And yet in much of industry a noise exposure 90 dBA for an eight hour workday is taken as the lower threshold of damage; this has gradually been and is being reduced to 87 or even 85 dBA. However there is a huge difference between sound exposure of 80 dBA, 85 dBA and 90 dBA for eight hours a day. Which is correct? What proportion of the population should be protected? Human studies will be difficult because any group wishing to undertake any prospective study will also be obliged to provide hearing protection! Questions remain and are important from the standpoint of hearing conservation practices in industry and social noise exposure levels.

Where high noise levels exist, the worker should be separated from it, either structurally or by use of personal protection (HPD). It is not necessary for workers to be exposed to loud noise in many industries, where the provision of sound proof control room would protect hearing, improve communication and in no way detract from the process. HPDs can be effective but to be so, must be offered, used and supervised. However, many find it uncomfortable, difficult to wear and suggest that they may be dangerous because they prevent the hearing of safety signals. With older devices this may be true. Quite recent developments have made them more comfortable, more effective and also enable communication to occur. Much more research is required in developing effective HPDs that WILL BE USED, and which allow communication including hearing warning signals in the direction from which they come. They have been in use in some industries for decades but few publications have ensued of the outcome of their use.

Unfortunately, many industries do not offer them in a consistent way, especially, the construction industry and industry with transient employees. Noise reduction and the use of HPDs amongst the largest group of the exposed population, those working in the developing world, barely exist. Legislation has been enacted in many parts of the world, but enforcement is largely absent. For these programs to gain traction requires an understanding both by workers and management that excessive noise produces hearing loss (something which is still too often ignored); that total health including good hearing is the right of worker, not just a privilege and that this can be achieved without bankrupting the industry. Much information exists, a great deal has been done in some industrialized countries; on a global scale much more remains to be done. It cannot be over emphasized that exposure to excessive levels of sound is the largest single preventable cause of hearing loss, the elimination of which would massively reduce the problem of presbyacusis in later life; this is the cumulative result of all previous problems including noise exposure.

Community noise is a closely related topic. Over the past 20 years the number of megacities has increased greatly and will continue to increase rapidly for another 20 years. The world is becoming more urban and nowhere more so than in the developing countries, such as India, Pakistan, China, Nigeria, and Brazil. The EU has issued directives of acceptable levels of community noise, focused particularly on transportation. It recognizes that it will not be possible to reach its recommended levels easily and has introduced interim levels. The directives also include maximum acceptable sound exposure. The minimum sound levels recorded in many developing world megacities exceed those maxima. Even if the sound levels in the cities are not high enough to produce hearing loss, and some of them are close to being damaging to the ear, they are certainly damaging to peace, tranquility, the ability to communicate and to rest. In many developing world cities the motorcycle, diesel engine and advertising sounds from bazaars are high enough to damage hearing, compounded by population densities unheard of in the industrialised countries. The prevention of the stress effects of excessive sound in those situations is very much an issue of social engineering, and presumably increasing wealth of society.

Legislation has the potential to play an important role in the reduction of harmful noise exposure, occupational, social and in the community. However legislation by itself is of little value; most countries in the world have some sort of legislation covering excessive industrial and community noise, if only in blanket environmental rules. Without regulations accompanying the laws and a means of enforcing them, these have no value in reducing noise levels. Even where very good legislation and regulations exist, the withdrawal of adequate inspection (as occurred in part in the United States) makes the regulations ineffective. The EU has developed excellent guidelines, in considerable detail, for the reduction of noise levels and for the appropriate levels in industry; unless these are adopted by the member nations, and enforced, they too remain empty promises.

In all instances it is better to reduce sound levels than to require protection; decades of hearing protector use have shown them to be difficult devices to use properly on a regular basis and for the majority of noisy work sites in the world, are not used at all. It is possible to reduce noise at source in industry, in the community and the individual listening but at present there is little incentive to do so. Here legislation, regulation and inspection can play an important part. Contrast the extreme efforts in the EU to reduce the sound of industrial machinery, with the US again refusing to enact similar regulations. In the long run the hearing of the worker in the EU will be by far better served than their transatlantic cohorts. However to do this requires commitment on the part of government. Similarly to reduce disco sound levels below those hazardous to hearing health, requires a system of inspection and enforcement.

The process of sound reduction is an iterative and reiterative one involving the community, legislators and those responsible for the enforcement. Until a community is sufficiently disturbed by, or enlightened about excessive sound and mounts protest and educational campaigns, legislators will not act. Once legislation, reinforced by the appropriate regulations, bylaws and ordinances are in place, the community must ensure that there are sufficient funds to monitor that they are observed. In the final resort, it is the population which decides where taxes are spent. There must be individual advocates and advocacy groups to initiate these processes and to see that they are maintained. Unless and until the population, workforce and community is sufficiently annoyed by excessive sound and its harmful effects, legislation will be filed and ignored. Without this sort of push excesses excessive noise will continue to be treated as an inevitable sequel of modern life – it need not be.

Probably the most important factor of all is the need to change attitudes about hearing. Everyone knows someone who is hard of hearing, everyone knows that this is a problem, even that it affects the quality of life of the hard of hearing adversely, sometimes a great deal. Sadly, people at large seem not care, there is a general complacency about hearing loss, it is just something that happens, about which nothing can be done. As this volume demonstrates, these views are wrong. There is much than can be undertaken now to prevent hearing loss from occurring and to mitigate its effects when it does. Until there is a public recognition of this, nothing will happen and the hard of hearing will continue to stand in the shadows of their normal hearing brethren.

Index

N

O

P

Q